Interventions for Mental Health

For Butterworth Heinemann:

Commissioning Editor: Heidi Allen
Project Development Editor: Robert Edwards
Project Manager: Jane Dingwall/Pat Miller
Design Direction: George Ajayi

Interventions for Mental Health

An Evidence-Based Approach for Physiotherapists and Occupational Therapists

Edited by

Tina Everett MSc MCSP

Head Physiotherapist, Oxfordshire Mental Healthcare Trust, Oxford, UK

Marie Donaghy PhD BA(Hons) FCSP ILTM

Head of School, Health and Biological Sciences, Queen Margaret University College, Edinburgh, UK

Sally Feaver MABA DipOT

Principal Lecturer, Oxford Brookes University, Oxford, UK

Foreword by

Phil Gray MSc FCSP

Chief Executive, Chartered Society of Physiotherapy, London, UK

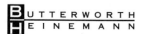

EDINBURGH LONDON NEW YORK OXFORD PHILADELPHIA ST LOUIS SYDNEY TORONTO 2003

BS

BUTTERWORTH-HEINEMANN
An imprint of Elsevier Science Limited

First published 2003

ISBN 0 7506 4965 8

British Library Cataloguing in Publication Data
A catalogue record for this book is available from the British Library

Library of Congress Cataloging in Publication Data
A catalog record for this book is available from the Library of Congress

Notice
Medical knowledge is constantly changing. Standard safety precautions must be followed, but as new research and clinical experience broaden our knowledge, changes in treatment and drug therapy may become necessary or appropriate. Readers are advised to check the most current product information provided by the manufacturer of each drug to be administered to verify the recommended dose, the method and duration of administration, and contraindications. It is the responsibility of the practitioner, relying on experience and knowledge of the patient, to determine dosages and the best treatment for each individual patient. Neither the Publisher nor the editors and contributors assumes any liability for any injury and/or damage to persons or property arising from this publication.

The Publisher

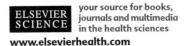

ELSEVIER SCIENCE your source for books, journals and multimedia in the health sciences
www.elsevierhealth.com

The publisher's policy is to use **paper manufactured from sustainable forests**

Cover design based on an original idea by Lee Haynes

Printed in China

11/17/03

Contents

Contributors

Diana Beaven Grad Dip Phys
Senior Physiotherapist, Barrow Hospital, Bristol, UK

Patsy Brodie Dip COT
Head of Occupational Therapy Service Adult Mental Health, Royal
Dundee Liff Hospital, Dundee, UK

Helen Buri MSc PGCert LT Dip COT
Senior Lecturer, Sheffield Hallam University, Sheffield, UK

David Carless MSc BA
Researcher in Exercise and Health Science, University of Bristol,
Bristol, UK

Sarah Childs BOcc THE
Head IV Occupational Therapist, Rehabilitation and Continuing Care,
Fair Mile Hospital, Cholsey, Berkshire, UK

Andrew Clyne Grad Dip Phys
Senior Physiotherapist, Adult Mental Health Service, Swindon, UK

Nicola Connolly D Clin Psych MA BA
Clinical Psychologist, Highfield Adolescent Unit Warneford Hospital,
Oxford, UK

Shelagh Creegan BSc (Hons) Health Studies, Dip COT
Head Occupational Therapist, Adult Mental Health, The Community
Workshop, Dundee, UK

Jennifer Creek MSc Dip COT FETC
Freelance Occupational Therapist

Pam Dawson PhD PGCED MCSP
Principal Lecturer in Allied Health Professions Research, Newcastle
upon Tyne, UK

Marie Donaghy PhD BA (Hons) FCSP ILTM
Head of School, Health and Biological Sciences, Queen Margaret
University College, Edinburgh, UK

Jonquil Drinkwater PhD AFBPsS
Head of Child and Adolescent Psychology, Oxfordshire Mental
Healthcare Trust, Oxford, UK

Edward A S Duncan	BSc (Hons) Dip CBT SROT Senior Occupational Therapist, The State Hospitals Board for Scotland, Carstairs, Lanark, UK
Tina Everett	MSc MCSP Head Physiotherapist for Oxfordshire Mental Healthcare NHS Trust, Warneford Hospital, Oxford, UK
Alice Farrington	DClin Psych Clinical Psychologist, The Park Hospital for Children, Headington, Oxford, UK
Guy Faulkner	BEd MSc PhD Lecturer in Exercise and Sports Psychology, University of Exeter, Exeter, UK
Sally Feaver	MABA DipOT Principal Lecturer, Oxford Brookes University, Headington, Oxford, UK
Kenneth Fox	BSc MSc PhD Professor and Head of Department of Exercise and Health Sciences, University of Bristol, Bristol, UK
Colin Godfrey	RGN SPSA Activities Development Nurse for Oxfordshire Mental Healthcare NHS Trust, Oxford, UK
Caroline Griffiths	MCSP Grad Dip Phys Clinical Specialist Physiotherapist, Northamptonshire Healthcare Trust, Northampton, UK
John Hall	PhD FBPsS Clin Psychol Head Clinical Psychologist for Oxfordshire Mental Healthcare NHS Trust and Senior Clinical Lecturer in Clinical Psychology, University of Oxford, Oxford, UK
Gita Ingram	Dip COT SROT Senior Occupational Therapist, Royal Hospital for Sick Children, Edinburgh, UK
Derek Jones	BA (Hons) Dip COT SROT Lecturer in Occupational Therapy, Queen Margaret University College, Edinburgh, UK
Mary Kavanagh	MSc BA (Hons) Dip COT SROT Cert. Couns. Lecturer in Occupational Therapy, Oxford Brookes University, Headington, Oxford, UK
Denis Martin	DPhil MSc (Applied Statistics) BSc (Hons) MCSP Grad Stat Director Scottish Network for Chronic Pain Research, Queen Margaret University College, Edinburgh, UK
Louise Montague-Jones	Dip COT SROT/Cert THE Senior Occupational Therapist, Oxfordshire Mental Healthcare NHS Trust, Oxford, UK

Nanette Mutrie   DPE, MEd PhD
Professor of Physical Activity and Health Science, University of Glasgow, Glasgow, UK

Margaret Nicol   Dip COT MPHIL PhD
Acting Head of Department, Occupational Therapy and Art Therapy, Queen Margaret University College, Edinburgh, UK

Gwyneth Owen   MSc MCSP
Professional Advisor, Chartered Society of Physiotherapy, London, UK

Catherine Pope   MA MCSP
Physiotherapy Manager, Nottinghamshire Healthcare NHS Trust, Nottingham, UK

Nick Rose   MB ChB MA FRC Psych
Consultant Psychiatrist and Honorary Senior Lecturer, University of Oxford, Oxford UK

Mick Skelly   MSc MCSP Dip Phys Dip AD SRP
Superintendent Physiotherapist, Rosslynlee Hospital, Roslin, Midlothian, UK

Linette Whitehead   BA MSc (Oxon)
Consultant Clinical Psychologist, Warneford Hospital, Oxford, UK

Emma Williams   BSc (Hons) MPhil (Clin Psychol) PhD
Consultant Clinical and Forensic Psychologist, Oxford Mental Healthcare NHS Trust, Oxford, UK

Foreword

Physiotherapy as a therapeutic intervention in the management of people with mental illhealth has come a long way since its small beginnings in the 1970s. It is now part of the central core of the profession, helping to further broaden the boundaries and scope of physiotherapy. Occupational therapy has a much longer history, almost since the inception of the profession in 1937 (in Scotland), occupational therapists have been providing a central therapeutic role in the rehabilitation and management of people with mental illhealth. Both disciplines are still advancing with the application to practice of the emerging evidence and the desire for more collaborative working. These wide developments are well covered in this text book, based on the solid evidence-base of real benefits to clients and the pioneering techniques that show promise for the future in treating particular conditions.

Mental health is a key priority for the modern NHS and social services. This is unsurprising considering that depressive disorders are the fourth most important cause of disability worldwide. In the UK, anxiety and depression are one of the major sources of visits to GPs, make a large component of the primary care drugs bill and result in over 80 000 working days lost annually, at a cost of at least £5.3 billion. The total cost of treatment in both primary and secondary care is huge. It is therefore unsurprising that governments have a major interest in care solutions that can help to improve mental health in its varied forms.

This is why mental health is an exciting and evolving area of work for physiotherapists and occupational therapists. It focuses on the reality that the mind and the body are one – they are not distinctive entities. People can become clinically depressed as a result of a physical disorder or those who have a mental disorder can develop a physical disorder as a consequence. The physical image of themselves that people with eating disorders have can be radically different from that of the rest of the world. Anxiety, depression or addictive behaviour can be heavily influenced by physical factors, self confidence or awareness.

As this book illustrates, physiotherapists and occupational therapists working in mental health are uniquely placed to provide an extensive range of physical approaches to treatment aimed at relieving symptoms, boosting confidence and improving quality of life. Interventions include physical activity, exercise and sport, balance, postural and movement education, useful occupation, creative therapy, achieving goals and life skills, management of chronic or acute pain, relaxation techniques, manual therapies, acupuncture and complementary therapies.

Available evidence suggests that exercise, training and increased goal-oriented physical activity produce definite improvement in reducing depression and anxiety, improved physical status, better cognitive function and can facilitate behavioural lifestyle changes. The enormous expansion of private gyms and sport facilities in the UK is testimony to the extent to which physical activity as a stress reducer has become accepted by the wider public.

More broadly, physiotherapists and occupational therapists are also involved in advice, guidance and education of users, carers and staff. The promotion of self confidence and self awareness, motivation and socialization are important components in this armoury. Increasing evidence suggests that interventions such as cognitive–behavioural therapy, counselling and exercise can reduce anxiety and depression and enhance psychosocial function either as an adjunct to therapy or as an alternative intervention. The psychological benefits of exercise in dealing with alcohol and other addictions is becoming better known.

The occupational therapist and physiotherapist in mental health are team players in a wider interdisciplinary team of social workers, psychologists, nurses and others. To this teamworking, occupational therapists and physiotherapists bring a breadth of assessment and treatment expertise that is often delivered alongside prescribed pharmacological or psychological interventions. This new textbook, written by experts in the field of mental health therapy, can only help to expand the horizons of the possible in improving mental health in the UK.

Phil Gray 2003

Introduction

The decision to write a new book for physiotherapists and occupational therapists working in mental health, rather than update the previous book *Physiotherapy in mental health: a practical approach* (Everett et al 1995) was taken to reflect current changes and trends in the delivery of services for people with mental health problems. These changes include the need to provide evidence-based interventions and the need for greater involvement of both physiotherapists and occupational therapists to promote and share best practice. The need for an integrated approach is emphasized in the standards of the National Service Framework for Mental Health and in the NHS Plan. Throughout the book we have attempted to stress the importance of working in partnership with the individual to whom we are delivering the service, with primary care and specialist mental health teams, voluntary agencies and social services. We support the concept that the person with mental illhealth should be placed at the centre of decision making, with the therapist as enabler. We appreciate the need to promote more interdisciplinary education and teamwork while recognizing the challenges that this can present.

The previous book evolved from the clinical interest group Chartered Physiotherapists in Mental Healthcare providing a standard text, with a global distribution, for physiotherapists working in this specialist field. This new book has been written as a key text by and for occupational therapists and physiotherapists, with notable contributions from other healthcare professionals, particularly clinical psychologists and academics in the sport and exercise sciences. It is hoped that the book will be of value to clinicians in other professions, particularly nursing and medical colleagues. A growing number of skilled technical instructors with degrees in sport and exercise science work within physiotherapy and occupational therapy teams and it is envisaged that this book will be a useful text for them also. The editors are very conscious of the fact that the authors are writing from a British perspective and that named government initiatives are mainly from the UK. However, attempts have been made to draw from research worldwide, and it is the intention that the book will be of value internationally.

Each chapter provides a description of the theoretical underpinning or a critique of theoretical issues and an inclusion of the research supporting the efficacy of the therapeutic intervention. It is our intention that this book will provide physiotherapists and occupational therapists and students with a scientific basis and an appropriate context in which decisions regarding the selection of intervention can be made.

When considering applying the evidence presented within the text to practice, it is important to distinguish between the efficacy of an intervention, i.e. the results achieved within the context of a therapeutic trial, and clinical effectiveness, i.e. the results achieved in everyday clinical practice. Research into therapeutic interventions involves a compromise between providing rigorous procedures to implement and evaluate the intervention and taking account of what normally happens during a therapeutic intervention, including the evolving and changing nature of the therapeutic relationship. There is a tension between the need to achieve high internal validity with an identifiable homogenized population and the extent to which these findings can then be generalized to other clinical settings where people with mental health problems differ in socioeconomic circumstance, psychological and physical function. The context in which the therapeutic intervention takes place also needs to be considered, particularly in relation to available resources that will impact on the frequency and length of treatment offered and on the quality of links with family and other professionals and services. The ability of physiotherapists and occupational therapists to provide a clinically effective service will be informed by an understanding and interpretation of the research evidence considered alongside a critical analysis of their own practice and the context in which they operate.

The content of this book has been organized into three sections. Section 1 provides background knowledge and sets the book in context for the reader. It includes: an introduction to mental disorder from different view points (Chapter 1), definitions and diagnostic categories of mental disorders including medical and psychological interventions (Chapter 2), the different contexts that inform the delivery of services including policy, service evaluation and accountability (Chapters 3, 4 and 5).

Section 2 takes a thematic and principles-based approach, with the emphasis firmly placed on activity and occupation. The intervention strategies presented were selected for their generic applicability across a range of mental health problems. The reader is presented with evidence and arguments to support the important role of physical self perceptions, in relation to self-esteem and personal identity. This provides theoretical links to the principles of and the evidence for physical activity as a legitimate intervention strategy for people with mental health problems (Chapters 6–9). Chapter 10 is dedicated to cognitive–behavioural strategies, this reflects the importance of this approach for occupational therapists and physiotherapists and signals that this approach is currently being integrated into a number of therapeutic interventions. Further chapters in this part of the book provide the reader with specific examples of the application of principles to deal with stress, aggressive behaviour and managing pain (Chapters 11–13). This part closes with chapters on enabling occupation and users' views on occupation (Chapters 14 and 15), stressing the importance of this therapeutic intervention within the rehabilitation process.

The third and final section of the book brings together for the reader a comprehensive knowledge of specific areas of physiotherapy and occupational therapy practice. Some of the chapters in this section are defined by population, for example children, adolescents and the elderly (Chapters 16 and 17), others are defined by nature of the specialist topic that is often associated with other symptoms and behaviours, for example eating disorders, chronic fatigue, sexual abuse and self harm (Chapters 21–24). These topics should not be viewed in isolation but are recognized for their association with other problems in mental health. Chapters 18, 19 and 20 introduce the reader to severe mental illness, forensic psychiatry and substance abuse. The final chapter, entitled 'Employment for health' is included to remind us that, for some people and their families, this is an important goal (Chapter 25). The reality, however, is that for many people it will be achievable but that for others it will not. For both physiotherapists and occupational therapists, an understanding of the process will inform realistic goal setting for other interventions

Some of the chapters contain case studies of clinical service user experience – these examples are generally created from clinical experience rather than being identified with one particular person. The names chosen bear no relation to any particular individual. Quotes from service users have either been published elsewhere or chosen anonymously from service audit. Identity has been hidden and, where necessary, permission has been obtained.

Complementary therapies, although referenced in some of the chapters, do not feature in this text. This is in recognition that complementary medicine is now an established therapy in its own right with several key texts published in this area.

This book is dedicated to Eirean Ricketts, a Fellow of the Chartered Society of Physiotherapy and editor of the previous text for physiotherapists, who sadly died of cancer. Eirean was a pioneer physiotherapist from Cardiff who, through vision and hard work with her occupational therapy colleagues, gained recognition for physiotherapy in the management of people with mental health problems.

2003

Tina Everett
Marie Donaghy
Sally Feaver

Reference

Everett T, Dennis M, Ricketts E (eds) 1995 Physiotherapy in mental health: a practical approach Butterworth Heinemann, Oxford

SECTION

1

1 Models of mental health disorder

Marie Donaghy

Introduction

Models are defined, for the purpose of this chapter, as representations of a particular body of knowledge, put forward as an explanation and interpretation of events. They are intended to give the reader insight into the application of different theoretical approaches to the clinical setting. Numerous models inform the work of physiotherapists and occupational therapists, and many of these are contained in other chapters of this book. Those selected for this chapter have been brought together to illustrate how knowledge from medicine and psychology provide different viewpoints of people with mental health problems and ultimately the interventions they are engaged in or prescribe. The biomedical and neurobiological models are presented alongside the family therapy, humanistic, psychodynamic and cognitive–behavioural models from psychology. Social models have also been developed to challenge and reject the established views of mental illness (Kovel 1982, Laing 1967, Szasz 1961). These were discussed by the author in an earlier publication (Donaghy 1995) and are not included here because they are perceived to be less relevant to the strategies currently used by physiotherapists and occupational therapists in the management of people with mental health disorders.

Mental health disorders

Mental health disorders can be studied from two major standpoints: (1) how the brain works; and (2) from knowledge about how man interacts within the environment (Goldberg & Huxley 1992). The first approach is from the biomedical perspective and considers the scientific discipline of the neurobiology of mental illness, including genetics. The other approach comes from the social sciences and considers methods of inquiry derived from epidemiology, sociology and psychology. A review of recent developments from the medical perspective suggests that although there have been advances in the field of neurobiology, progress is lagging behind other medical advances. The excitement over the genetic breakthrough in schizophrenia and manic depression in the 1980s has been replaced with the recognition that, to date, explicit psychiatric disease genes have not been identified (Peroutka 1997), nor has the precise aetiological and pathophysiological basis of mental disorders been delineated (Charney et al 1999). The prediction that molecular genetics will revolutionize our understanding of psychiatric disorders and human behaviour has not been realized, despite the unfolding of the sequence of the human genome (Owen et al 2000). There is, however, no doubt that the role of medicine in the treatment of people with mental health problems has become more prestigious, in the undertaking of successful research (Cowan et al 2000, Weller & Eysenck 1992) and in the application of increased therapeutic efficacy (Roth & Fonagy 1996).

The development of therapeutic models by different schools of psychology provide a focus for clinical treatment, e.g. psychodynamic, cognitive–behavioural therapy (CBT) and family therapy. Two types of research are necessary to test therapeutic models. Initially, research attempts to establish efficacy. This usually compares one approach against another (e.g. CBT versus relaxation in the treatment of panic disorder). The other type of investigative inquiry is designed to test a specific hypothesis (e.g. is the reduction of panic attacks contingent on changing cognitions?). Although the efficacy of different models has been developed, enabling us to make technological advances in the application of interventions, our scientific understanding of why things work is still poor (Salkovskis 1996).

Biomedical model

The medical model has existed since the fourth century BC. It was at this time that the Greek physician Hippocrates attempted to explain behaviour disorders such as depression and epilepsy as physical diseases (Bernstein et al 2000). Hippocrates' views were further developed by Greek and Roman physicians into what became known as mental illness or psychopathology. This model is dominant in psychiatry today and is based on assumptions that health can be defined by the absence of disorders, and that mental disorders are discrete disease entities that can be defined categorically into distinct conditions with recognizable symptoms (Cloninger 1999). Classification is made under the International Classification of Disease ICD-10 (WHO 1992) or the *Diagnostic and statistical manual of mental disorders* (DSM-IV) (American Psychiatric Association 1994). Within psychiatry it is recognized that these conditions might or might not respond to medical intervention, e.g. the use of antidepressant drugs to treat unipolar depression. Success in treatment is therefore not seen to be imperative to sustaining the model. In medicine it is generally accepted that there are major diseases that defy explanation in terms of aetiology, favourable prognosis and successful outcome.

The way in which people become defined as having mental health problems and reach mental health services has been illustrated in a five-level framework by Goldberg & Huxley (1980). This framework suggests that a large number of the population will suffer minor bouts of mental illness lasting less than 2 weeks. This has been identified as levels 1 and 2 within the framework and medical intervention is not always required. The majority of distressed people will consult their doctor, but often they will do so for associated physical symptoms. At level 3, mental disorders are identified and treated by primary care physicians, with only a small minority of the population (those at levels 4 and 5 in the framework) being seen by mental health professionals. These higher levels contain the more severe illnesses such as schizophrenia and bipolar affective disorders, with unipolar depression and anxiety disorders being more prevalent at levels 1, 2 and 3.

Definitions of mental illness that are based entirely on symptoms can be entirely appropriate for severe illnesses such as psychotic depression and schizophrenia (Goldberg & Huxley 1992) but are less appropriate for short-term bouts of anxiety or depression. For these illnesses, Williams et al (1986) offer a triaxial model consisting of symptoms, personality and social functioning, as a more appropriate definition. To assess whether someone has a mental disorder, the physician will need to discover whether the person has experienced a discernible number of symptoms from an identified constellation of symptoms, within a known timeframe (see Chapter 2 for examples of classification).

The biomedical model can be criticized for failing to establish neurobiological pathogenesis for every category of mental health disorder. Instead, most diagnostic information derives from the subjective report of people with mental health problems and their relatives. This occurs within powerful cultural and social influences that include a history of superstition, emotional and illogical reasoning, and metaphorical explanations (Ussher 1991). This poses a threat to reliability of classification on at least two counts: (1) variance by the person reporting the symptoms, e.g. fluctuating intensities and range of symptoms; and (2) variance by the evaluator, e.g. different conceptual biases influencing interpretation and differences in style of questioning.

In summary, the problems with the biomedical model in regard to classification can be identified at three levels: (1) assessing mental ill-health via a constellation of symptoms; (2) assessing and determining neurobiology; and (3) evaluating the complex interaction between neurobiology and behaviour (Heninger 1999). On the last point, it has been suggested that genes and the environment have an ubiquitous influence. If we accept the premise that the interaction between an individual and the environment is person specific, then it follows that the potential value of molecular genetics lies in the elucidation of causal processes because they apply both to brain systems and to nature—nurture interplay (Rutter & Plomin 1997).

It is worth considering whether advances in genetics will improve diagnosis and lead to better interventions or whether they will increase discrimination and stigmatization (Chadwick 2000). The premise that all psychiatric illnesses are linked to genetic factors was formed and nurtured in the 1930s by the eugenics movement (Ussher 1991). Over 70 years on, there are still concerns that developments in this field will lead to stigmatization and discrimination (Gill 1991). At this time, knowledge on both genetic and environmental causal factors are still fragmentary, although progress has varied among diagnostic categories. Specific gene–environment interaction seems likely to be important in relation to neuropsychiatric syndromes, e.g. obsessive compulsive disorder (OCD), and less important in relation to susceptibility to environmental stress linked to triggering common mental health disorders, e.g. anxiety (Cooper 2001). The only disease gene that can be located in psychiatry at the present time is Huntington's disease. The growing body of evidence for a genetic link with other disorders is complicated by the multifactorial nature of these illnesses.

The neurobiological model will now be examined briefly in an attempt to gain a better understanding of the rationale underpinning this approach.

Neurobiological model

Although the difficulty in relating mental health problems to the specific underlying neurobiological abnormalities involved in the pathogenesis of disease has led to criticism of the biomedical model, there is optimism for the future. Many neurochemical pathways, and how drugs influence these, are now known and advances have been made in molecular genetics, offering the potential for identifying abnormalities that lead to mental health problems (Heninger 1999). In addition, specific non-invasive methods such as single photon emission computed tomography (SPECT), positon emission tomography (PET) and magnetic resonance imaging (MRI) allow neurochemical processes to be measured.

In regard to the most common severe mental illness, schizophrenia, there is ongoing debate with regard to the causal links of the disease with advances in knowledge of altered brain structure and neurochemistry informing the field. Structural brain abnormalities such as ventricular enlargement have been found to be robust correlates of schizophrenia (Bruton et al 1990), with more recent research providing evidence of greater deviation for cortical and left hemisphere measures of cerebrospinal fluid space enlargement than previously reported (Zorilla et al 1997). Advances in the neurochemistry of schizophrenia provide a growing awareness that the role of dopamine is more complex than originally thought. It is now established that dopamine interacts with a variety of neurotransmitter systems, which include complex feedback circuits with neurotransmitters mutually influencing each other (Byne et al 1999). This is further complicated by findings that indicate that dopamine and other neurotransmitters are regulated differently in different brain regions. For example, Davis et al (1991) suggest that the cortical hypodopaminergic state underlies the negative symptoms of schizophrenia, whereas the subcortical hyperdopaminergic state underlies the positive symptoms. Findings from molecular genetics have been slow to emerge; although D_2 and D_3 receptor genes have been indicated, no region has yet emerged that has been replicated at every attempt (Kendler 1999).

There has been notable progress in determining molecular genetic links for susceptability to mood disorder. It now seems unlikely that a single major locus genetic model can account for this. The evidence suggests that, in relation to bipolar disorder, susceptibility loci reside on chromosomes 18, 21 and X (Sanders et al 1999). Drug intervention is at present based on efficacy of treatment from clinical observations. Developments in molecular genetics offer the potential for advancing our understanding of the pathophysiology of the illness, which in turn should lead to pharmacotherapeutic developments in the future.

For the majority of psychiatric illnesses, neurotransmitters have been investigated as the possible root of psychological illness (de Fonseca 1989). Synaptic conductive agents such as noradrenaline, 5-HT, dopamine and acetylcholine have been singled out for attention. In depression and anxiety, also, the cerebral monoamines have been linked with the aetiology of the illness. Goldberg & Huxley (1992) propose that general psychological processes such as reward, punishment, attention and memory are related specifically to these chemicals. For example, dopamine is related to reward systems, noradrenaline is associated with attention and memory, and might transmit information with regard to the magnitude of reinforcement. These findings should be regarded with caution. Although there is unequivocal support for biochemical changes associated with depression, anxiety and schizophrenia (Charney et al 1999), a causal relationship has yet to be established.

Influence on treatment

The focus of research within the field of neurobiology and genetics has been to look for a biologically identifiable problem that resides within the individual, this has inevitably led to physical treatments, such as pharmacology, being seen as the most appropriate. Whereas past treatments have included lobectomy, insulin therapy and electroconvulsive therapy (ECT), the treatment of choice today is invariably pharmacological. Psychiatrists also use psychological interventions, but these are invariably seen alongside other treatments such as physiotherapy and occupational therapy, as adjuncts to pharmacological intervention. However, there is a growing body of research in psychology to suggest that this is a legitimate approach, in its own right, for the treatment of people with mental illness (Roth & Fonagy 1996).

Typically, physiotherapists and occupational therapists have worked in psychiatry alongside psychiatrists, and their role has therefore been shaped by this relationship. Generally, therapists see their role as supportive. Exercise regimens used within psychiatry have been, and will continue to be, justifiable on biomedical grounds. However, recent research, in the use of exercise as an intervention strategy for mental health problems (see Chapter 7), suggests that, in the future, exercise might be considered an important psychological intervention in its own right for the management of anxiety and depression (Biddle et al 2000).

Despite its widespread influence, the biomedical model has been criticized for its failure to take into account cultural and other sociological and psychological perspectives. Critiques of the model have continued, with much of the criticism coming from psychologists and sociologists. The majority of the psychological models view mental health problems as arising within the individual because of interactions with the family, the workplace and wider society, with an emphasis on the relationship between environmental triggers and illness. The viewpoints from psychology presented have been selected for their relevance to physiotherapy and occupational therapy in the management of people with mental health problems.

Family therapy model

Laing & Esterson (1964) were among the first British writers to express the view that individuals with mental illness were the victims of a pathological family process. Fundamental to their theory, which has its roots in psychoanalysis, is the notion that those aspects of the human psyche denied legitimate expression in the value system of a family will manifest themselves in other ways (Skynner 1976). Family therapy usually begins by an approach that encourages all members of the family to work together in resolving the conflict. The process is designed to identify and change relationships where necessary. The therapist pays attention to family interactions, especially to alignments and discord and the engagement and disengagement of the different group members (see Chapter 16, Part A). The aim of treatment is often to engineer changes in communication (Minuchin & Fishman 1981). For example, parents could be taught to engage in conversation without interruption or to delineate boundaries. Whatever the strategy employed, the treatment approach is based on modifying the present situation, not on exploring or interpreting the past. The overall goal of family therapy is not just to resolve an existing problem but to assist families in gaining a better understanding of interactions within the family and the problems they create (Gurman et al 1986). The success of this approach is dependent on the full cooperation of key family members, and any sustained resistance to the efforts of the therapist is likely to result in failure of this approach. The other barrier to success is where a key family member has a psychological disturbance, such as a paranoid personality, that prevents that person gaining insight into his or her own situation, or that of another family member. Occupational therapists and physiotherapists involved in the treatment of patients with anorexia nervosa and bulimia can find it useful to be informed of family therapy sessions to gain an understanding of the family dynamics. The treatment approach adopted by the occupational therapist and physiotherapist can include other family members.

Humanistic psychology

The humanistic model sees mental health problems as a signal that an individual is failing to reach his or her potential and that psychological growth has stopped (Bernstein et al 2000). This model informed the philosophy of client-centred therapy, developed from the work of Carl Rogers, and is based on caring and equal respect for others. It was suggested that if mental illness was recognized within a therapeutic setting, and the distress was acknowledged and understood, the person would progress in recovery.

This model has been influential in forming the foundation of counselling (Rogers 1980) and, as such, has been a useful model for dealing with problems in everyday living. It aims at increasing peoples' autonomy to enable them to take greater control over their lives. The approach requires the therapist, who is acting as a counsellor, to be able to listen intently to what is being said and to help the individual recognize and clarify the feelings being experienced. The counsellor, in a non-directive manner, offers a safe environment where the individual can talk freely and explore these feelings, while still maintaining a sense of control. Critics of the approach argue that therapists, although portraying a non-directive approach, can in fact lead their clients more than they think by reflecting selectively on the things that the therapist deems to be important (Gray 1991).

This model would seem less appropriate for dealing with more serious problems of mental illness such as severe depression, obsessive compulsive disorders and schizophrenia.

The humanistic model is one that physiotherapists and occupational therapists can find useful in their everyday communication with people with mental health problems and in the application of specific counselling techniques. It requires a relationship between the therapist and the individual that is based on trust and the sharing of information. The knowledge possessed by the therapist is shared with the individual, thus establishing a partnership in the therapeutic relationship.

Psychodynamic therapy

Sigmund Freud (1856–1939), undoubtedly the most influential of all psychoanalysts, developed his classical theory in response to his clinical work with neurotic patients. The treatment was intensive and was aimed at attempting to restructure the entire personality by establishing a therapeutic relationship between therapist and patient allowing the resolving of conflicts at the root of distress through facing and accepting repressed feelings in the security of the analytical setting. Behaviour is interpreted symbolically and it is the therapist's role to interpret and explore its meaning with the patient. Modern psychoanalysis is no longer aimed at pervasive transformations of the personality but assumes that symptomatic change will come about through developing an understanding of personal problems through either exploratory or focused approaches (Roth & Fonagy 1996). Treatment can span a year or longer.

Classical psychoanalysis has led to many different psychotherapies – the term defined as any systematic treatment that is theory based and utilizes psychological rather than physiological means for the treatment of mental disorders. During the twentieth century, it is estimated that over 400 different psychotherapies have appeared, each with a different name (Karasu 1986)

Psychotherapy has been influential with regard to physiotherapy practice. One example of this has been in the development of psychomotor therapy (Bunkan & Thornquist 1990), a specialist branch of physiotherapy that has its roots in psychotherapy, merging psychotherapy with knowledge about patterns of breathing and movement. It is used by physiotherapists who have trained in psychomotor therapy as a treatment approach for a wide range of problems, but with a particular application to people with mental health problems.

Cognitive–behavioural model

This model, which combines elements of behavioural and cognitive theories, suggests that mental disorder occurs as the result of a combination of maladaptive learning and through thought disturbance. The theory has developed from the initial work of Pavlov on classical conditioning, into Wolpe's (1958) systematic desensitization approach for anxiety and panic, and the work of Skinner (1953), who used operant conditioning techniques to modify the behaviour of psychotic patients. The early approaches of Skinner and Wolpe ignored the influence of cognition. Maladaptive cognitions were later recognized as a cause of anxiety and depression (Beck 1976) and implicated in schizophrenia (Frith 1979). Beck proposed that negative thoughts are stored in memory in the form of schemata based on prior experience. These schemata are activated when similar events occur, resulting in automatic negative thoughts and corresponding emotional responses. Ellis (1962) developed an approach that he called rational–emotive therapy (RET). Meichenbaum (1977) was also interested in helping individuals to identify irrational beliefs and negative thoughts. His approach differs in that he is more concerned with the internal dialogue (what people say to themselves before entering stressful situations) that serves to maintain behaviour. This treatment approach involves the identification and modification of negative self-statements and can involve some training in coping and problem-solving skills. The role of the therapist is to assist in this training process by providing the necessary guidance and reinforcement. These cognitive approaches remain influential in guiding therapeutic interventions (Newell & Dryden 1991).

There is some overlap between approaches. For example, cognitive therapies share with psychodynamic therapies the assumption of irrational thought processes, the difference being that cognitive–behavioural approaches suggest that these thought processes are learned and maintained through reinforcement, and so can be challenged directly rather than through unconscious determinants, as implied by psychodynamic therapy (Roth & Fonagy 1996). Other examples of overlap include the notion of helplesness, which includes feelings of low self-efficacy and self-esteem. This can be observed by therapists when working with people with mental illness. The tendency is to avoid painful cognitions through denial, and therapists might see this in patients who have had recent news of terminal illness. This coping mechanism allows the person to deal with feelings that cannot be dealt with in any other way and is a means of protecting one's self-concept. Cognitive–behavioural therapy is described in detail in Chapter 10 and is used extensively by occupational therapists in their work with people with mental health problems. Physiotherapists are increasingly integrating cognitive–behavioural strategies into the management of people with mental illness with skills acquired through attendance at postgraduate courses. The application of this model in the management of pain by occupational therapists and physiotherapists has been emphasized in Chapter 12. Cognitive–behavioural strategies such as motivational interviewing and joint goal setting are routinely used in promoting both the uptake and adherence to physical activity programmes (see Chapter 8 for examples) and other social integration activities.

Conclusion

Although advances have been made in molecular genetics and identifying neurochemical pathways, there has been general disappointment that the pathophysiology of mental illness has not yet been delineated. It is perhaps, naïve of the medical fraternity to expect that causal explanations will be fully accounted for within the brain when the explanations offered to account for mental health disorders are multitudinous and include strong support for environmental and psychological factors. These diverse explanations provide a range of models that influence and direct current approaches in the treatment and management of people with mental health problems. The dominance of the biomedical model is increasingly being challenged by other professional groups such as psychologists, psychotherapists, nurses, occupational therapists, physiotherapists and social workers (Ussher 1991), all of whom are increasing their expertise and proficiency in the care of people with mental illhealth. The contribution by these professional groups is recognized within the National Health Service Framework for Mental Health (Department of Health 1999). With an emphasis on multiprofessional and interdisciplinary team working, providing support for both the individual and the family within the community setting, facilitating social integration and providing equity in access to treatment for people from all cultures and all social classes.

An evidence-based approach is generally advocated in deciding which therapeutic model to base interventions upon. The efficacy of the different models of psychotherapy have been established through controlled research studies, with sufficient evidence to indicate that more than one type of therapy seems to be effective in alleviating symptoms for the majority of people (Roth & Fonagy 1996). There is a growing body of evidence to support cognitive–behavioural interventions (Donaghy & Durward 2000). However, our understanding as to why these different approaches work is still poor. The placebo effect and the influence of the therapeutic relationship have not been controlled for in the majority of studies that have looked at the efficacy of therapy. Future research should attempt to address these issues. It might be that the benefits of therapy are due to contact time and the enthusiasm of the therapist. Hence, it would seem appropriate that, where the evidence is equivocal, the most appropriate way forward is to use the approach that best fits with the identified needs of the person. It is important to ensure that the philosophy underpinning the model is consistent with the individual's own view of his or her condition and is in keeping with the skills of the professional. Consideration should be given to the patient's views with regards to treatment and in deciding whether to work with the individual, with the group or with the family.

Historically, physiotherapists have worked within the biomedical model and occupational therapists within a psychodynamic or cognitive–behavioural framework. However, increasingly other models are being applied in approaches to treatment, e.g. the client-centred approach as a way of communicating with people and specifically as applied to counselling. Intuitively, physiotherapists might find they are applying a cognitive–behavioural approach in treatment, with the use of strategies such as diary keeping to facilitate motivation in activity and adherence. Training in the cognitive–behavioural approach can inform the treatment of anxiety management and depression, social skills training and in working with people with enduring mental illness. Multiprofessional working requires the physiotherapist and occupational therapist to work alongside the clinical psychologist and community psychiatric nurse. The roles might overlap but there are boundaries of delineation and each profession has a different knowledge-base and clinical skills. Eclecticism encourages a diversity of therapeutic process; however, the goals should be clearly identified for each individual and for all professionals involved in the management plan.

Current trends in delivery of care emphasize a collaborative team approach. It is likely that in the future physiotherapists and occupational therapists will influence existing theoretical models by evaluating practice, undertaking research and debating the issues pertinent to the health-care provision alongside other members of the team, including the people with mental health problems receiving the therapeutic intervention.

Summary

- Different models are used to give specific perspectives to the understanding of mental health disorder.

- The models originate from both medicine and social sciences and broadly reflect two major standpoints: how the brain works and knowledge about an individual's interaction with the environment. The biomedical viewpoint focuses on neurobiology and genetics, whereas social science is influenced by epidemiology, sociology and psychology.

- Therapeutic models influencing interventions are also informed by different schools of thought, usually from psychology. These include psychodynamic, cognitive–behavioural and humanistic.

- Therapists working in the field of mental health are informed by these models and are increasingly challenging the dominance of the biomedical approach and asserting their clinical expertise in this field.

- With increasing emphasis on evidence-based practice, therapists are selecting models according to the efficacy of intervention.

- The need for more interprofessional teamworking signalled by current mental health policy, ensures that therapists will use the approach that best fits the needs of the individual within the context of his or her environment.

- Continued research is needed into cognitive–behavioural therapy to ensure that the growing body of evidence to support these interventions is unequivocal.

References

American Psychiatric Association 1994 Diagnostic and statistical manual of mental disorders, 4th edn. APA, Washington DC

Beck A T 1976 Cognitive therapy and the emotional disorders. International Universities Press, New York

Bernstein D, Roy E, Srull T, Wickens C 2000 Psychology, 5th edn. Houghton Mifflin, Boston, MA

Biddle S J H, Fox K R, Boutcher S H 2000 Physical activity and psychological well-being. Routledge, London.

Bruton C, Crow T, Frith C et al 1990 Schizophrenia and the brain: a prospective cliniconeuropathological study. Psychological Medicine 20:285–304

Bunkan B H, Thornquist F 1990 Psychomotor therapy: an approach to the evaluation and treatment of psychosomatic disorders. In: Hens T, Sveram M (eds) Psychological and psychosomatic problems. Churchill Livingstone, Edinburgh

Byne W, Kemether E, Jones L et al 1999 The neurochemistry of schizophrenia. In: Charney D S et al (eds) Neurobiology of mental illness. Oxford University Press, New York, p 263–245

Chadwick R 2000 Ethical issues in psychiatric care: geneticisation and community care. Acta Psychiatrica Scandinavica Supplementum 399: 35–39

Charney D S, Nestler E J, Bunney B S (eds) 1999 Neurobiology of mental illness. Oxford University Press, New York

Cloninger C R 1999 A new conceptual paradigm from genetics and psychobiology for the science of mental health. Australian and New Zealand Journal of Psychiatry 33(2):174–186

Cooper B 2001 Nature, nurture and mental disorder: old concepts in the new millennium. British Journal of Psychiatry Suppl 40:S91–S101

Cowan W M, Harter D H, Kandel E R 2000 The emergence of modern neuroscience: some implications for neurology and psychiatry. Annual Review of Neuroscience 23:343–391

Davis K L, Kahn R S, Davidson M 1991 Dopamine in schizophrenia: a review and reconceptualisation. Americal Journal of Psychiatry 148: 1474–1486

de Fonseca A F 1989 Psychiatry in the 1990s. In: Hindmarsh I, Stoner P (eds) Human psychopharmacy: measures and Methods, vol. 2. Wiley, New York

Department of Health (DoH) 1999 National service framework mental health. Modern standards and service models. Department of Health, London

Donaghy M 1995 Models of mental disorder. In: Everett T et al (eds) Physiotherapy in mental health. Butterworth Heinemann, Oxford

Donaghy M, Durward B 2000 A report on the clinical effectiveness of physiotherapy in mental health. Chartered Society of Physiotherapy, London

Ellis A 1962 Reason and emotion in psychotherapy. Springer-Verlag, New York

Frith C D 1979 Conscious information processing and schizophrenia. British Journal of Psychiatry 134:225–235

Gill M 1991 Ethics, molecular genetics and psychiatric disorders. In: Sram R J et al (eds) Ethical issues of molecular genetics in psychiatry. Springer Verlag, London

Goldberg D, Huxley P 1980 Mental illness in the community: the pathway to psychiatric care. Tavistock, London

Goldberg D, Huxley P 1992 Common mental disorders: a bio-social model. Tavistock, London

Gray P 1991 Psychology. Worth, New York

Gurman A S, Kniskem D P, Pinsof W M 1986 Research on marital and family therapies. In: Garfield S L, Bergin A E (eds) Handbook of psy-

chotherapy and behavioural change, 3rd edn. Wiley, New York

Heninger G R 1999 Special challenges in the investigation of the neurobiology of mental illness. In: Charney D S et al (eds) Neurobiology of mental illness. Oxford University Press, New York, p 89–99

Karasu T B 1986 The specificity versus nonspecificity dilemma: toward identifying therapeutic change agents. American Journal of Psychiatry 143:687–695

Kendler K S 1999 Molecular genetics of schizophrenia. In: Charney D S et al (eds) Neurobiology of mental illness. Oxford University Press, New York, p 203–213

Kovel J 1982 The American mental health industry. In: Ingelby D (ed) Critical psychology: the politics of mental health. Penguin, Harmondsworth, UK

Laing R D 1967 The politics of experience. Penguin, Harmondsworth, UK

Laing R D, Esterson A 1964 Sanity, madness and the family. Tavistock, London

Meichenbaum D 1977 Cognitive behaviour modification. Plenum Press, New York

Minuchin S, Fishman C 1981 Family therapy techniques. Harvard University Press, Cambridge, MA

Newell R, Dryden W 1991 An introduction to the cognitive–behavioural approach. In: Dryden W, Rentoul R (eds) Adult clinical problems: a cognitive–behavioural approach. Routledge, London

Owen M J, Cardno A G, O'Donovan M C 2000 Psychiatric genetics: back to the future. Molecular Psychiatry 5(1):22–31

Peroutka S J 1997 The medical utility of genomics data in neuropsychiatry: mutational genetics versus association genetics. Current Opinion in Biotechnology 8(6):688–691

Rogers C R 1980 A way of being. Houghton Mifflin, Boston, MA

Roth A, Fonagy P 1996 What works for whom? A critical review of psychotherapy research. Guilford Press, New York

Rutter M, Plomin R 1997 Opportunities for psychiatry from genetic findings. British Journal of Psychiatry 171:209–219

Salkovskis P M 1996 Trends in cognitive and behavioural therapies. Wiley, Chichester, UK

Sanders A R, Sevilla Detera-Wadleigh S D, Gershon E S 1999 Molecular genetics of mood disorders.

In: Charney D S, Nestler E J, Bunney B S (eds) Neurobiology of mental illness. Oxford University Press, New York, p 299–316

Skinner B E 1953 Science and human behavior. Macmillan, New York

Skynner R 1976 One flesh: separate persons. Trowbridge and Esher, London

Szasz T 1961 The myth of mental illness: foundations of the theory of personal conduct. Secker, London

Ussher J 1991 Women's madness: misogyny or mental illness? Harvester Wheatsheaf, London

Weller M, Eysenck M 1992 The scientific basis of psychiatry, 2nd edn. W B Saunders, Philadelphia

Williams P, Tarnopolsky A, Hand D, Shepherd M 1986 Minor psychiatric morbidity and general practice consultations: The West London Survey. Psychological Medicine 16(Suppl):1–37

Wolpe J (1958) Psychotherapy by reciprocal inhibition. Stanford University Press, Stanford, CA

Wood R J 1987 Brain injury rehabilitation: a neurobehavioural approach. Croom Helm, London

World Health Organization 1992 International classification of diseases, 10th edn (ICD 10). WHO, Geneva

Zorilla L T E, Cannon T D, Kronenberg S et al 1997 Structural brain abnormalities in schizophrenia: a family study. Biological Psychiatry 42:1080–1086

2 Mental health disorder: a biomedical approach

Nick Rose

Introduction

One in four people experience a mental health disorder at some point in their lives, and the risk is particularly high for those who have chronic physical disability or illness. Occupational therapists and physiotherapists, therefore, are very likely to be working with individuals who have specific mental health disorder and, as symptoms often go undetected, this might not be recognized. In keeping with a biomedical approach, patient and psychiatric illness are terms that are used in this chapter.

When people are physically ill it is sometimes difficult to distinguish between normal emotional responses to stress and psychiatric illness. Yet this is important, because psychiatric illnesses are generally treatable, thus making it much easier to help with the underlying physical problem. Correspondingly, failure to recognize and help a patient's psychiatric problem is likely to slow down that person's physical recovery, particularly where active participation in therapy is needed.

This chapter will explain what is meant by the term 'psychiatric illness' and will describe the main types you are likely to encounter as a physiotherapist or occupational therapist. It will then highlight the reasons why particular individuals become ill, and how common this is. Finally, the recognition of psychiatric illnesses, the awareness of particular risk factors, the importance of personality and ways in which people can be helped are described.

What are psychiatric illnesses?

Individual psychiatric illnesses consist of particular clusters of symptoms that recur in different people at different times and places. These symptoms typically consist of a combination of abnormal thoughts and bodily sensations, usually called cognitive and somatic symptoms. For example, in the psychiatric illness of depression the cognitive symptoms include thoughts of guilt, worthlessness and hopelessness, whereas the somatic symptoms include loss of energy, sleep and appetite disturbance, and tiredness. Similarly, in the illness of anxiety state the cognitive symptoms include fearful thoughts of dying, suffocating, collapsing or making a fool of oneself, whereas the somatic symptoms can include palpitations, breathlessness and sweating.

To recognize a psychiatric illness one must detect the cluster or pattern of symptoms. Unlike physical medicine, there is rarely a laboratory test to confirm the diagnosis. This is because with most psychiatric illnesses we have yet to find any single underlying physical cause such as a virus. Thus, diagnosis of psychiatric illness is usually determined by whether sufficient key symptoms of a recognized cluster are present.

When does a symptom cluster become an illness?

In psychiatry, there is often a continuum between normality and illness. For example, after major loss or trauma it is natural to develop symptoms of sleep and appetite disturbance, features that are also found in depression. How then can one distinguish between the two?

Three things tend to point towards a diagnosis of illness. First, the presence of a full cluster of symptoms. Therefore, in someone coping with a major loss, a diagnosis of depression would need the presence of symptoms of guilt or hopelessness, together with a number of the somatic symptoms summarized in Table 2.1.

Second, symptoms would normally be persistent, often over a period of weeks if not months.

Third, the intensity of symptoms is likely to impair daily living to some degree.

Thus, where an individual is experiencing psychiatric symptoms, the diagnosis of mental illness depends on whether there is a sufficient clustering of individual symptoms, and on the duration and intensity of these symptoms. If a psychiatric illness is thought to be present this is likely to have specific treatment implications.

What different types of symptom clusters are there?

Broadly speaking, there are two groups of psychiatric illnesses. The first comprises those with symptoms that represent a gross exaggeration of experiences that many of us are familiar with; examples include depression, anxiety and obsessional illness. These are sometimes called neuroses. The second comprises those with symptoms totally different from normal experience; examples include schizophrenia and bipolar affective disorder (manic depression). These are sometimes called psychoses.

Less frequently, psychiatric illness can be caused by physical factors, such as in drug or alcohol withdrawal, endocrine disorders or steroid use. These are usually called organic psychiatric disorders.

In addition to psychiatric illnesses, some people suffer from abnormalities of behaviour and personality. If these abnormalities are enough to cause serious persistent disruption in relationships and in employment, then a personality disorder might be present. People with personality disorders are often distressed and needy, are more likely to seek medical attention and can pose particular difficulties during treatment.

Table 2.1 *Diagnosis of psychiatric illness*

Diagnosis	Main symptoms	Comments
Depression	Depressive thinking: sadness, thoughts of guilt and suicide Physical symptoms: hopelessness (worse in mornings); waking early; loss of energy, interest, appetite, weight and concentration In less severe forms of depression: symptoms more variable, physical symptoms less prominent, often associated with irritability, anxiety and/or tension	A very common disorder, especially among the physically ill Physical symptoms can predominate and be attributed to physical illness Diagnosis often missed Antidepressant medication generally effective Beware of suicide risk
Anxiety	Anxious thinking: irrational fears of dying, falling, looking foolish Physical symptoms: palpitations, sweating, breathlessness, 'pins and needles', gastrointestinal symptoms Can be acute (weeks/months) or chronic (years) Can be associated with avoidance of situations that trigger anxiety, e.g. crowded places (agoraphobia) or social situations (social phobia) Often associated with coexistent depression	Very common disorder Physical symptoms can predominate and can be attributed initially to cardiac or gastrointestinal disorder Acute anxiety is usually self limiting, even without treatment Anxiety management and relaxation techniques used in preference to minor tranquillizers (e.g. valium), which can cause dependency Phobic avoidance behaviour might indicate the need for specialized psychological treatment
Anorexia nervosa	Characteristic overconcern about shape and weight Active maintenance of unduly low weight by excessive dieting, exercise and less commonly self-induced vomiting Amenorrhoea and physical effects of starvation Associated depression, anxiety and obsessional symptoms	Uncommon Reluctant to seek or engage in help Mainly affects young women aged 16 to 35 years Might present to physician with associated medical problems such as fainting or weight loss Can be life-threatening
Bulimia nervosa	Characteristic overconcern about shape and weight Normal body weight (usually) Frequent bulimic episodes (bingeing) involving consumption of large amounts of food in out-of-control way	More common than anorexia Most cases never come to medical attention Some people have combined symptoms of anorexia and bulimia

Table 2.1 *Cont'd*

Diagnosis	Main symptoms	Comments
	Use of extreme behaviour to control shape and weight	Specialized psychological help usually needed for both anorexia and severe bulimia
	Associated depression and anxiety, sometimes with substance abuse	Long-term outcome (years) of anorexia and bulimia: less than half remain well
Schizophrenia (acute form)		Uncommon
	Bizarre false beliefs often of persecution (delusions)	Individuals might not believe they are ill and so not seek or engage in help
	Often hear frightening voices (auditory hallucinations)	Compulsory treatment sometimes necessary if person poses serious risk to self or others
	Sometimes bizarre disturbed or aggressive behaviour	
	Can be triggered in vulnerable individuals by stress, e.g. surgery, accident, childbirth	Effective help usually comprises social, psychological and pharmacological interventions
Schizophrenia (chronic form)	False beliefs and voices can persist	Families and carers often under stress
	Negative features such as poor motivation and social withdrawal	
	Associated chronic social, occupational and personal dysfunction	
Hysteria	Disturbance of motor sensory or cognitive function in which:	Uncommon in severe form
	■ There appears to be no physical cause	Can be associated with coexistent depression
	■ Symptoms usually correspond to patient's level of understanding about illness, with resultant discrepancies between hysterical signs and symptoms and those of organic disease	Often chronic, presenting to physicians rather than psychiatrists
	■ Patients can gain advantage from symptoms (secondary gain)	Treatment often slow and only partially effective, involving reduction of secondary gain resulting from illness
	■ Patients can be unconcerned by symptoms (*belle indifference*)	
	■ Dysfunction can include limb weakness/ paralysis, loss of sensation, loss of memory	

Table 2.1 *Cont'd*

Diagnosis	Main symptoms	Comments
Obsessions	Obsessional thinking: compulsively repetitive thoughts, images or impulses that are out of character with the person, and recognized as being nonsensical (e.g. quite conscientious mother has obsessional impulses to harm her child)	Uncommon Can be associated with coexistent depression and anxiety Treatment can involve intensive psychological therapy, sometimes combined with medication Often of chronic duration (years)
	Obsessional behaviour: usually associated with obsessional thoughts, e.g. thoughts of contamination might be associated with repeated cleaning Can also be in the form of repeated behaviour, such as pacing in particular ways, gestures, arranging objects, etc.	
Mania	Grandiose thinking, overactivity, sleeplessness, irritability, disturbed behaviour	Uncommon
	Can be triggered by stress, as in schizophrenia and severe depression	Reluctant to seek help because of lack of insight Compulsory treatment might be necessary
	Usually occurs in individuals who are vulnerable to severe recurrent depression (manic depression)	Long-term prophylactic medication, such as lithium, might be needed to reduce the risk of recurrent manic and depressive episodes
Acute (organic) mania	Consciousness impaired, with confusion, disorientation in time, place and person	Can be caused by a variety of agents, including alcohol and drug withdrawal, toxaemia and septicaemia
	Person might experience voices, persecutory beliefs, visual hallucinations	Disturbed, often fearful, behaviour
	Usually acute onset	Can occur following surgery, childbirth, dialysis, etc.
Dementia	Global intellectual impairment	Most common pathological cause is Alzheimer's disease
	Preservation of clear consciousness	Depression with associated slowed thinking can mimic organic dementia

Table 2.1 *Cont'd*

Diagnosis	Main symptoms	Comments
	Might be progressive, depending on cause Usually slow, insidious onset associated with uncharacteristic behaviour	Some dementias are treatable, e.g. vitamin B12 deficiency Dementia might not come to medical attention until relatively late Families and carers often under great stress

In any one individual, a psychiatric illness and personality disorder can coexist, making the outcome of treatment for the psychiatric illness less favourable. Likewise, personality disorder and physical illness or disability can coexist and result in difficulties during the rehabilitation phase of the illness.

More commonly, dominant personality traits can influence the clinical picture. These traits are of insufficient severity to cause the level of dysfunction associated with personality disorder but can nevertheless present clinical management difficulties, particularly in the diagnosis and care of physical illness.

Thus, influential personality characteristics can vary across a spectrum from mild (personality trait) to severe (personality disorder). Some of the more commonly encountered personality characteristics likely to be encountered in physical medicine are described later in this chapter.

What are the characteristics of psychiatric illnesses?

Eight important characteristics of psychiatric illnesses are described below.

Common Psychiatric illnesses are particularly common among general hospital inpatients and general practice and hospital outpatient clinic attenders. Up to one-third of attenders have significant psychiatric symptoms and up to one-fifth have a specific psychiatric illness, most commonly depression or anxiety. This is significantly higher than would be expected from a general population sample and in part reflects the stressful nature of physical illness.

Those at particularly high risk of developing psychiatric disorders include people with chronic physical disability or pain, people who have life-threatening illnesses and people who have lost a significant part of their bodily functioning, e.g. after a stroke, an amputation or a mastectomy. (By contrast, women undergoing hysterectomy appear to have a particularly low risk of developing psychiatric disorder after surgery.)

Recurrence   Once a person has suffered from a psychiatric illness the risk of recurrence is greater than if they had never had that illness. For example, the risk of a psychotic illness after childbirth increases from 1 in 500 to 1 in 5 if the mother has had a previous psychotic illness. Likewise, a man who has had a history of depression during his life is at particular risk of developing depression following a major health problem such as a heart attack.

Hidden   The presence of a psychiatric illness is often missed, even by experienced clinicians. At least a half of depressive illnesses are missed in hospital and GP clinics, for example. Alcohol dependence and eating disorders, particularly bulimia, are also likely to be missed.

The reasons why certain common psychiatric disorders are so readily missed are various: depressed patients might fail to recognize their illness, feel unworthy of asking for help, or attribute symptoms to physical illness; bulimic patients might be too ashamed to seek help; patients abusing alcohol might deny the problem not only to others but to themselves.

Varied presentation   Psychiatric illness can present in different ways. This is partly because individuals attach differing importance and meaning to certain symptoms.

Psychiatric disorders presenting with physical symptoms   Both anxiety and depression can present with predominantly physical symptoms. In anxiety, for example, some patients will almost exclusively focus on physical symptoms such as palpitations, interpreting these as evidence of a failing heart. Such patients might eventually be referred to cardiac clinics, and it can be hard to reassure them that their problem is psychological. Similarly, patients suffering from depression might focus on physical symptoms such as tiredness, lack of energy or weight loss. Because they do not complain of sadness or hopelessness, physical illness might be assumed to be the cause and a treatable depression missed.

Psychiatric disorders can sometimes present as a failure of the patient to progress as expected through a physical rehabilitation care plan, particularly when the cognitive symptoms of illness are not conspicuous enough to alert carers to the possibility of psychiatric disorder.

Psychiatric disorders presenting with behaviour change   Sometimes it is not the symptoms of psychiatric disorder that present, but their behavioural consequences. For example, a depressed or anxious person might uncharacteristically shoplift or drink heavily; an anxious person might become increasingly housebound for fear of having a panic attack when not at home; a depressed person might underfunction at work or at home; or a manic depressive person during a manic phase of the illness might behave in a highly disinhibited overactive fashion, perhaps spending recklessly and getting into trouble with the law.

Stress related

Most psychiatric illness is triggered by stress. This is particularly true of the more acute illnesses. Stress usually arises from loss or threatened loss, conflict of some sort, change or relationship difficulties. It can therefore be seen that the onset of physical illness, particularly of a chronic or disabling type, can act as a potent source of stress, especially in those vulnerable to psychiatric illness. A stroke or heart attack, for example, represents a loss of good health and can impose substantial changes in the person's lifestyle, employment and relationships.

Distressing to patient and carers

Most psychiatric illnesses are unpleasant to experience. The degree of distress caused can be considerable, with little relief. Because much of the distress comes from the associated preoccupying thoughts, it is particularly invasive. For example, constant preoccupation with anxious thoughts of impending disaster, obsessional thoughts of dirt and cleanliness, distressing thoughts about bodily image (eating disorders) or persecutory thoughts (paranoid disorders) can be intensely preoccupying and exhausting. Such thoughts, when combined with other symptoms, can lead to ideas of suicide as the only escape route. Indeed, the suicide rate in most psychiatric disorders is in excess of 10 times that of the general population.

The distress for families and carers is also great. This is particularly true of the more chronic disabling illnesses such as obsessional and agoraphobic disorders, schizophrenia and bipolar affective disorders. It is also true that stressful and overcritical home circumstances can increase the relapse rate of some of these disorders, thus creating a vicious circle of family stress contributing to illness relapse, which further increases stress on the family.

Impair personal functioning

Most psychiatric illnesses have a serious effect on the individual's day-to-day functioning, whether at work, socially or in the family. Sometimes the impairment is found in just one area of functioning, e.g. a patient with bulimia might be able to perform well at work but has considerable difficulty socializing because of his or her eating habits. More often than not, however, the impairment is global. For example, the patient with depression or an acute anxiety state is likely to find problems in most, if not all, areas of functioning.

Associated with high risk

Psychiatric illnesses, as noted previously, are associated with a high suicide risk. This is particularly true of depression but is also true of many other psychiatric conditions, such as schizophrenia, eating disorders, alcohol dependence and personality disorder. Patients who self-harm, for whatever reason (usually relationship problems) also have a high risk of eventually killing themselves.

Some psychiatric disorders are associated with other forms of risk. Risk of extreme self-neglect can occur in depression and schizophrenia. Risk of harming others through assault can occur in schizophrenia and in paranoid or manic states, either as a result of patients believing that others are against them in some way, or as a result of frightened and disorganized behaviour. More rarely, patients with very severe depression might believe that both they and their family would be better off dead and act accordingly. This can be a particular risk in severely depressed mothers who have recently had a baby (puerperal depression).

Why do people get psychiatric illnesses?

Although psychiatric illness is common, most people do not succumb. What then predisposes particular individuals to become ill at particular times? There is no simple answer, because illness usually results from a complex dynamic interaction between a person's vulnerability and the sources of stress in his or her current life situation.

Personal vulnerability

Certain people are particularly likely to develop psychiatric illness during their lives, given the right circumstances. Vulnerability comes from four main sources. First, many psychiatric disorders appear to be familial. For example, the risk of developing schizophrenia or severe depression appears to be increased at least 15-fold if a first-degree relative has the disorder. Thus, whereas the risk of developing schizophrenia at some time during life is 1%, this increases to about 15% if a parent or sibling has the disorder. This is true even if the relatives were separated from birth, thus ruling out shared experience as the cause of the increased risk.

Second, there is evidence that some psychiatric disorders, particularly depression, occur more often in those who have had a deprived or traumatized upbringing.

Third, certain enduring forms of personality and temperament can predispose in some cases to psychiatric disorder. For example, those with lifelong marked anxiety traits might go on to develop anxiety illnesses, whereas those with lifelong overmeticulous or melancholic temperaments might develop depressive disorder.

Fourth, there is some evidence that psychiatric disorder, especially depression, is more likely to occur in those who are in unfavourable social circumstances: people who are unemployed, socially isolated or looking after young children with little support are all at particularly high risk of depression.

Sources of stress in current life situations

As mentioned previously, stress usually arises from loss or threatened loss, conflict, change or relationship difficulties. Sometimes, the development of psychiatric illnesses can be understood as resulting from the impact of a major life event such as bereavement, major illness or redundancy on a vulnerable individual. At other times, less conspicuous stresses can accumulate until one of them finally 'breaks the camel's back'. The relationship between personal vulnerability, stress and any resulting psychiatric illness thus depends on a number of interacting factors. For example, the greater a person's vulnerability, the more sensitive that person is to stress, even minor sources of stress; the less a person's vulnerability, the more resilient that person is likely to be.

It is probably true to say, however, that everyone has a breaking point, and massive stress can trigger psychiatric illness even in the absence of obvious personal vulnerability factors. It is also true that psychiatric illness can develop in the absence of clear stressors, particularly in very vulnerable individuals.

The relevance of an individual's personality

As already described, certain personality traits can be a risk factor for certain psychiatric illnesses. In a more general way, however, an individual's personality and temperament can be an important factor in influencing how that person presents and copes with physical illness, irrespective of whether a psychiatric illness is present. Four personality traits are particularly likely to be important in helping those with physical problems. These will be described separately, although in reality many individuals have features from more than one of the groups.

Somatization

The tendency to respond to life's difficulties by developing a range of physical complaints. This can result in repeated presentation of physical symptoms, with persistent requests for medical investigations despite repeated negative findings and reassurances that symptoms have no physical basis. If physical illnesses are present, they do not explain the nature and extent of the symptoms or the distress and preoccupation of the patient. Any attempt to discuss the possibility of psychological or social factors causing the symptoms is usually resisted. Such patients can become chronic clinic attenders (see Case study 1 in the Appendix, p. 31). The term 'hypochondriacal' is usually used when patients develop a persistent preoccupation with the possibility of having one or more specific serious and progressive physical disorders.

This tendency to express emotional stress through physical complaints might be acutely exaggerated by superimposed depressive or anxiety illnesses. When this is the case, the depression or anxiety should be treated and this might relieve the somatization symptoms.

In its severe form, persistent somatizing behaviour can be regarded as an illness in itself, the two main forms being somatization disorder characterized by multiple bodily symptoms and hypochondriacal disorder characterized by preoccupation with a specific disease. Specialized psychological treatment for these disorders can be of benefit in some cases.

Anxiety

The tendency for the individual to experience persistent and pervasive feelings of tension and apprehension, often associated with poor confidence, sensitivity to rejection, and restricted lifestyle. Individuals can be especially at risk of developing fears and physical symptoms of anxiety when medically ill. Reassurance, careful provision of relevant information and relaxation techniques are likely to help.

Over-dependency   The tendency to allow others to take over, often at the expense of their own needs. This includes powerful feelings of helplessness when alone or abandoned because of patients' exaggerated fears of being unable to care for themselves. Individuals can find everyday decisions difficult without an excessive amount of advice and reassurance from others, and they might also regress to an immature level of functioning when faced with what to them can feel overwhelming difficulty. Often tolerance to loss, particularly of a partner, is poor, and the sick role can be particularly rewarding (see some of the aspects of Case study 2 in the Appendix, p 31).

Antisocial   The tendency to antisocial behaviour, with poor ability to keep friendships, impulsivity, and low tolerance to frustration. Also the tendency to be demanding, blame others and not feel guilty themselves. Individuals might present with fictitious illnesses and other attention-seeking behaviours. Firm boundaries as to what behaviours are acceptable and what are not, together with social and personal support can help.

How to recognize that someone has psychiatric illness

Given the tendency for psychiatric illness to remain hidden, is it worth trying to detect it and, if so, how should this be done? Most psychiatric illnesses are treatable and, because they are associated with suffering, with reduced ability to engage in physical rehabilitation and, in the case of depression, with risk of deliberate self-harm, then detection is clearly worthwhile. How should you go about this?

Three things are important: first, you should develop a low threshold of suspicion. This is particularly important if you see people who are at a special risk of psychiatric illness, e.g. young mothers, those with chronic physical illness or those coping with very stressful circumstances. It is important always to consider the possibility of a psychiatric disorder even when the individual is not complaining of psychiatric symptoms specifically. In some circumstances it might be worthwhile using a screening questionnaire to detect the most commonly ocurring illnesses. The self-report Beck depression inventory, which takes about 5 min to complete, can be used in this way. Patients who score highly could then be assessed in more detail for possible depressive illness. Similarly, the Spielberger anxiety questionnaire can be used to screen for anxiety. It can be particularly useful to do this before and after surgery, because high anxiety levels are associated with increased postoperative complications such as chest infection.

Second, you need to have a working knowledge of the range of symptoms and features that occur in the more common psychiatric disorders. You are then more likely to recognize the symptom patterns involved, understand their significance and mobilize relevant help or advice. A brief description of the psychiatric illnesses you are likely to encounter is given in Table 2.1 (p. 18) together with a commentary on key points to note.

Third, you need to develop the necessary listening and interview skills to enable your patients to disclose their feelings and problems. For example, GPs who give their patients little opportunity to talk about difficulties in their own way are particularly likely to miss treatable underlying psychiatric disorders such as depression.

Listening skills involve the capacity to show interest and sympathy towards the other person, encouraging the person to talk in confidence about things that he or she find worrying, and providing sufficient quiet and confidential 'space' for this to be possible.

Interview skills refer more to the capacity to elicit particular areas of relevant information through a process of careful probing and questioning. Important information to establish would include the nature of any stress or personal vulnerability factors, and the presence of specific psychiatric symptoms. In this way, the likelihood of psychiatric illness and the possible causal factors, together with any associated risk factors such as suicidal thoughts, can be ascertained. An example of a structured interview covering a patient's recent circumstances, past history, current behaviour and state of mind is given in Box 2.1. A more detailed version of this framework would be used by a psychiatrist when doing a formal psychiatric assessment.

What help is available for those with psychiatric illness?

The treatment of psychiatric illness usually involves a combination of psychological, physical and social approaches.

Psychological help

Psychological help is most often in the form of support, together with problem-focused counselling that aims to understand and tackle any difficulties that might have triggered the illness in the first place. Explanation about the nature and effects of the psychiatric symptoms can be important, particularly where physical symptoms of anxiety and depression are prominent. The teaching of relaxation techniques in anxiety, and distraction techniques when preoccupying thoughts and worries are present, can also be useful. These forms of help can be given by a variety of health professionals.

More specialized psychological treatment might be needed in certain conditions. For example, cognitive–behavioural psychotherapy for those with eating disorders, exposure therapy for those with phobic avoidance disorders such as agoraphobia and psychodynamic

Box 2.1
*Example of
structured interview*

Recent events and symptoms
- A 57-year-old man, physically well, working and living alone until having a mild stroke 2 months ago.
- Slow progress in physical rehabilitation, when he was noted to be increasingly irritable and socially withdrawn. He denied problems and subsequently took a massive overdose one weekend, from which he only just recovered.
- Closer enquiry revealed increasingly low mood over a period of 6 weeks; mood was particularly low in the early part of the day. There was also early-morning waking together with general loss of energy and interest.

Relevant past history, focusing on vulnerability factors
- Lifelong dependency on capable spouse who died a year ago. Has few close friends to turn to for support.
- Previous depression treated by GP after patient's mother died 8 years ago.
- Father died of a stroke in his early 60s and patient fears same outcome for himself.

Current behaviour and state of mind
- Able to 'put on a brave face' but cannot sustain this, with his underlying sad expression emerging. Poor self-care, 'letting himself go'.
- On persistent enquiry, reveals he is preoccupied with joining his dead wife, believing he has lost his health, his job and his only friend, and now has nothing to live for. Also feels guilty and worthless, believing he is beyond hope. Regrets surviving the overdose. Unable to see that he is ill and in need of help.

Opinion
- A man with a number of vulnerability factors who succumbed to a severe depression following a stroke. The depression remained hidden because of his reluctance to disclose his feelings, and the way his symptoms were attributed to the physical consequences of his stroke. This resulted in him taking a near-fatal overdose.

Lessons to be learnt
- Awareness that depression is common in the physically ill but can remain hidden; thus vigilance is important.
- Early detection of and intervention in depression can reduce the risk of serious self-harm.
- People who have increased vulnerability to developing mental illness should be observed particularly carefully.

---

counselling for those with certain types of persistent difficulties in relationships.

Psychological help is usually given on a one-to-one basis but can also be given to groups (e.g. learning anxiety management or exploring relationship difficulties) and to families or couples. A family or couple approach is especially valuable if domestic problems have contributed to the illness.

Physical help

Physical help is usually in the form of medication, although in very serious intractable or life-threatening depression, electroconvulsive therapy (ECT) can be given under a brief general anaesthetic. Medication for the treatment of psychiatric illnesses can be divided into antidepressants (including mood stabilizers), antipsychotics and minor tranquillizers.

Antidepressants

These will help about 70% of those who have a depressive illness. However, they do take 1–3 weeks to be effective, some have unpleasant side-effects and care must be taken when prescribing for people who have physical illnesses, especially those of the heart, liver and kidneys. Although tricyclic antidepressants such as amitriptyline are effective and have been available for over 30 years, newer antidepressants such as paroxetine and fluoxetine (selective serotonin reuptake inhibitors, or SSRIs) or venlafaxine (a serotonin and noradrenaline reuptake inhibitor, or SNRI) are now more likely to be prescribed because they are safer in overdose, have fewer side-effects and can be used with fewer problems in many physical illnesses, particularly cardiac ones.

Where a person appears resistant to a trial of antidepressants, alternative medication strategies are available that are usually, although not always, successful. Antidepressant-resistant depression is a common reason for referral to a psychiatrist.

Antidepressants have two purposes. First, to shift depression and second, to prevent depression returning. It is for the latter reason that antidepressants are continued for at least 6 months after the illness has resolved, because to discontinue them sooner increases the risk of relapse. However, some people need to continue taking prophylactic antidepressant medication for many years. In addition to antidepressants, mood stabilizers such as lithium and sodium valproate can be used for the treatment and long-term prophylaxis of manic depressive disorder.

Antipsychotics

These are used to treat the acute symptoms and associated behavioural disturbance of psychotic illnesses, particularly schizophrenia and mania. They can also be used in severe agitated depression. The older antipsychotics such as chlorpromazine and haloperidol cause sedation and can also cause unpleasant muscular side-effects. Where sedation of disturbed or agitated behaviour is not needed, newer antipsychotics such as risperidone and olanzapine can be used, because they produce fewer side-effects. Whatever medication is used, the antipsychotic action will take at least 1–4 weeks before being effective in resolving the underlying symptoms of illness, such as delusional ideas or the hearing of voices. Like antidepressants, antipsychotics have two purposes: initial treatment of the acute illness and prevention of relapse.

During the prevention phase, antipsychotics can be given in intramuscular depot form, usually on a fortnightly basis.

Minor tranquillizers   These are used less and less because of the ease with which people can become physically dependent on them. They are sometimes valuable, however, for brief interventions of up to 3 weeks in severe acute anxiety, after severe trauma or loss, and in combination with antipsychotics in the management of acute psychotic illness.

One of the most common reasons for the failure of any medication treatment is that some patients do not take their tablets. Compliance is better if the purpose of medication is continually reinforced and side-effects can be kept to a minimum either by careful dosage control or, where appropriate, choosing medication with the fewest side-effects.

Electroconvulsive treatment is used in life-threatening depression (either because of very serious suicide risk or failure to take fluids and food) and can also be used when medication treatments have failed. A brief electric shock is given while the patient is lightly anaesthetized. The underlying antidepressant mechanism is almost certainly the same as for antidepressant medication but the effectiveness might be slightly greater, particularly in the most severe depression, and the speed of action faster. Side-effects include a short-lived headache and temporary memory problems for a week or so. There is no evidence of any lasting side-effects or damage, and the temporary side-effects that do occur are usually more acceptable to patients than those of high doses of medication.

Social help   Just as social stress factors can predispose to or trigger psychiatric illness, so help with social difficulties can aid recovery and reduce the risk of relapse. Help with housing, physical problems, finance, social supports, links with self-help groups, and the building-up of structured day activities can all have a part to play. Support to families and carers is also very important and can greatly reduce the risk of the patient's illness relapsing.

How to deliver help to those with psychiatric illness   Often, help can be provided by a number of different people. A GP or psychiatrist can prescribe and give support; a counsellor, health visitor, occupational therapist, physiotherapist, psychologist or nurse can give psychological help; and a friend, family member, social worker, pastor or employer can help with social interventions of one sort or another.

Two things are particularly important. First, it is important for all those professionally involved to establish a trusting therapeutic relationship with the patient. Without this, the helping potential will be greatly undermined. Indeed, a poor relationship can actually make things worse, particularly if it is rejecting in anyway.

Second, and especially if a number of people are involved in helping, it is important to have a clear care plan so that there is no conflict. The care plan should be agreed jointly between the patient, carers or relatives where appropriate and the relevant professionals. A key worker is usually responsible for ensuring that the care plan is carried out and that it is reviewed from time to time.

Summary

- Psychiatric illnesses are recognized by a cluster of symptoms rather than a laboratory test.

- Mental health problems are particularly common in general hospital inpatients and outpatients and people with chronic pain or physical disability.

- Depression and self harm are associated with high suicide risk, as are other psychiatric conditions.

- Intervention needs to psychological, social and physical, and this might include medication and/or ECT.

- Each individual has a right to trusting therapeutic relationships, a clear care plan and a key worker who coordinates the involvement of the multidisciplinary team.

Appendix

Commentary

Case study 1: the chronic somatizer

A 55-year-old with a 10-year history of severe low back pain. Retired on medical grounds 5 years ago from a stressful job	No objective evidence of severe physical dysfunction
Increasing dependency on family, use of walking aids, hospital transport, analgesia, etc.	Secondary gain from sick role includes retirement on medical grounds, attention of the family, no responsibilities
No objective evidence of deterioration on physical examination and investigation	Gain from continued sick role sabotages motivation to improve through progress with physiotherapy and other medical interventions
Regular physiotherapy meets with no progress	Recovery must be based on advantages of health outweighing those of sickness

Case Study 2: overdependent self harmer

A 25-year-old woman who jumped 10 feet (3 metres) and sustained bilateral fractured ankles in an intentional self-harm attempt	Self-harm not clearly suicidal, and might have been, in part at least, a cry for help to ensure subsequent medical care and attention.

Long history of failed relationships, impulsivity, overdoses, and poor ability to live independently or to take full responsibility for herself

Resistant to physiotherapy and attempts to help her mobilize, yet frequently demanding of attention and constantly managing to get nurses to do things for her that she in fact could do for herself

Very slow physical progress towards eventual discharge from hospital to returning to live alone in her isolated bedsit

Isolated impulsive individual who relates to others in a childlike fashion and has high dependency needs

Gain of sick role includes constant professional attention, and the shifting of her responsibilities onto others. Thus poor motivation to become well and poor capacity to become truly independent

Management must:

■ Emphasize advantages of progress to full mobility (e.g. by helping with more supported accommodation, befriending schemes, day activities, etc.)

■ Not collude with dependency by never doing for her the things that she can reasonably do for herself, thus increasing her sense of control and self-esteem

■ Consider contract approach (e.g. appropriate behaviour could be reinforced by regular talking sessions with a member of staff)

3 Policy into action

Gwyneth Owen

Devolution has had an impact on health and social policy in Great Britain: each nation is developing its own unique strategy to address the needs of its population. Reflection on the current situation suggests that there are common principles underpinning the policy agenda; the main differences will be around the organization of service delivery.

Policies are influenced by political, cultural and economic ideologies, and also reflect dominant public opinion and act as pointers to preferred services structures and interventions. Epidemiological statistics identify mental illness as a priority public health problem in Europe, yet less than half the countries in Europe have declared national policies on mental health (Henderson & Van Remoortel 1997).

Throughout the text of this chapter, reference will be made to the English policy documents.

Henderson & Van Remoortel (1997) draw attention to the work of the European Regional Council of the Work Federation for Mental Health (ERCWF-MH). ERCWF-MH notes that a range of issues, including long-term unemployment, homelessness, breakdown of family structures and the emergence of multicultural societies, will have a significant impact on the incidence of mental illness within a population. The Council's recommendations reflect the need for a multifaceted approach to address mental health issues. Health organizations should:

- tackle stigmas
- involve the community
- confront old practices with the use of an evidence-based approach
- assess the quality of services.

This chapter focuses on how the British government is responding to this agenda by reflecting on the health and social policies aimed at improving the quality of care available to people with mental health-care needs.

Mental health policy in Britain

Since coming into power in 1997, the Labour government has actively pursued policies that aim to increase social inclusion, such as *Welfare to work, Saving lives: our healthier nation* and the agenda around homelessness (Department of Health 1999a).

Government policy at the start of the twenty-first century recognizes the interrelationship of health and poverty/social exclusion:

> *The vicious cycle of poverty, social exclusion, educational failure and illhealth is mutually reinforcing. It needs to be broken. It can be broken...Just as good education is a route out of social exclusion and into economic prosperity, so too is good health. By intervening in the poverty cycle, health services can effect what Giddens calls the 'redistribution of possibilities'.*
>
> (Alan Milburn, Secretary of State for Health, 8 March 2000)

Mental health: a public health issue

During the 1980s and 1990s the health inequalities (gender, race and social class) in Britain were ignored, the government of the day preferring to talk about health variations. *Saving lives: our healthier nation* (Department of Health 1999a) represents a shift in ideology and language. It is a 10-year strategy aimed at 'tackling poor health and improving the health of everyone in England, especially the worst off'.

The government has highlighted a range of risk factors for mental illness including poverty, unemployment, social isolation (including that stemming from discrimination), major life events and drug and alcohol misuse (Department of Health 1999a): these complement the position held by ERCWF-MH.

Suicide has been targeted as a marker for the nation's mental well-being: the strategy aims to reduce the number of deaths from suicide and undetermined injury by one-fifth. This target will evaluate the impact of policy changes on health rather than their impact on health inequalities. It could be argued that health is a better measure than health inequalities for a number of reasons including:

- data collection and consistency (mortality is quantitative, morbidity is qualitative)
- political desirability (an overall reduction in mortality rather than morbidity may be achievable over 10 years)
- political sensitivity (reduction in health inequalities implies a redistribution of wealth).

Meeting the target will demand the development of a new three-way partnership between government, local communities and organizations, and the individual, which will be formalized via the Health Improvement Programme (HImP) as illustrated in Fig. 3.1.

Saving lives: our healthier nation proposes a range of action:

- promoting good mental health and reducing risk
- early recognition
- access to effective treatment.

Figure 3.1
Tripartite relationship between the government, communities and the individual

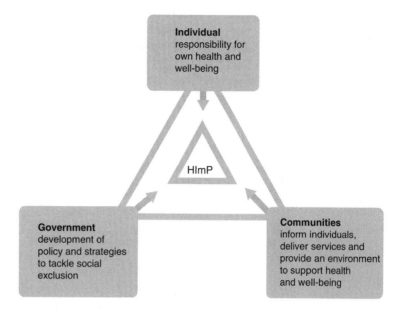

Individual
responsibility for own health and well-being

HImP

Government
development of policy and strategies to tackle social exclusion

Communities
inform individuals, deliver services and provide an environment to support health and well-being

Integrated action across the government departments at a national level should be reflected locally by the development of partnerships across the statutory, independent and voluntary sectors. Such partnerships could be developed and formalized by a range of mechanisms including the Health Improvement Programme and Joint Investment Plans.

The strategy also provided services with flexibility to set their own strategy and milestones for public health, based on the health needs of their population: an early example of the government's drive towards devolving power from a national to a local level. The target-setting process is a means of performance management and will also enable some form of benchmarking, e.g. the creation of performance league tables.

The National Service Frameworks: a model mental health service

National Service Frameworks (NSFs) are a significant element of the standard-setting machinery referred to in *A first class service: quality in the NHS* (Department of Health 1998). NSFs will ultimately determine service configuration in England and Wales (Scotland is developing a separate model of managed clinical networks) around a particular client group/care setting, and will set standards of service delivery for implementation at a local level.

The NSFs are a performance management tool; implementation of the NSF will standardize services as summarized in Fig. 3.2.

The standards and goals set by the NSF have milestones for implementation; these will be used to assess whether the service is moving towards the changes required by the NSF. The service models described

Figure 3.2 *National Service Frameworks – a performance management tool*

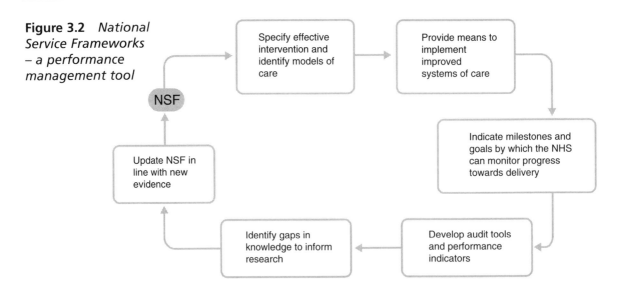

aim to enable services to reflect the need of their local population while ensuring that services across England and Wales meet an agreed standard.

Performance will be monitored by the Commission for Health Improvement, the NHS Performance Assessment Framework and the programme of service-user surveys. Gaps in the current evidence-base will be used to inform the research and development agenda, which will in turn be used to ensure that the NSF is updated to reflect the best-available evidence.

The Mental Health NSF (Department of Health 1999b) covers all elements of mental health for the working-age population, including health promotion, assessment and diagnosis, treatment, rehabilitation and care. The underpinning principles of the NSF include:

■ user involvement in planning and delivery of care
■ non-discriminatory, user-focused services
■ accessibility and continuity of care
■ safety: users, carers, staff and the wider public
■ choices that promote independence
■ interagency collaboration
■ accountability.

The standards from the Mental Health NSF are shown in Box 3.1. Implementation of the NSF is being directed at three levels:

1. A mental health 'czar' has been appointed to oversee the national implementation of the NSF.
2. There are named officers within the Strategic Health Authorities with responsibility for the implementation of the NSF within their region.
3. Implementation teams have been set up locally to develop a programme of change to meet the milestones set by the NSF.

Standard 7 of the recently published NSF for Older People (Department of Health 2001a) aims to address the needs of older people with mental healthcare needs. Its content reflects the ethos of the standards within the Mental Health NSF in terms of promoting good mental health, early recognition and management of mental health problems and access to specialist care.

Box 3.1
*National Service Framework for Mental Health – standards.
(Department of Health 1999b)*

Standard One
Health and Social Services should:
- promote mental health for all, working with individuals and communities
- combat discrimination against individuals and groups with mental health problems, and promote social inclusion.

Standard Two
Any service user who contacts their primary health care team with a common mental health problem should:
- have their mental health needs identified and assessed
- be offered effective treatments, including referrals to specialist services for further assessment, treatment and care if they need it.

Standard Three
Any individual with a common mental health problem should:
- be able to make contact round the clock with the local services necessary to meet their needs and receive adequate care
- be able to use NHS Direct, as it develops, for first level advice and referral on to specialist helplines or to local services.

Standard Four
All mental health service users on the Care Programme Approach (CPA) should:
- receive care which optimizes engagement, anticipates or prevents a crisis, and reduces risk
- have a copy of a written care plan which:
  - includes the action to be taken in a crisis by the service user, their carer and their care coordinator
  - advises their GP how they should respond if the service user needs additional help
  - is regularly reviewed by their care coordinator
- be able to access services 24 hours a day, 365 days a year.

Standard Five
Each service user who is assessed as requiring a period of care away from their home should have:
- timely access to an appropriate hospital bed or alternative bed or place which is:
  - in the least restrictive environment consistent with the need to protect them and the public
  - as close to home as possible

Box 3.1 (Continued)

- a copy of a written care plan agreed on discharge which sets out the care and rehabilitation to be provided, identifies the care coordinator, and specifies the action to be taken in a crisis.

Standard Six
All individuals who provide regular and substantial care for a person on CPA should:
- have an assessment of their caring, physical and mental health needs, repeated on at least an annual basis
- have their own written care plan which is given to them and implemented in discussion with them.

Standard Seven
Local health and social care communities should prevent suicide by:
- promoting mental health for all, working with individuals and communities (Standard One)
- delivering high quality primary mental health care (Standard Two)
- ensuring that anyone with a mental health problem can contact local services via the primary care team, a helpline, or an A&E department (Standard Three)
- ensuring that individuals with severe and enduring mental illness have a care plan which meets their specific needs, including access to services round the clock (Standard Four)
- providing safe hospital accommodation for individuals who need it (Standard Five)
- enabling individuals caring for someone with severe mental illness to receive the support they need to continue caring (Standard Six)

and in addition:
- support local prison staff in preventing suicide among prisoners
- ensure that staff are competent to assess the risk of suicide among individuals at greatest risk
- develop local systems for suicide audit to learn lessons and take any necessary action.

The NHS Plan: partnerships, patients and professionals

The NHS Plan (Department of Health 2000) is the Labour government's 10-year strategy for reforming the NHS in England. Scotland and Wales have developed separate plans – they have themes in common with the plan for England but also reflect the healthcare needs of the population and the organization of services in both these countries. This Plan, together with the NSFs, offers a real opportunity to transform services and respond to the needs of users and carers.

The NHS Plan reiterates the principles of the NHS (equity of access, universal provision, free at the point of delivery and funded by taxation) before outlining a strategy to modernize the service and the investment (staffing and resources) required to achieve this. The themes running through the Plan can be seen in previous policy documents and include:

■ partnerships
■ patient focused care
■ performance management
■ prevention
■ professional boundaries.

The Plan promises an extra annual investment of over £300 million by 2003/04 to fast-forward the (mental health) National Service Framework. The strategy contained within the Plan specific to mental health outlines new service components in the spirit, but beyond the boundaries of, the NSF. The implementation of these proposals should address the needs of people with mental healthcare needs and their carers in primary care and community settings, high security hospitals and prisons (shown in Box 3.1).

In addition to the milestones shown in Box 3.1, the NHS Plan contains a number of other proposals of significance to therapists. The Plan recognizes the current shortage of therapy staff within the NHS and proposes year-on-year increases in the numbers being trained. Implementation of the Plan will also create a new clinical career structure by the creation of consultant therapy posts and opportunities to develop advanced clinical practice posts (clinical specialists and extended scope practitioners). It is likely that the delivery of service will also change, with plans for greater integration of health and social services and the development of new Care Trusts (which will be able to commission and provide primary, community and social care).

Modernization Action Boards (including one for mental health) have been set up at a national level to pioneer the implementation of the NHS Plan. Modernization Teams have been set up regionally and locally, which is where the real opportunities will arise to change the shape of the service for the benefit of patients while ensuring that services are configured appropriately and that they are adequately resourced.

The Labour government's public health strategy stressed the added value of exercise as a means of improving health and well-being. This is formal recognition of the impact of exercise on mental well-being and supports 'exercise on prescription'. This theme is continued across the NSFs and the NHS Plan and has been formalized by the publication of *Exercise referral systems: a national quality assurance framework* (Department of Health 2001b). The framework makes specific reference to the added value of exercise for the management of anxiety and depression. The aim of the policy is to raise the standard of exercise schemes available to the public and to improve the quality of services provided. The framework focuses primarily on the most common model of exercise referral system, where the individual is referred to facilities such as leisure centre gyms for a supervised exercise programme (see Chapter 8).

Mental health policy: an international perspective

Mental health is a global challenge. In Europe alone, one in ten people is known to have a mental illness; 62% of these have psychoses, depression and major psychiatric problems (Walsh 1987). Suicide is the tenth leading cause of death worldwide, and mental illhealth accounts for 10.5% of the 'total global burden of disease' (Sayce 1997).

A long-term survey of 21 European countries undertaken by the WHO Regional Office for Europe (Walsh 1987) concluded that the organization and finance of mental health services in the countries studied was diverse. Institutional care was generally available to all who lived in the countries studied, although the funding of the service varied (either insurance-based, provided by the state or privately funded, or – in the majority of cases – a combination of both the latter). What was common to all 21 countries was the declaration (either explicitly or implicitly) that the policy objective was an integration of mental health services with those at primary care level.

Seven years later, Hall et al (1994) reported an increased worldwide discharge of formerly institutionalized people with mental health problems into the community and an increased focus on alternatives to traditional large psychiatric hospitals. The authors highlighted their concern that the increased contact between people with mental illhealth and the general public, without paying attention to issues of tolerance within the community, could have an adverse effect on the mental health of both parties.

This issue of reducing stigma and discrimination on mental health grounds is becoming an increasingly high policy priority in a number of countries. The Australian government has developed a public education campaign, the New Zealand government has introduced an antidiscrimination strategy based on lessons from other marginalized groups who have achieved change, such as people with HIV/AIDS (Sayce 1997).

Despite common foci (such as reducing discrimination, or de-institutionalization), the organization and delivery of mental health services continues to vary from one country to the next. Jones (2000), in her comparative study of mental healthcare reforms in Britain and Italy, concludes that such variations are considered to be the result of the different national experiences of mental health reform. This is somewhat inevitable given the international diversity in terms of public attitude towards mental health, the underpinning philosophical, professional and legal frameworks, and the organization and funding of health and welfare services.

From ideology to action

A fortnight after the publication of the Mental Health NSF, an editorial in the *British Medical Journal* (Tyrer 1999) stated that implementation was key in determining whether it was a support or a gallows. The author supported the standards in principle, but questioned whether they were achievable.

The Sainsbury Centre for Mental Health (2000) notes that the NSF set seven standards of good practice, but did not specify a precise model to be implemented nationally. Local implementation teams were made responsible for developing the required service with a degree of flexibility: the exceptions being the national milestones around assertive outreach teams, the removal of mixed sex wards, 24-hour staffed beds and more secure beds. Reflection on the proposals for the implementation of the NSF for Older People would suggest that government has recognized the need for a more prescriptive approach in ensuring the local implementation of the NSFs.

The NHS Plan provides a timetable of action for implementation of targets to enhance the Mental Health NSF. This should ensure that stakeholders (service users, providers and commissioners) will know what they can expect, but it could be argued that this prescriptive approach might reduce innovation and responsiveness to local need (Sainsbury Centre for Mental Health 2000).

One consistent theme underpinning health and social policy in Britain is that of partnership. The notion of working together has been reflected in health and social policy since the 1970s. However, the concept of 'partnership' is more than working together because it implies a level of equality between the collaborating parties (Basset 2000). The following barriers are likely to challenge true partnership in a mental health context:

- paternalism of the professions
- stereotyped images of the professionals involved in mental health
- health/social services divide
- mixed messages from the government, e.g. strong language on social inclusion ('involvement', 'stakeholders', 'inclusion') versus messages that non-compliance, especially with regard to medication, will not be tolerated.

Therapists have been actively engaged in developing services that are meeting the government's agenda on mental health care. All the examples listed involve an interprofessional approach; many of the models involve other agencies. This would suggest that therapists are being enabled to articulate their added value and that other professional groups/organizations are aware of the role played by therapists in mental health care.

Vocational
rehabilitation

An assessment and training unit provides a vocational work programme for people with mental illness seeking routes back into employment. People are assessed and offered opportunities to learn new skills in a multiprofessional, supported environment via an occupational action plan. The therapists assess for fitness to work, offer appropriate programmes, run activity groups and use local sport and leisure centres to enhance physical and mental health and social interaction.

The scheme involves work development teams liaising with the Employment Service, local New Deal initiatives, voluntary organizations and Further Education Colleges to improve and develop vocational services.

Prison services

Examples from the prison service, which has formed a partnership with local trusts to ensure that any prisoner needing mental health care is offered this by a specialist mental health multidisciplinary team. The team includes psychiatrists, psychologists, nurses, occupational therapists and qualified counsellors. It has close links with the local primary healthcare providers, thereby improving the equity of access and quality of health care available to prisoners. A therapeutic programme provided from a day unit has been developed in collaboration with prison staff for those prisoners with mental health concerns.

Older people: mental health services in the north of England

The Trust offers an interprofessional approach to the management of older people with mental healthcare needs. The aim of the service is to support clients in the community as long as possible. On receipt of a referral, a psychogeriatrician will complete a home visit to assess the needs of the client and carer(s). A day hospital service is available (offering nursing, occupational therapy, psychology and physiotherapy assessment and intervention) to support and enable service-users to remain in the community; this service has developed links with social workers, community psychiatric nurses (CPNs) and community occupational therapists. More intensive intervention can be offered, if needed, in an inpatient setting, where the ultimate aim is to return the client safely to the community. The team supports a carer's group that meets on a monthly basis. The service is tailored to meet individual needs and has successfully enabled people to be supported at home for many years after initial diagnosis.

Exercise prescription scheme

An exercise referral scheme for people with mental healthcare needs has been running in a northern English town for a number of years. People can be referred to the scheme by any professional involved in their care. The physiotherapist then screens the person and discusses which programme would be most suited to his or her needs. A range of options are available including: multigym and exercise sessions led by the physiotherapist in a primary care rehabilitation centre and swimming sessions in the hydrotherapy pool led by a trained physiotherapy assistant. The physiotherapist is available to see anyone with physical problems; multigym, aerobics, badminton, squash and swimming facilities in the local leisure centre are available for one morning a week. These sessions are supervised by a trained physiotherapy assistant and the leisure service staff. People whose mental state prevents them from accessing any of the above sessions will be given one-to-one sessions with the physiotherapist or trained physiotherapy assistant, depending on the individual's need.

Health promotion: a mother and baby unit

In a regional unit for mothers suffering from postnatal mental health problems, the physiotherapist works alongside the interprofessional team and offers exercise, relaxation and baby massage to enable mother–baby bonding, together with other appropriate interventions.

It is unclear whether these models have evolved as a result of the Mental Health NSF or whether they are examples of models of best practice to which the NSF aspires. Involvement of therapists in the local implementation of the Mental Health NSF would appear to be patchy, although there are examples where therapy involvement in the development of local protocols has changed the nature of the services accessible to clients.

Challenges and opportunities

The mental health agenda, as articulated in *Saving lives: our healthier nation*, the NSFs and the NHS Plan, offers a range of opportunities and challenges to therapists.

The Labour government's focus on mental health will demand that a wider range of professionals develop skills in addressing the needs of this group. Feedback from physiotherapists highlights the high levels of stigma experienced by people with mental health problems. For example, there are instances of referrals for low back pain being passed on to physiotherapists specializing in mental health from musculoskeletal specialists because the prospective client had a secondary diagnosis of schizophrenia. Although this can sometimes be appropriate for a particular individual, it should not be routine. It is hoped that implementation of the Mental Health NSF will go some way to addressing the training needs of staff working outside mental health services, so that individuals are able to access the service most appropriate to their primary needs.

The local implementation of the NSFs and the NHS Plan will demand that therapists become actively involved in the process; otherwise services will become obsolete. There is a growing evidence-base to underpin the role of physiotherapy and occupational therapy in mental health: this should be utilized to inform commissioning of services.

Opportunities exist to develop a clinical career structure with the creation of the consultant therapist. It is hoped that consultant therapy positions will be created within mental healthcare, as this would be one means of attracting therapy staff into this specialism. Furthermore, the promise of additional therapists outlined by the NHS Plan should provide opportunities to consolidate existing services and develop innovative models of service delivery, e.g. services to meet the needs of homeless people, mental health promotion in schools. The career structure for non-professional members of the therapy team also needs attention to attract and retain sports and gym instructors of high calibre.

To maximize the new opportunities, therapists will need to develop their generic skills, notably:

■ communication and networking skills
■ leadership
■ managing change
■ negotiation within a commissioning framework
■ promoting the added value of therapy
■ working across traditional boundaries
■ working in partnership – with service-users and other agencies
■ providing training in mental health awareness to colleagues in other specialties.

Summary

There are some common principles underlying mental health policy across the four countries, with the main difference around service delivery:

■ Policy is influenced by political, cultural and economic ideology and reflects dominant public opinion.

■ Mental health is a priority for national health targets and more recent policy changes reflect an increasing understanding of the multifaceted approach needed to tackle the problem: specifically unemployment, poor housing, social exclusion and breakdown of family structures.

■ Suicide has been targeted as an indicator of the national mental health well-being; the aim to reduce the number of deaths from suicide by one fifth underpins the overall aim of the National Service Framework for Mental Health.

■ Meeting this aim will involve a three-way partnership between the individual, the government and communities.

■ Therapists will need to develop their generic skills in order to continue to impact on the nation's mental health well-being. Those skills include: leadership, working across traditional boundaries, providing mental health training and communication and networking skills.

■ There are some excellent examples of therapists working together to meet the government's agenda of health care that involve a range of interventions and that take place in a range of contexts.

References

Basset T 2000 Is partnership possible? Openmind 104 July/Aug 2000 12–13

Department of Health 1998 A first class service: quality in the NHS. The Stationery Office, London

Department of Health 1999a Saving lives: our healthier nation. The Stationery Office, London

Department of Health 1999b National service framework: mental health. Modern standards and service models. Department of Health, London

Department of Health 2000 The NHS plan: a plan for investment, a plan for reform. Department of Health, London

Department of Health 2001a National service framework for older people. Department of Health, London

Department of Health 2001b Exercise referral systems: a national quality assurance framework. Department of Health, London

Hall P, Brockington I, Eiseman M, Madianos M 1994 Tolerance of mental illness in Europe. In: Sensky T et al (eds) Psychiatry in Europe: directions and development. Gaskell, London, p 171–179

Henderson J, Van Remoortel J 1997 Mental health. The poor relation in Europe. Eurohealth 3(3): 8–10

Jones J 2000 Mental health care reforms in Britain and Italy since 1950: a cross-national comparative study. Health and Place 6:171–187

Milburn A 2000 A healthier nation and a healthier economy: a contribution of a modern NHS. LSE Health Annual Lecture, 8 March 2000. Online. Available: http://www.doh.gov.uk/speeches/index

Sainsbury Centre for Mental Health 2000 Briefing 11: An executive briefing on the implication of the NHS Plan for mental health services. Sainsbury Centre for Mental Health, London

Sayce L 1997 Stigma and social exclusion: top priorities for mental health policies. Eurohealth 3(3):5–7

Tyrer P 1999 The national service framework: a scaffold for mental health. British Medical Journal 319:1017–1018

Walsh D 1987 Mental health services models in Europe. In: Mental health services in pilot study areas: report on a European study. WHO Regional Office for Europe, Copenhagen, p 53–75

4 Service evaluation

John Hall

Everyone engages in a wide range of activities in their own everyday life. From the moment they wake up in the morning, they turn off the alarm clock (maybe!), go to the bathroom, go down the stairs or corridor, search for (and hopefully find) the coffee and bread, put on the kettle and switch on the toaster. Within 5 min they have carried out, unaided, a wide range and sequence of activities involving the integrated use of motor, sensory and cognitive processes – and they aren't even fully awake!

People with mental health problems need to carry out just the same range of activities. They need to be able to carry out a range of desired activities according to the demands of the environment, or the need to fulfil any social, work or domestic role required of them such as:

- fine and gross motor activities, such as dressing oneself or children and the use of handtools
- physical activity, such as shopping, walking or using public transport
- skilled occupational activities, such as using a word processor
- social and recreational activities, such as keep-fit classes, joining in a discussion group or reading.

People with mental health problems can also engage in activities that are undesirable – either to them or to others with whom they share their lives:

- physically aggressive and threatening behaviour
- bizarre or inappropriate speech or behaviour.

The skills of occupational therapists and physiotherapists – and other therapists – are required when patients are unable to carry out everyday activites unaided or at the speed or degree of coordination needed to function. But are those skills used effectively? All therapists are likely to want to know whether their work benefits their patients – and most healthcare funders, whether private insurance companies or national healthcare systems, such as the National Health Service (NHS) in the UK ask the same question. The pressure is now on all healthcare staff to demonstrate the effectiveness of their treatments, and in the NHS the management systems involved in clinical governance require that demonstration (Evans & Haines 2000, Muir Gray 1997).

This chapter outlines some methods of demonstrating the effectiveness of activities carried out by therapists in the mental health field, and shows how a simple evaluation project can be carried out. It focuses on approaches to evaluation that are applicable in normal clinical practice and that can be carried out by internal evaluators – by staff within a clinical service.

The task of a therapist is not just to improve functional performance but to increase the frequency and the degree to which the activity is performed skilfully, thus enabling a sense of efficacy leading to a sense of mastery and a more fulfilling life. Therapeutically, it can also be helpful to reduce the rate of some unwanted activities.

There might be complex interrelationships between these two contrasting goals, so that, for example, an overenthusiastic attempt to engage a socially withdrawn psychotic patient might actively contribute to the exacerbation of positive symptoms. This means that a key professional skill (and an essential skill in designing an evaluation study) is to specify in advance which are the most significant positive changes, and reductions in undesired behaviour (the target behaviours), expected as a result of any therapy, and also to anticipate which adverse changes might occur.

There might be equally complex relationships between a patient's level of activity and his or her internal thoughts and, for example, level of self-esteem. Specific psychiatric disorders can affect some activities but not others, so that depression can selectively affect those activities that depend on speed or concentration. It is often important to assess the consequential changes in mood and patient beliefs arising from therapeutic engagement in activity, but the emphasis of this chapter is on interventions, the main objective of which is to change levels and quality of activity.

It is only possible to know if professional skills are producing an effect if the desired outcome can be defined, and if the expected nature of the change in those activities can also be defined – the target outcome. Treatment evaluation is then, stated simply, the determination of the effectiveness, efficiency, and acceptability of a planned intervention in achieving stated objectives (Holland 1983). This is often stated more fully by such definitions as:

Evaluation is attributing value to an intervention by gathering reliable and valid information about it in a systematic way, and by making comparisons, for the purposes of making more informed decisions or understanding causal mechanisms or general principles.

(Øvretveit 1998. p 9)

This definition adds an emphasis to the importance of conducting the evaluation carefully, of considering standardized measures (if possible) and of comparing with other services or intervention. In practice, several therapists might be treating the same patient at once – a physiotherapist carrying out a physical therapy, a psychologist or counsellor carrying out a psychological therapy and a psychiatrist prescribing pharmacological treatment. It can be very difficult to evaluate the effectiveness of one treatment if other treatments are going on concurrently. So the effectiveness of either a single intervention or a package of interventions – the whole service provided to the patient – may be evaluated.

Research studies on single treatments often involve controlled research designs, where everything except the variables of interest are controlled as far as possible and where patients are assigned randomly to the active treatment and control conditions (a randomized controlled trial [RCT]). In clinical practice, this degree of control is usually unattainable. The impact of new or redesigned specific treatments in routine clinical circumstances can be evaluated, over perhaps longer timescales than research trials, and not necessarily using outside staff, with the potential for seeing how generalizable the results of research trials are to local services.

Service evaluations examine the impact of whole services, or packages of concurrent interventions from a number of different professionals. Audit tends to have a more limited focus, often making use of data collected over a shorter timescale, and which is fed back to practitioners relatively quickly. Rather than seeing these as three separate processes, it is better to see treatment evaluation, service evaluation and audit as overlapping approaches, so the general points made in this chapter are applicable to all three approaches.

It is also important to be clear about who wants to know about effectiveness – who are the 'stakeholders'? Is it the health professional? Is it the service user – the patient? Or is it the managers of the service? Presumably, any professional will want to know how to do their job better, but a professionally led evaluation will focus on outcomes of interest primarily to professionals. Managers could have a prime interest in the cost-effectiveness of a treatment.

Users of services will have different concerns. Whenever possible, any evaluation study should include some assessment of user satisfaction – a symptomatic improvement of interest to a psychiatrist might not be of so much interest to users as their ability to occupy themselves meaningfully. Taking user views into account demands careful thought, and should be done as early as possible in designing a study. Users may justifiably complain if a study has been designed in some detail before they have had any opportunity to contribute, as this carries the risk of untested assumptions by professionals about user views becoming embedded in the project. The World Health Organization (1988) proposed that all projects in their initiative to support people disabled by mental illness should be guided by principles that empower service users, and should avoid the use of value laden terminology. Box 4.1 summarizes these basic elements of any evaluation project.

Box 4.1
The basic elements of an evaluation project

What are the key objectives of the study?

Who are the stakeholders – given the objectives, whose views must be taken into account?

Set objectives:

- specify the desired positive changes
- consider if there are any desired reductions in undesirable behaviour
- consider if there are any desirable secondary consequences of the main predicted changes.

Choose an appropriate focus – single-intervention or whole-service – and design for the study, depending on the resources available.

Choose the data and measures to be collected – the outcomes.

Carry out the study – collect the data.

Analyse the data.

Compare the outcome you have found with outcomes from similar studies or services.

Consider what decisions could be made as a result of this study to improve the service – be an evidence-based, reflective practitioner!

Different conceptual approaches to audit and evaluation

A number of different conceptual models have been developed to articulate the evaluation process. Donabedian (1966) made the classic and simple distinction between three elements of a programme or service: describing the structure (the resources available), the processes (the application of resources, such as the delivered clinical treatment), and the outcomes – or end results.

Shadish et al (1991) suggest that there are five components to evaluation theory:

1. The nature of the programme (that is, the treatment or service) to be evaluated, including theories about how it functions and how change occurs.
2. What type of knowledge about the programme is considered valid.
3. What values are implicit in the evaluation (such as the differing values of staff and users).
4. Ideas about the practice of evaluation and the role of the evaluator.
5. How the knowledge arising from the evaluation can then be used to improve treatment or the service.

Thinking about these components at the outset of a study will guide an evaluator's choice of method, and analysis of results. Dalley (1999) presents an interesting discussion of the tension between client and staff concerns in promoting the idea of client-centred approaches to evaluation, from the author's experience as a physiotherapist. She points out that whereas clients might be seeking a broad-based approach to evaluation, this might not allow attributions of outcome to the specific physiotherapy treatment. On the other hand, professional requirements might be too specific to be truly client-centred. She considers the impact of increasingly complex outcome measures in permitting more holistic measures of health and rehabilitation, but not measuring the specific physiotherapy outcomes. Her article is a helpful overview of how to balance the views of different stakeholders.

A number of different perspectives to evaluation can be adopted, which have implications for both the methodology and content of a project:

- An experimental evaluation is concerned to establish not only *whether* an intervention is effective, but *why* it is effective. This perspective usually requires a precisely stated hypothesis, a careful experimental design and independent external evaluators; it usually focuses on outcomes.
- A variant of this approach is the semi-experimental evaluation, where a non-randomized series, or cohort, of patients is observed or assessed, or where cases are examined retrospectively.
- A developmental evaluation uses systematic methods to enable service providers to develop and improve services. This perspective can focus on process, and might involve qualitative as well as quantitative methods. Examples of this approach would be feedback to the staff of an occupational therapy department about the satisfaction of users with the department, or describing the different patterns of flow of patients through the physiotherapy service.
- A managerial or economic evaluation is concerned with performance management and cost-effectiveness, with a concern for inputs, processes and outcomes. Unless presented carefully, this type of evaluation can appear semi-inspectorial; and the positive benefits need to be emphasized if staff are not to feel defensive.

The semi-experimental, developmental and managerial evaluation perspectives are most relevant to readers of this chapter.

Practical steps in carrying out an evaluation project

The first step in an evaluation project is to agree, with the relevant stakeholders, the desired changes that the intervention or service is expected to bring about. There are limits to what can be achieved in any one evaluation – what are your key objectives? Time and resources will be limited – what can you achieve with the resources you have?

The next steps are then the interconnected ones of choosing a project design, and selecting what data need to be collected. A small pilot study – sometimes just involving one or two patients – can be very helpful in checking the feasibility of a project.

Choosing a design

Descriptive evaluation

This type of evaluation simply answers the question: What happens? For example, the project might answer the questions:

- What resources (e.g. staff, fixed equipment and consumable materials) are actually used to provide the service?
- Who are the users of the service? (e.g. referral criteria, age range and range of presented needs and diagnosis)
- What is the process of providing the service? (e.g. hours of access, size of groups, length of sessions)
- What are the communication routes for both record keeping, and informing referrers and others of outcome?

To expand on two of these points: first, when describing the treatment or service process, it is important to describe what actually happens. It is not sufficient to say the patient engaged in art therapy. How many sessions? What form of art therapy? How experienced was the therapist? What check was made to ensure that the therapy conformed to accepted standards of art therapy? In general, the treatment offered should be described as carefully as possible, including details of therapist competence. In formal research trials it is standard practice to check that the therapists conform to a detailed research protocol – this is known as treatment fidelity.

Second, the characteristics of the patients must also be described carefully. To take a common condition such as depression, the responsiveness of a group of patients to treatment is likely to differ according to the severity and duration of depression, and this is likely to differ depending on how the patients to be studied have been referred. Are they attending a self-referral group run at a health centre, are they being treated at an outpatient clinic held at the Community Mental Health Centre, or are they being treated at a specialist day programme for patients with multiple needs arising from their psychiatric condition?

Carrying out a simple descriptive evaluation can highlight some uncomfortable gaps in knowing what actually happens and would, for example, be an important step in preparing to make a competitive bid for new funding to a manager who does not know the service.

Audit

An audit compares what a service *actually* does, with what it *should* be doing for patients (as stated in a policy or clinical practice guideline). This requires the service to have objectives or procedures specified in writing, which then become the standards that will be checked. In setting standards, account should be taken of the differing views of patients, carers, and professional staff. Standards should be:

■ Relevant – matching standards to the needs of your patients
■ Achievable – be within reach of reasonably resourced competent staff
■ Specific – clearly defined.

Standards set by a national or regional health commissioning or accrediting body are non-negotiable and are mandatory for every service. In England, standards can be set by the National Institute of Clinical Excellence (NICE) or might be set for specific services, as in the National Service Framework for Mental Health. Standards can also be set by a professional registration body, or by local management, where there is some scope for negotiation.

Audit lends itself to the use of simple checklists, remembering that each category must be specific and mutually exclusive of any other category, but the method is not sensitive to the relative value of different items on a checklist. Again, the method can show up where a service is economically poor. This author was involved in a simple audit of the extent to which a key Trust handbook of clinical procedures, kept on every ward and clinical department, was actually updated when new or replacement procedures were distributed – only 3 out of 35 handbooks had been properly updated!

Before-and-after evaluations

Before-and-after studies compare the effectiveness of a treatment or service on the same group of patients. In this design, the data to be collected must be able to be repeated with the same patients. The Rivermead Behavioural Memory Scale (Wilson et al 1985) is a good example of a standard memory scale where there are parallel (psychometrically similar) different forms of the scale, in circumstances where patients might remember the exact wording of an item of the scale. An evaluation study of this design can help to judge the broad effectiveness of an intervention and can suggest factors that might need more detailed study, but it cannot be used to attribute cause-and-effect relationships. In clinical practice, a number of factors can confound the interpretation of results. Thus, it is common for some patients to drop out of treatment or to fail to complete outcome measures, so the drop-out rate, or non-completion rate, from any study should always be noted – and of course could itself warrant evaluation.

Comparison of treatment evaluations

Treatment or service comparison studies compare the effect on two or more groups of patients of different treatments. Whenever a new version of treatment is introduced it is good practice to check that the new form of treatment is better than the one it replaces! It is then important that nothing else changes during the evaluation study, so that, for example, there are no changes in the entry criteria to treatment and both groups have equal exposure to the treatments, in terms of number of sessions or length of treatment sessions. If outcome data have been collected routinely for some time, then the introduction of new procedures in a department can allow a 'natural experiment', whereby the effectiveness of the previous procedure over a fixed period – say, 1 year – can then be evaluated retrospectively and compared with the new programme.

What data should be collected?

Thornicroft & Tansella (1999) discuss three levels of outcome: (1) at the national or regional level where population morbidity rates are known, especially for high-profile conditions such as suicide; (2) outcome indicators for local community use can be derived by interpolating from national figures or by measuring directly at the local level; or (3) by aggregating information collected from individual patients. Therapists' main concern will be at the third level – with individual patient outcomes.

The outcomes of most concern to patients are likely to be:

- Quality-of-life – is their life more satisfying as a result of more activity?
- Effectiveness – has the treatment increased their level and range of activity?
- Confidence – are they willing to carry out the activity on their own without fear of failure?
- Safety – have there been any untoward side-effects or consequences of the treatment?
- User satisfaction – were all the circumstances around the treatment, such as the quality of decoration of the buildings, and friendliness of staff, satisfactory?

Professional staff might also be concerned about:

- Equity – was the treatment equally available to patients, irrespective of where they lived in the catchment area of the service and irrespective of the ethnic origin of the patient?
- Cost-effectiveness – how much staff time equipment time and consumable materials were used to obtain the outcome?
- Appropriateness – even if the patient was satisfied with the service, was there another treatment that could have been used but that was not deliverable?

Identifying the content of the desired outcome then leads to the data categories that need to be collected. In an occupational therapy or physiotherapy service, desired changes might include:

- dealing with referrals more quickly
- offering a wider range of treatments
- having clearer treatment plans.

For these three examples, a simple audit or evaluation data category, or measure, for each of these respectively could be:

- Time elapsed between initial referral and the first contact with the patient.
- Recording the number of specific treatment(s) actually provided within a specified period of time.
- Agreeing a checklist of aspects of a treatment plan that need to be known, and that could be checked by an independent rater.

The above examples all use measures that yield a simple count or number. With the widespread use of electronic patient contact systems, it is quite possible that routinely collected data could answer some of these questions, without the need to collect any additional data. It is easy to design a simple chart or checklist, as already outlined. However, the desired change might require a more subjective (qualitative) measure – such as the satisfaction of the patient with the treatment – or complex measure – such as the change in the pattern of the patient's symptoms. The central issue is to select a method of data collection that is useable in your circumstances. How long will it take to collect the data? What level of professional training or education is needed to understand the measure? How robust is the measure to the realities of service delivery, such as staff absences and sick leave?

There are a number of helpful guidelines to producing a rating scale or questionnaire (Streiner & Norman 1995), but it is unwise to design a complex rating scale without expert advice. It is acceptable to add a few questions of special concern to a project to a standard scale, using the same item format, as long as the standard scale is used intact without revision.

There are a number of useful summaries of commonly used standard measures (Bowling 1995), but often the best way to choose a standardized scale is to read published articles on the topic you are investigating and select a commonly used measure. For example, the Lancashire Quality of Life Profile, developed by Oliver and his colleagues (Oliver & Mohamad 1992) is an interview-based rating specially developed for use in mental health settings. It covers eight 'life-domains': health, social relations, law and safety, living circumstances, leisure, family, work and finances, and religious concerns, and also includes a self-esteem measure and a measure of positive and negative mood. As it has been developed in and widely used in Britain, and is also derived from a well-known American scale (Lehman 1983), it is a good example of a quality-of-life measure that has wide applicability. The 12-item Health of the Nation Outcome Scale (HoNOS) (Wing et al 1996), with accompanying variants for use with young people (HoNOSCA) and with older adults (HoNOS-65), has been promoted as a simple outcome measure for general use. However, the individual items are not sufficiently change-sensitive to evaluate specific treatments.

The level of pain is an issue in a number of activity therapies, and the management of pain is a common task for many therapists. However, the experience of pain is multidimensional, so considering the possible different domains of assessment of pain illustrates the potential use of multiple measures in a study. These might include:

■ Pain or exertion intensity, using a simple numerical rating scale of pain intensity (such as the widely-used Borg Property Scale, or Ratio of Perceived Exertion (Borg 1982)).

■ Level of disability, using a questionnaire measure such as the Sickness Impact Profile (Bergner et al 1981).

■ Subjective distress, assessed by the level of depression, using the widely used Beck Depression Scale (Beck et al 1961).

■ Beliefs or fears about pain, assessed by a cognitively based scale such as the Pain Catastrophizing Scale of Vienneau et al (1999).

■ Use of health care, using the number of visits to the GP, or use of medication.

Most mental health services have a high demand for their services with consequent high demands on those who provide them, so it might be useful to examine the impact of a treatment on staff. For example, it has been shown that there are high staff turnover rates in assertive outreach treatment programmes and, when it is difficult to recruit experienced staff, this has an impact in its own right. Professional staff can thus themselves be the subject of evaluation projects – and managers!

Special issues in evaluating mental health treatments and services

There might be variables that confound treatment outcomes with the consequences of other factors. For example, some psychiatric patients will be taking prescribed medication and some will be taking illicit drugs – or both. Psychotropic medication can cause, as unwanted side-effects, some tremor or unsteadiness. When evaluating the effectiveness of therapeutic activity in mental health it is thus important to consider whether there has been any change in medication over the period of therapy, as these can account for some of the changes seen. Similarly, a patient might have smoked cannabis or, more noticeably, have drunk a substantial amount of alcohol, just before a treatment session; and will usually not admit to either. Whereas inpatient wards can have policies and procedures to limit substance abuse, it is often more difficult to achieve this in day-care or community settings.

In the mental health field an additional factor is not just whether a person can do an activity but whether they are motivated to start and continue an activity by virtue of their current psychological or psychiatric state. If they are severely depressed they might find it difficult to maintain their concentration on a task. They might also judge themselves as performing less well than in fact they do, so their self-evaluation of their performance will tend to be poorer than that of the therapist working with them. It is, then, important to check that patients are engaged with their therapists and their treatment, before including them in an evaluation study. This might mean, for example, that patients would be included in a study only if they had completed at least four sessions, to exclude those who dropped out before any possible benefit could have been achieved.

Making it happen   The initiative for carrying out an evaluation study can come from staff or from managers, themselves driven by external requirements. It takes time and resources to carry out an evaluation project, so the support of a local manager might be needed to negotiate release from some other duties. It could be necessary to gain some funding, so it is then important to find out local sources of research or audit funding and support. It is usually helpful to read and appraise existing practice publications and research, both before carrying out a project and before interpreting the results, so easy access to library facilities and electronic databases will be useful. The numerical or statistical analysis for a simple evaluation project is well within the scope of a hand-held electronic calculator.

The responsibility for an audit and evaluation project could rest with managers outside a therapeutic service but, wherever the pressure comes from, clinical staff might not cooperate willingly in a study unless they can see the benefit of the study for their patients or themselves. Making it happen includes engaging all staff in the potential benefits of the project, and telling all staff, well in advance, about the project and what they will be expected to do.

The best way to start in this field is often to become involved in a project being carried out by an experienced evaluator, and then to ask for supervision from such a colleague. Some services, especially those with high costs or with high-risk patients or treatments, routinely audit and evaluate their services, so ready-made examples of ongoing practice evaluation and audit might already exist. Since the 1990s, there has been increased emphasis in the NHS on demonstrating effectiveness and on applying research. Most areas usually have some form of local Public Health Audit or Resource Unit, or R&D Support Unit, whose job it is to help beginners and who might offer short audit or evaluation training courses. As part of what is called clinical governance, each NHS Trust is required to have a Clinical Governance Committee, which is often linked to a Trust Audit group, whose primary function is to ensure that the lessons learned from projects do lead to improved practice. In all of these contexts, terms such as 'evidence-based', 'clinically effective', and 'good outcome' are common currency. This links the evaluation and audit activities of therapists to other forms of enquiry, such as action research, qualitative and narrative research and service innovation – and the maintenance of innovation (Parry & Watts 1996).

Conclusion   An example of a service evaluation by therapists is provided by Bassett et al's (2001) account of an innovative programme run by occupational therapists in the fastest-growing city in Australia. The group-based programme was designed for adults with a major mental illness, who were also parents of 'under-fives' children. The programme aimed both to consolidate the parent–child relationship and to enable the parents to improve their parenting skills. Six specific objectives were set for the group, including providing a safe environment for discussion of parents' concerns, and providing an opportunity for parents to interact with their children through play and to develop ideas for stimulating their children. Outcomes of the project were based on staff observational data, client self-report, readmission rates and access to community facilities. Thirty-four parents were referred to the programme over 2 years, and observed outcomes have included parents becoming more responsive to their children, increased treatment compliance and a decrease in the number of children in temporary foster care. The article is a fascinating example of an evaluation of an innovative programme, leading to suggestions on how to further improve the programme.

The main purpose of evaluation and audit methods is to inform the ways in which we make clinical decisions, to monitor and justify the use of resources and to improve clinical practice. There is little point in evaluating services unless the knowledge and information we obtain can then be used to improve the quality of services. Users, carers and professional staff should all be involved in choosing those objectives, and the outcomes that will be relevant to a local service. The experience of carrying out an evaluation study successfully can be a valuable entry into a more critical awareness of relevant literature, and an encouragement to carrying out both better evaluation studies, and more formal research studies.

Summary

- The main purpose of evaluation and audit is to inform the ways in which clinical decisions are made, to monitor and justify the use of resources and to improve clinical practice. The outcome from evaluation must then be used to improve the quality of the service.

- Users, carers and professionals must all be asked to help define the objectives and outcomes of service.

- Evaluation is simply the determination of effectiveness, efficiency and acceptability of a planned intervention in achieving stated objectives.

- Different stakeholders (patients, professionals and managers) in mental health might have different priorities in relation to outcomes.

- The main elements involved in evaluation are: defining the key objectives of the study; identifying the stakeholders; setting the objectives; choosing the appropriate focus, e.g. single intervention or whole service; choosing data to be collected; collecting data; analysing the data; reflecting on the outcome and influencing change if appropriate.

■ Different perspectives on evaluation have implications for both methodology and content: experimental evaluation, developmental evaluation and managerial or economic evaluation.

■ Specific issues in mental health service evaluations include the variables that confound treatment outcomes, such as effects of prescribed medication.

References

Bassett H, Lampe J, Lloyd C 2001 Living with under-fives: a programme for parents with a mental illness. British Journal of Occupational Therapy 64: 23–28

Beck A T, Ward C H, Mendelson M, et al 1961 An inventory for measuring depression. Archives of General Psychiatry 4:561–571

Bergner M, Bobbit R A, Carter W B, Gilson B S 1981 The sickness impact profile: development and final revision of a health status measure. Medical Care 19:787–805

Borg G 1982 Psychophysical bases of perceived exertion. Medical Science Sports Exercise 14: 377–381

Bowling A 1995 Measuring disease: a review of disease-specific quality of life measurement scales. Open University Press, Buckingham, UK

Dalley J 1999 Evaluation of clinical practice. Physiotherapy 85:491–497

Donabedian A 1966 Evaluating the quality of medical care. Millbank Memorial Fund Quarterly 44: 166–206

Evans D, Haines A 2000 Implementing evidence-based changes in healthcare. Radcliffe Medical Press, Abingdon, UK

Holland W W 1983 Evaluation of health care. Oxford University Press, Oxford

Lehman A F 1983 The well-being of chronic mental patients: assessing their quality of life. Archives of General Psychiatry 40:369–373

Muir Gray J A 1997 Evidence-based healthcare: how to make health policy and management decisions. Churchill Livingstone, Edinburgh

Oliver J P J, Mohamad H 1992 The quality of life of the chronically mentally ill: a comparison of public, private and voluntary residential provision. British Journal of Social Work 22:391–404

Øvretveit J 1998 Evaluating health interventions: an introduction to evaluation of health treatments, services, policies and organisational interventions. Open University Press, Buckingham, UK

Parry G, Watts F N 1996 Behavioural and mental health research: a handbook of skills and methods. Lawrence Erlbaum Associates, Hove, UK

Shadish W, Cook T, Leviton L 1991 Foundations of programme evaluation: theories of practice. Sage, London

Streiner D L, Norman G R 1995 Health measurement scales: a practical guide to their development and use. Oxford University Press, Oxford

Thornicroft G, Tansella M 1999 The mental health matrix: a manual to improve services. Cambridge University Press, Cambridge

Vienneau T L, Clarke A J, Lynch M E, Sullivan M J L 1999 Catastrophising, functional disability and pain reports in adults with chronic low back pain. Pain Research & Management 4:93–96

Wilson B A, Cockburn J, Baddeley A D 1985 The Rivermead Behavioural Memory Test. Thames Valley Test Company, Titchfield, UK

Wing J K, Curtis R H, Beevor A S 1996 HoNOS: Health of the Nation Outcome Scales. Royal College of Psychiatrists Research Unit, London

World Health Organization 1988 Initiative of support to people disabled by mental illness. Division of Mental Health, World Health Organization, Geneva

5 Conceptual frameworks for community care and working with carers

Mick Skelly

Introduction

There are two fundamental themes to this chapter: one is community care – the sociopolitical context, history and intention of care in the community (Busfield 1997, Pilgrim 1997, Pilgrim & Johnson 1997, Walker 1997); the second is working with 'users', including carers – here primarily conceived of as 'informal carers', i.e. family, friends and neighbours. It should be remembered that six million informal carers – 14% of the population – provide care across all 'disabling' conditions (Parker 1992).

The focus of this chapter will be on carers and the summary of key ideas. The Care Programme Approach (CPA) provides a conceptual foundation for care planning that is relevant to the needs of all stakeholders. Current systems of mental health care have been criticized for tending to provide interventions that primarily see the 'problem' in terms of deficits in the diagnosed individual (Johnstone 2000). Decontextualized, the service-user and their carers' behaviour, feelings and thoughts often appear unreasonable, and it can appear legitimate to seek a return to 'normality', or prevention of 'abnormality' through medication (Brown & Walmsley 1997). Furthermore, we should differentiate between care *in* the community and care *with* the community. 'Collective care' should be considered more rigorously, especially regarding tensions between 'people with disabilities, including the long-term mentally ill, pursuing independence and empowerment and carers pursuing help regarding the "burden of caring"' (Dalley 1997).

The Community Care Act of 1990 made commitments for both Health and Social Services. The current National Service Framework for Mental Health strongly reinforces this message. Services will increasingly be committed to working in a multiagency way with a greater responsibility and responsiveness to service users. Any process of 'normalization' is to be sought primarily through 'social inclusion' and in terms of more local 'norms' negotiated between providers and users. Barriers to closer working between agencies and to interprofessional working will be dismantled, as will unjustified professional boundary setting. Evidence-based practice (EBP) can be seen either as a method of disciplining the professions by replacing 'professional opinion' with objective evidence, particularly research, or as a means by which each profession and its service users can be empowered, through research and objective evidence, both to fight for resources and to ensure that 'best practice' is delivered to patients and carers alike.

Since the inception of community care there has been an implicit risk that needs will tend to be determined by professionals who also hold a brief to contain costs (Walker 1997). This risk is being increasingly mediated by the policy of gradual reduction of professional status and the greater availability of medical information via the internet, etc. It is also mediated through greater user/carer expectations, involvement and (self-) empowerment. The 'fragmentation' of, and friction within, theoretically comprehensive services tends to be along fault-lines best understood in terms of a comparison between biomedical and social–constructionist perspectives. These reflect philosophies connected to theories of: (1) scientifically agreed diagnoses identifying definite medical conditions; and (2) social care, including the concept of 'social capital' (Harding & Palfrey 1997, Johnstone 2000).

The Care Programme Approach (CPA) attempts to resolve potential conflicts and shortfalls in provision by aiming to identify the needs of the person inclusive of carer needs, and provide multiagency services that are comprehensive enough to meet these needs. The CPA follows logically from the aims of Community Care (Box 5.1).

Philosophy and structure for working with users: the overall service context

Mental health services have a statutory obligation to provide interventions within the structure provided by the CPA. Trusts will have needs-based protocols for who requires a formal and full CPA.

The CPA is a 'process-led', 'ecological' system attempting to provide a service that fits the individual person's needs within the local environment. A high level of interpersonal skill will be necessary in such a

Box 5.1
Aims of community care (adapted from Ritchie 1994)

- Enable people to live as normal a life as possible in their own homes or in a homely environment in the local community.
- Provide the right amount of care and support to help people achieve maximum possible independence and, by acquiring or reacquiring basic living skills, help them achieve their full potential. (The concept of providing support is also extended to informal carers.)
- Give people a greater individual say in how they lead their lives and the services they need to help them do so.
- Ensure continuity of care through all involved 'agencies': health, social, voluntary, 'informal'.
- Provide services within a philosophy of social justice and acknowledging the local socioeconomic environment.

system (Klaber-Moffett & Richardson 1997); high technical skills are also required. A process-led system is person-centred and global, attempting to meet all the case needs within the 'package of care'.

This approach ideally requires a comprehensive, unified, multidisciplinary team, possessing access to adequate resources, which is authoritative yet works collectively with the person, their carers or advocate. If anything, its orientation is educational, promoting informed choices and providing appropriate practical support.

Within the Community Mental Health Team (CMHT), the therapists are considered to be specialists, each providing a particular perspective and approach to intervention. Their primary function is to provide specialist assessment of the users'/carers' needs and the tensions between these needs, to suggest possible interventions that might meet these needs and to identify who might best provide these interventions. Certain interventions might be provided only by the therapist, whereas many interventions can be provided by educated/supported carers and/or care staff. The primary role of the therapist is assessment in a 'needs' or 'process-led' system, the secondary role is educational.

The underlying philosophical premise for the physiotherapist in particular is that body and mind are one, that the neurophysiology of the brain is thought/emotion and vice versa; that thought/emotion modulate neurostructure over time, changing the physiology of the body and therefore the body itself. This is a dynamic 'dialectical' relationship, so that changes of body are also changes of mind. This might make most sense in terms of phenomenology (Merleau-Ponty 1967) and Organic Unity Theory (Goodman 1991; see also Chapter 1).

Service quality should primarily be conceptualized in terms of user and carer perceptions. A key dimension for intervention is in the realm of stress management and enabling the evolution of appropriate networks of support (Figs 5.1 and 5.2).

Working with carers

The critical issue for both the person with mental illhealth and for their carers is most probably stress (Cassidy 1999; see also Chapter 11). Parker (1992) asserts that informal carers experience a higher level of stress than the population at large and notes that there are few clear indicators to the specific factors that cause increased stress. Perhaps one clue is that the highest levels of occupational stress are reported amongst voluntary workers. Besides personal factors, the main causes of stress are usually related to perceived lack of control or disempowerment, the perception of poor social support, the perception that formal support via service provision is inadequate to needs and the lack of designated – 'guilt free' – time for themselves. Stress-related problems appear to be greatest for those carers who live with the person whom they care for, yet in this situation the individual concerned often receives the least input precisely because they have someone at home (Parker 1992).

Figure 5.1
Physiotherapy roles in the community care/multidisciplinary team context

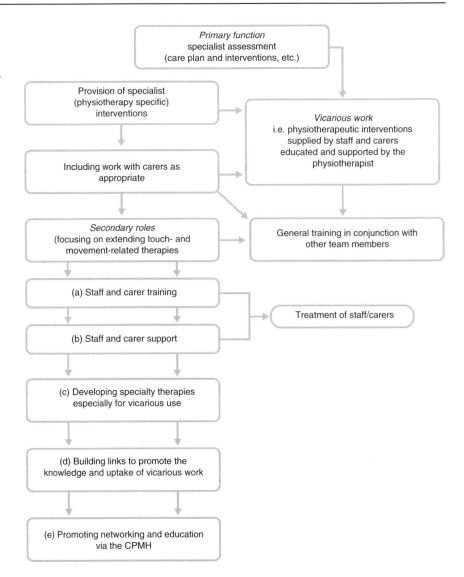

Fifty-eight per cent of carers will develop mental health or other health-related problems as a result of the impact of caring (Pitkeathley 1994).

In structural terms, carer needs might best be dealt with by involving them in every step of the evolution of the care plan and checking that it also meets their needs. In this context it might be best if the care plan is expressed in terms of choices, as a menu, not as a programme dictated by the professionals.

There is also the fundamental need for high quality information, clear without being simplistic, which informs the carer of the condition/needs of the person and helps to put the overall care plan into a rational context. Understanding is a form of empowerment.

Figure 5.2
Multiagency support team (MAST)

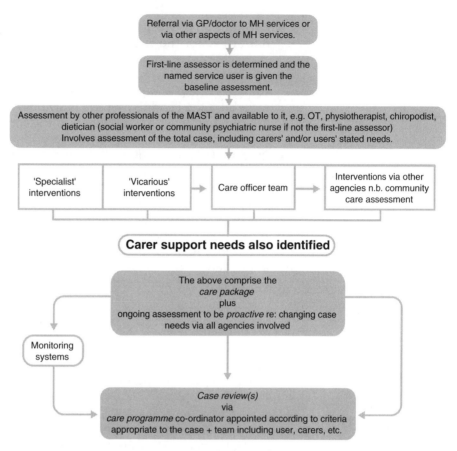

N.B. the case = Named clients + carer(s) + identified relevant 'others' with support or educational needs around the quality of client care. Monitoring systems include all types of outcome and quality assurance measures being used plus the various types of audit.

N.B. 'Vicarious' interventions are interventions provided by one member of the team for another; e.g. a Carer

In terms of service provision, it is the user's/carer's perception of the appropriateness and practical usefulness of the interventions that is important not the professional's 'objective' conceptualization of what is effective.

The care plan should also be focused on recruiting further informal social support and/or upon providing formal alternatives. Individual stress management, addressing all four dimensions of stress (see Chapter 11), is a probable need for all carers. Respite care, holiday cover and/or support is a key need for carers.

The carer might be both angry and guilty, as well as grieving for the person they are caring for and the life they might have otherwise lived. Caring largely takes place in poverty (Pitkeathley 1994) and, in a society where value is largely expressed via remuneration, carers are likely to feel devalued and discounted. Carers are also more likely to be isolated from their sources of community support, including their families. In this context, counselling might be less crucial than more direct forms of intervention. Primarily, carers need practical solutions for practical problems (Box 5.2).

Box 5.2
*Key carer needs
(Pitkeathley 1994)*

- **Recognition (status).** Respect for the carer's opinions and narratives, for the value of what he or she does and for the stress that he or she is under.
- **Information**. First, regarding services, including all possible sources of help and practical support in accessing help. Second, regarding the condition of the individual he or she is caring for and the best ways of working with this individual (this could involve access to training for the carer).
- **Practical help**. Regarding all the practical aspects of care from moving and assisting to continence care, domestic support, aids and adaptations, equipment, transport, respite – including respite that enables the maintenance of a working and/or social life. That practical help should involve rapid access and support for 24 hours per day, 7 days per week, 52 weeks per year.
- **Emotional support**. Dealing with issues of isolation, guilt, anger, fear, etc.

Case study: Reg

Reg was a 76-year-old man with a diagnosis of dementia and anxiety and a history of low back pain, mobility problems and falls. His wife, Irene, was 72. She was Reg's main carer, and was also very anxious and had a history of back pain caused by assisting husband. Their nearest family were over 70 miles away.

Day care was provided and input included exercises for mobility, balance and strengthening under the direction of the physiotherapist. Functional activity was incorporated into the occupational therapy programme. Irene was encouraged and supported in structuring her social life during this 'free' time so as to extend her informal social support network by renewing old friendships. Home visits by the physiotherapist focused on relaxation and massage related to back pain and stress, both for Reg, the service-user, and for Irene as carer. Irene was also given advice and training on moving and assisting her husband. This was the last visit of day so as to be able to have a prolonged 'tea break' with the couple and engage Reg in conversation regarding his old hobbies, information that he remembered well and could talk about at length. This also cheered Irene, and she felt that she had 'regained' her husband for a short while.

During residential respite, home visits to Irene were continued to help her deal with the stress and guilt regarding the separation, and support was provided around continued intervention for the back pain.

After Reg died, Irene was supported by the team for several months until she moved to be closer to her son and his family.

Case study: George

George was 58 years old and suffered from depression. He had a three-and-a-half year history of steady deterioration, increasing medication, reduced social contacts and increasing dependence. His 54-year-old wife, Sue, continued in work and this, plus visits from family, provided her social support. She was considering giving up work to focus on caring for George but did not know what to do for the best. Both were very anxious and could only imagine things getting worse.

The primary issue was that no one had explained the neurophysiology of depression, the purpose of medication or the potential of other forms of intervention, including diet, in the light of the research/evidence base. Over two lengthy visits this was explained and a programme for change negotiated. Carer support simply focused on validating Sue remaining at work and on her extending her own social activities.

Support for George focused on physical activity/exercise at the local leisure centre, in which he was able to involve his sister-in-law, and on relaxation training. Extended support was provided through involving his sons in the weight-training programme and his grandchildren with swimming. He was supported in taking up a hobby by help with shopping for a computer (on a Saturday morning). He now attends a computer class, 'Computers for the Terrified!', where he has renewed a relationship with an old workmate. Further social interaction and mutual support is provided through an informal fitness network, involving service-users of all ages at the local leisure centres.

Although subject to occasional bouts of depression, George states that he is much better, feels more in control, more confidant and optimistic about the future, and is seeking to reduce his medication. Sue also reports less stress and increased optimism.

George was discharged by the psychiatrist to the care of his GP with a view to progressive reduction of medication. This took 5 months from the first visit.

Therapists should try to remember that they are not working simply with the named client, rather, that they are working with the 'case', including all those 'significant others' who can impact on the well-being of the named person. Pre-eminently this involves the carers. The case studies above intend to provide examples of this way of working.

Conclusion

There is a clear rationale for comprehensive community care assuming a requirement for variations in services to meet the needs of clients and carers. There is also a need for a structure formalizing interagency partnerships, user-centred services and social inclusion. The structure should balance variations in service provision to meet the needs of service-users and their carers.

Summary

- For those who are most at risk within the community, a 'needs'-led, client-centred system of care/intervention has to be in place to attempt to create the best possible equity of service provision.

- The concept of 'equity' proposed is that those who need more get more and that needs are more likely to be determined by social (resources) and interpersonal factors than by the diagnosed condition.

- Intervention must be based on a comprehensive assessment of needs involving client and carers.

- Some people will always need 'asylum' from a hostile environment and some people will need continuing care, neither of which necessarily needs to be provided from a hospital base or primarily in terms of medical intervention.

- The CPA philosophy commits all staff to a 'needs'-led system working *with* the community.

References

Brown H, Walmsley J 1997 When 'ordinary' isn't enough: a review of the concept of normalisation. In: Bornat J et al (eds) Community care, a reader, 2nd edn. Open University Press, Buckingham, UK, p 227–236

Busfield J 1997 Managing madness: changing ideas and practice. In: Bornat J et al (eds) Community care, a reader, 2nd edn. Open University Press, Buckingham, UK p 237–244

Cassidy T 1999 Stress, cognition and health, 1st edn. Routledge, London

Dalley G 1997 The principles of collective care. In: Bornat J et al (eds) Community care, a reader, 2nd edn. Open University Press, Buckingham, UK, p 153–159

Goodman A 1991 Organic unity theory: the mind–body problem revisited. American Journal of Psychiatry 148:553–563

Harding N, Palfrey C 1997 The social construction of dementia: confused professionals. Jessica Kingsley, London

Johnstone L 2000 Users and abusers of psychiatry, 2nd edn. Routledge, London

Klaber-Moffett J A, Richardson P H 1997 The influence of the physiotherapist–patient relationship on pain and disability. Physiotherapy Theory and Practice 13:89–96

Merleau-Ponty M 1967 The structure of behaviour. Beacon, Boston MA

Parker G (1992) Counting care: numbers and types of informal carers. In: Twigg J (ed) Carers research and practice. HMSO, London, p 6–29

Pilgrim D 1997 Mental health services in the twenty-first century: the user–professional divide. In: Bornat J et al (eds) Community care, a reader, 2nd edn. Open University Press, Buckingham, UK, p 245–253

Pilgrim D, Johnson J 1997 Anthology: policy. In: Bornat J et al (eds) Community care, a reader, 2nd edn. Open University Press, Buckingham, UK, p 173–184

Pitkeathley J 1994 Safeguarding the carers. In: Davidson R, Hunter S (eds) Community care in practice. Batsford, London, p 142–152

Ritchie P 1994 Community care – a quick look at some of the big issues. In: Davidson R, Hunter S (eds) Community care in practice. Batsford, London, p 7–15.

Walker A 1997 Community care policy: from consensus to conflict. In: Bornat J et al (eds) Community care, a reader, 2nd edn. Open University Press, Buckingham, UK, p 196–220

SECTION

2

6 The physical self

David Carless and Kenneth Fox

Introduction

Understanding people and the way they react to their past, current and future circumstances is at the heart of successful therapy. It has long been recognized that how people view themselves and their place in the world – their self-perceptions – is fundamental to the explanation of their behaviour. Campbell (1984), for example, suggested that the greatest human need, once physiological necessities such as warmth, hunger and thirst were satisfied, was the affirmation of self through enhanced self-esteem. The need to feel good about ourselves is a universal characteristic and hence the self has been studied as a central theme in a wide range of disciplines, including philosophy, sociology, psychology, psychiatry, theology and education. In this chapter, the significance of key concepts regarding the self and, in particular, one of its key components – the physical self – will be discussed in the context of the rehabilitative process.

The self system

Through the early work of James (1892) and, more recently, that of Epstein (1973), Markus & Wurf (1987) and Harter (1996), it has been realized that the self is not a single static entity but a working dynamic system. Since the 1980s, theoretical and clinical research have moved us forward considerably in our understanding of the structure and functioning of this system. Although some psychologists still disagree, there is now consensus that there are two separate elements of the self. The directive (actioned or subjective) self can be distinguished from the described (or objective) self. The directing self or, as James referred to it, the 'I', has executive properties and has been likened to the chief of a large corporation whose job it is to manage the corporate properties, assets and structure of the described self, or, in Jamesian terms, the 'Me'. This distinction helps sort out the difference between the terms self-concept and self-esteem, which are often confused and used interchangeably in the literature. Self-concept is best viewed as the self-description of the abilities, activities, qualities, traits, personal philosophies, morals and values, and roles adopted by the self. Murphy (1947, p. 996) described the self-concept as 'the individual as known to the individual'. The term identity, which is often adopted in the sociology or educational psychology literature (see Erikson 1968, Marcia 1980, Stryker 1987) extends the notion of self-concept to include the self's attempt to integrate the various described components into consistent and coherent parts (seeking or developing identity). Self-esteem or self-worth is quite different. It is often termed global self-esteem because it takes into account the range of activities of the self and provides the summary statement from the equivalent of a balance sheet on how well the self is doing. Whereas self-concept is essentially descriptive, self-esteem is evaluative and Campbell (1984, p. 9) defines it as 'an awareness of good possessed by self'.

Organization of the self system

With this view of the self as a system has emerged strong evidence to support its multidimensionality. Under a multidimensional view it is possible to conceive how experiences across diverse areas of life have the potential to make unique and independent contributions to global self-esteem. This theoretical conception is reflected by the development of psychological measures specifically designed to assess self-ratings in different life domains. Examples of these measures are Harter's self-perception profiles for children, adolescents and adults (Harter 1996) and Marsh's series of Self-Description Questionnaires (Marsh 1992). These instruments take life domains or subdomains thought to be consequential to the intended population and provide subscales to assess self-perceptions of competence in each of them, hence forming a profile. With advancing maturity, profiles become more complex, with more subscales as individuals become able to discriminate with more precision their performance in each area. Added to the profile is a global measure of self-esteem or worth so that the relationships among the different constructs can be investigated as well as individual scores assessed.

A subsequent development is the awareness that components of the self-system are organized into a hierarchical structure of which global self-esteem forms the apex. The key domains of life such as social, emotional, physical and work-related aspects of self create a second level, which subsequently splits into more and more increasingly situation-specific subdomains. For example, the social self can be subdivided into same sex or opposite-sex relationships. Thus, the components of the self-system are seen to be a network of finer and finer roots, the finest of which represent quite specific self-perceptions where the self interfaces with daily life contexts. These experiences are akin to self-efficacy expectations, which have been widely researched in several aspects of health behaviour (Bandura 1997). The view is that these perceptions, if repeated with sufficient power and frequency, will generalize to higher more stable levels of self-perceptions, and perhaps eventually feed into the global self-esteem of the individual. The direct relevance of this model of the self-system is that it provides a framework by which we can visualize and investigate different layers and contexts of self-perceptions and the way in which life events influence them.

Self-esteem and its origins

Because of its evaluative nature, self-esteem is seen to be the self-construct that is critical to both mental health and the explanation of choice and persistence in behaviours. High levels of self-esteem have been linked with desirable psychological traits such as subjective well-being and happiness (Diener 1984), emotional stability (Sonstroem 1997), and stress resilience, independence and adaptability (Wylie 1989). The breadth of accumulated evidence has led health organizations to emphasize the importance of self-esteem as a central component of mental health in its own right (US Department of Health and Human Services 1999). Conversely, low levels of self-esteem are consistently associated with a range of mental disorders such as depression (Baumeister 1993), and a goal of therapeutic interventions is often to bring about an increase in self-esteem (Rogers 1951). The importance of self-esteem is such that it has crossed academic, clinical and educational boundaries and is one of only a few psychological constructs to have acquired meaning among the general public. It is, therefore, a broad umbrella construct that potentially summarizes factors across the entire human experience.

The criteria on which self-esteem is based vary among individuals. The dominant values of the culture in which the individual exists will exert influences. Athletic abilities, educational attainment, job performance, physical appearance (particularly slimness), social and financial success are often particularly valued. Self-ratings in these highly valued attributes in westernized societies are closely associated with self-esteem (Harter 1996). Therefore, in many senses, we are at the mercy of societal values and rules for the determination of our level of well-being. However, people also ascribe to the value of the subcultures to which they belong, and this membership allows some scope to modify the agenda. For example, belonging to a sports club, a gang of soccer hooligans, a religious or spiritual group, a circle of friends or family can help individuals achieve a value system that is more coherent with their personal needs. Finally, some individuals are relatively independent of societal value systems, are more free spirited and express 'individualism' or even 'eccentricity' as opposed to submissive conformity. We see these effects changing across the lifespan: whereas the majority of adolescents resort to the security of the peer group, which produces an unwritten uniformity and slavery to fashion, older populations seem released from these inhibitions and have the confidence of life experiences to take on greater character. The point is that what counts towards our self-esteem is, to varying degrees, determined by a value system that is derived from the cultures to which we ascribe. It is important, therefore, when trying to understand people's motives and reactions, that we analyse their central aspirations and the origins of those aspirations.

Self-enhancement processes

The task of the self-director is to make the best of performance in self-roles or competencies that are personally highly valued components of the self-system. Because self-esteem is so central to mental well-being, a range of strategies is used to compliment this process. Examples include the following:

- Self-serving bias is applied to information used in self-evaluation. It is a relatively healthy strategy to filter out or modify negative information and make the most of successes and acclaim. Attributing success to effort and ability and failure to external factors such as luck and lack of control appears to be highly beneficial (Blaine & Crocker 1993).

- To prevent low competence from having a negative influence on self-esteem, there is some evidence that the attachment of low importance through discounting the significance of that competence is effective in preserving a higher level of self-esteem. It is difficult for some areas, such as physical attractiveness, to be discounted because of the high cultural value assigned to it.

- The public self is often enhanced through the use of self-presentation strategies, such as developing a confident style or using humour (Leary 1995). This, in return, is more likely to produce positive reflections from others, such as smiles or compliments, or even preferential treatment.

Absence of the use of self-serving strategies is a strong predictor of low self-esteem (Blaine & Crocker 1993) and therapists should consider techniques to encourage their use where self-esteem is a problem. However, overuse of the strategies can also be a problem, as it can be accompanied by delusion, boastfulness or arrogance, and defensiveness, and this can curtail socialization and prevent progress to full mental health. Establishing and maintaining self-esteem is therefore a complex dynamic process. Although there seems to be an intrinsic drive to explore and develop the self, there is also a need to establish and protect a coherent base from which to operate. Stability across time and consistency across situations in patterns of behaviours and emotional reactions provide the sense of identity and predictability that ties the self together. This stability, in turn, equips the individual with the roots necessary for the challenges of personal learning and growth. The balance between the two seems vital and the self is left with a delicate balancing act between consolidation and change. It is perhaps not surprising that this often goes wrong.

The physical self

The focus of this chapter is the physical self, or the view that the individual has of his or her physical attributes and capabilities. We live in times when there is a high cultural value attached to physical appearance and physical competencies for almost all sectors of society. Harter (1996) has suggested that the physical self is more than a domain of the self. It functions as the public self because it acts as the visible and audio interface between ourselves and the world, and is therefore highly salient to people's lives. Body shape, size, proportion, mannerisms, style and the physical skill with which it operates provide the first social projection of our personality, sexuality, confidence and prowess. The physical self therefore acts as an 'observable currency' that can carry negative or positive consequences. How we feel about our public image can therefore determine and reflect how we feel about ourselves in general, and this is reflected in strong associations between self-ratings of the physical self and global self-esteem across the lifespan (Fox 1997).

Although there has been interest in singular aspects of components of the physical self, such as body image or sport competence, during the 1990s attempts were made to incorporate the theoretical developments of multidimensional and hierarchical structuring into instrumentation. We now have two reliable and well-validated instruments that allow the simultaneous measurement of multiple aspects of self-perceptions in the physical domain. These are the Physical Self-Description Questionnaire (PSDQ; Marsh et al 1994) and the Physical Self-Perception Profile (PSPP; Fox & Corbin 1989). In the case of the PSPP, which is a 30-item inventory, four self-perception subdomains of sport competence, physical attractiveness, physical strength and physical condition were identified through open-ended questionnaires and interviews and subscales developed around this content. An additional, superordinate measure of global physical self-worth was also added to the profile, providing two levels of the hierarchical structure. The 70-item PSDQ contains subscales assessing strength, body fat, activity, endurance, sport competence, coordination, health, appearance and flexibility, and also the superordinate measures of general physical self-concept and self-esteem.

Research with these instruments has confirmed the hierarchical structure of the physical self. It has also shown clearly that physical self-perceptions are closely tied to related behaviours such as sport and exercise participation. The PSPP, for example, was able to closely predict level and type of exercise engaged in by American college students (Fox & Corbin 1989). Although there are some exceptions, people tend to gravitate to domain-specific behaviours where they are able to exhibit high competence, hence a positive association between domain-specific behaviours and perceptions. In addition, the literature indicates that positive physical self-perceptions are weakly associated with positive physical attributes such as being athletic, fit and slim. This relationship is weak because perceptions are not always accurately based in reality but are more predictive of behaviour as they often underpin motives.

The PSPP has recently demonstrated that physical self-perceptions are independently associated with indicators of mental well-being and emotional adjustment. This is the case even when responses are controlled for self-esteem and socially desirable responding (Sonstroem &

Potts 1996). Furthermore, the role of physical self-perceptions in the mental health of depressed patients receiving treatment has recently been established (van der Vliet et al 2002). It seems that physical self-worth in particular is a valuable target in its own right for interventions where improved mental well-being is a target.

Exercise, Physical Self and Self-Esteem

The majority of reviews that have considered all available evidence for the effects of participation in physical activity on global self-esteem have reported at best a weak positive impact (Fox 2000, Sonstroem 1984, 1997, Spence & Poon 1997). These reviews have identified a surprisingly small number of well-designed studies that use a range of instruments that are often outdated and of limited quality. For example, Fox (2000) identified only 36 randomized controlled trials (RCTs) that had been reported since 1970 that involved a wide range of populations and exercise programmes. The findings of this research can be summarized as follows:

- 78% of studies reported a positive effect on some aspect of physical self-perceptions or self-esteem/self-concept, indicating that exercise participation generally helps people see themselves more positively. The strongest effects were found for physical self-perceptions, such as body image, and physical self-worth in general.
- Approximately 50% of the studies reported an improvement in global self-esteem. Evidence suggests that increases in self-esteem do not occur reliably through exercise participation and that they do not necessarily accompany improvements in physical self-perceptions.
- Among middle-aged adults, the better studies provide evidence for a range of self-perception improvements that are likely to complement the physical health benefits of exercise that are particularly important for this age-group.
- Although no RCTs were located for older adults, non-randomized studies suggest that strength and fitness programmes might be effective for this age group and are worthy of further investigation.
- The greatest improvements in self-esteem and physical self-perceptions are found in those, usually the inexperienced and unfit, who begin with the lowest scores. This would include middle-aged to older populations, as well as those with a mental disorder or physical disability.

This limited literature suggests that improvement in self-esteem is possible through increased exercise participation but that its effects are inconsistent. This finding should not be surprising. Global self-esteem is based on a variety of more specific self-domains and it is perhaps unrealistic to expect exercise interventions that typically last 8–10 weeks to have a substantial influence on self-esteem in everyone taking part. A more likely proposition, and one that has been investigated by recent research, is that physical activity participation will influence physical self-perceptions and that these might generalize to change in global self-esteem or well-being under certain circumstances with certain people.

Currently, too few well-designed trials have been conducted with the newer theory-driven instruments to be able to make precise recommendations. Further studies are required to find optimal conditions for self-perception and mental health improvement, perhaps utilizing the relatively neglected modified Exercise and Self-Esteem model (Sonstroem et al 1994), which documents physical self-perception change at three levels in the self hierarchy.

However, the exercise experience is likely to be highly personalized, producing diverse psychological responses to similar exercise stimulus. The randomized controlled trial masks these ideosyncracies and tells us little about the mechanisms in operation at the individual or subgroup level. Different approaches that emphasize individual change and individual needs will be needed before the mechanisms can be truly unraveled. Furthermore, there exists important self-theory that has not been addressed to date in the exercise intervention literature or that has not been fully accommodated in the physical self-perception/self-esteem instrumentation.

Exercise and self-esteem: further considerations

One potentially effective alternative is to investigate the more pronounced self-perception changes experienced by people faced with serious physical challenges such as disability, injury or illness. Traumatic changes such as major health events are likely to exaggerate the impact of the self on mental well-being compared to the more gradual and insipient effects found in the general population. Therefore, changes might be more visible and informative for the practitioner and researcher in addition to having a more profound impact on the individual. For example, a serious physical health event might be expected to affect an individual's physical self-perceptions to the extent that changes generalize to global self-esteem. In therapeutic contexts, therefore, changes in physical self-perceptions can be both an important outcome of the physical challenge and a determinant of subsequent adaptation.

Existing disability research suggests that understanding the self-perceptions held by people with disabilities is far from straightforward. Sherrill (1997, p. 269) has suggested that 'physical disability is so complex and variable that no generalisations can be safely made about self-esteem'. Research repeatedly finds that individuals with a diverse range of disabilities report inconsistent and unpredictable self-perception change. For example, a recent study of stroke patients (Ellis-Hill & Horn 2000) used a multidimensional self-rating measure to compare stroke patients' current self-concept with their self-concept prior to the stroke. Although the authors concluded that overall self-concept deteriorated significantly following the stroke, not all dimensions deteriorated. Specifically, patients reported being less capable, independent, in control, satisfied, interested, confident, active and of value following their stroke. However, no change was found in other dimensions of self-concept, where patients reported being just as calm, caring, friendly and hopeful as prior to their stroke.

Physical appearance is perhaps the single most important factor for global self-worth among adolescents (Wichstrom 1998), yet studies typically find no differences in self-esteem between healthy adolescents and those with chronic physical disorders (Lavigne & Faierroutman 1992). However, Aasland & Diseth (1999) report global and specific dimensions of self-worth in 23 adolescents with juvenile chronic arthritis that were *higher* than the general population. Llewellyn & Chung (1997) reported similarly contradictory findings in the literature on the self-esteem of children with physical disabilities. Two studies of young people (with spina bifida and physical disabilities) reported that certain aspects of self-worth and self-concepts were lower than the general population, whereas four studies reported self-concept and self-worth differences to be marginal or non-existent. One further study reported self-concept to be higher in children with spina bifida than in healthy controls.

Although the reasons for these seemingly incompatible findings have yet to be resolved, research clearly shows that change in self-perception is not simply a function of severity of disability or disorder (see Sherrill 1997). Although we might expect more negative psychological changes in those who experience the most serious health challenges, this does not seem to be the case. This robust finding has been reported across several health contexts, such as cardiac events (Denollet & Brutsaert 1998) and strokes (Ellis-Hill & Horn 2000). These findings suggest that, among people who have experienced a major health event, mental well-being is more dependent on individual psychological factors than on the severity of disability or disorder. In other words, subjective interpretation of the disability or disorder is more important in self-perception change than the actual disability or disorder itself.

It is impossible to understand self-perception change without recognizing the diversity of factors that are involved. Contextual (age of onset, parental influence, gender), social, environmental and psychological factors will influence self-esteem development and also the extent that the individual interprets the disorder as a disability (Imrie 1997, Sherrill 1997). These considerations have often been neglected in previous research. The diverse range of potential influences suggests that self-perceptions of people with disabilities will be just as varied as among the general population. The presence of a physical disability does not in itself imply any specific psychological or personality factors (Sherrill 1997) that separate these individuals from the general population. It is more likely that the individual's unique combination of psychological factors determines whether the disability has a positive or negative impact on self-perceptions and self-esteem. The result is that, at one extreme, successful wheelchair athletes experience growth through adversity and regard their disability as no more than the kind of challenge they needed. This could produce higher self-esteem than might be expected, whereas at the other extreme, individuals might simply not be able to override the social stigma attached to disability resulting in low self-esteem.

Understanding self-esteem change

It is only through developing new approaches to understanding psychological factors at the individual level that we will be able to answer the practical questions of when and under what circumstances people benefit in terms of self-esteem from physical activity. Some recent developments in related fields of psychology and psychiatry might offer some interesting and relatively untested hypotheses.

Several theorists have begun to investigate the nature of self-esteem in greater depth and have provided initial evidence to suggest that mental health is not simply dependent on the *amount* but the *nature* of self-esteem an individual possesses (Deci & Ryan 1995, Kernis 1993, Roberts & Monroe 1994). Almost all self-perception instruments focus heavily on self-estimates of competence, adequacy or level of desirable attributes. Other factors might be important to sense of self (but have been largely neglected in the empirical literature).

Deci & Ryan (1995) have recently proposed a broader conception of self-esteem to better explain individual variation in psychological health. They define *true* self-esteem as being dependent on the satisfaction of three fundamental psychological needs: competence, autonomy and relatedness. Optimal mental health, they suggest, is achieved when the requirement for these three needs is balanced in the individual, and psychological problems occur when one or more of these needs are unmet. Their theory suggests that the accepted human desire for feelings of competence, or effectance, is a necessary but insufficient condition for achieving mental well-being. To achieve high levels of true self-esteem, and hence mental health, the individual must also experience a degree of personal responsibility for his or her achievements while at the same time maintaining fulfilling social relationships and interactions. Factors such as autonomy and relatedness are not addressed by most self-perception measurement techniques. Therefore, potentially important contributors to the self-system are being ignored. For example, the availability of unconditional social support is likely to improve relatedness and the maintenance of a belief in one's own ability to take control over rehabilitation could produce a sense of personal mastery or autonomy. In the case of mental or physical disorder or disability, exercise therapy might buffer or even counteract any decrease in perceived competence resulting from the disorder or condition. Exercise and sport are also social events and their potential to influence mental health through changes in relatedness and affiliations and changes in the social self has rarely been investigated. This could be particularly critical in groups such as the elderly where social isolation is related to depression.

In the field of psychiatry, parallel progress has been made by Cloninger and colleagues (Cloninger 1999, Cloninger et al 1994). The psychobiological theory of personality proposes that three specific components of the self-concept mediate between personality traits and mental health and function. Although personality traits predispose towards certain psychological outcomes and behaviours, the individual's self-concept exerts a powerful influence on whether these outcomes become a health threat. Two key dimensions of personality identified by Cloninger and colleagues mirror Deci & Ryan's true self-esteem theory. *Self-directedness* closely relates to the concept of autonomy, and *cooperativeness* is similar to relatedness. Cloninger and colleagues (1994) consistently find through their empirical research that these dimensions are positively linked to mental health. Because these two dimensions are thought to be consciously influenced and modifiable across the lifespan, they represent a potential route for the improvement of self-concept, and subsequently mental health, through planned therapeutic interventions. If these possibilities are established by future research, this theoretical framework offers the potential for a comprehensive explanation of the influence of the self-system on mental health. The role of exercise in mental health enhancement might then be more clearly established (see Chapter 7 for further discussion).

Practical implications

The discussion in this chapter has focused on the potential benefits to the physical self that are possible through exercise participation. The strengths and weaknesses of the existing literature have been highlighted. Whereas it is clear that exercise has real potential for improving perceptions of the physical self, the mechanisms through which it might promote self-esteem or improvement in other aspects of self are not yet fully understood. This makes definitive recommendations for professionals utilizing exercise as a therapy impossible at the current time. However, existing findings and consideration of contemporary psychological theories make it possible to offer some guidelines.

Summary

- The literature suggests that aerobic exercise that is moderately demanding (the equivalent of brisk walking) or weight training is likely to be successful in improving self-perceptions. However, programmes that concentrate on physical skills should not be ruled out.

- Some empirical research and theory suggests that the activity setting should be designed to produce a sense of mastery and self-determination. This requires an approach where ownership for success is handed over to the person undertaking the activity. The therapist should take on a facilitative rather than a directive role using techniques that underpin exercise counselling.

- It is not clear whether individual or group exercise is the most effective. Personal choice might be important. Group sessions have the advantage of offering a social environment that can be manufactured to encourage social interaction and support. This could provide a powerful mechanism for change that, to date, has not been adequately tested out.

- Those who are currently inactive, recovering from physical health problems, depression, body image concerns or who have a disability are most likely to do well.

- Particularly in the case of global self-esteem, existing evidence suggests that interventions of at least 12 weeks are required to result in measurable change. Therefore, programme adherence is critical if self-perception improvements are to be experienced. Any exercise intervention should therefore primarily be designed to be attractive to participants and facilitate continued participation and monitoring of goals.

In summary, knowledge of the nature of the self system will help therapists understand the needs and problems facing people with mental health problems. In particular, the values and strategies that the individual adopts are critical to interpreting how that person will react to various therapies including exercise. The physical self appears to play a key mediating role in the exercise/self-esteem relationship. Current theory suggests exercise might be most effective if it is presented in a way that it satisfies fundamental psychological needs such as autonomy, competence and relatedness or affiliation.

References

Aasland A, Diseth T H 1999 Can the Harter Self-Perception Profile for Adolescents (SPPA) be used as an indicator of psychosocial outcome in adolescents with chronic physical disorders? European Child & Adolescent Psychiatry 8(2):78–85

Bandura A 1997 Self-efficacy: the exercise of control. Freeman, New York

Baumeister R F 1993 Self-esteem: the puzzle of low self-regard. Plenum Press, New York

Blaine B, Crocker J 1993 Self-esteem and self-serving biases in reactions to positive and negative events: an integrative review. In: Baumeister R F (ed) Self-esteem: the puzzle of low self-regard. Plenum, New York, p 55–86

Campbell R N 1984 The new science: self-esteem psychology. University Press of America, Lanham, MD

Cloninger C R 1999 A new conceptual paradigm from genetics and psychobiology for the science of mental health. Australian and New Zealand Journal of Psychiatry 33(2):174–186

Cloninger C R, Przybeck T, Svrakic D, Wetzel R D 1994 The Temperament and Character Inventory (TCI): a guide to its development and use. Center for Psychobiology of Personality, Washington University, St Louis, MO

Deci E L, Ryan R M 1995 Human autonomy: the basis for true self-esteem. In: Kernis M (ed) Efficacy, agency, and self-esteem. Plenum Press, New York

Denollet J, Brutsaert D L 1998 Personality, disease severity, and the risk of long-term cardiac events in patients with a decreased ejection fraction after myocardial infarction. Circulation 97(2):167–173

Diener E 1984 Subjective well-being. Psychological Bulletin 95(3):542–575

Ellis-Hill C S, Horn S 2000 Change in identity and self-concept: a new theoretical approach to recovery following a stroke. Clinical Rehabilitation 14(3):279–287

Epstein S 1973 The self-concept revisited or the theory of a theory. American Psychologist 28:405–416

Erikson E 1968 Identity, youth, and crisis. Norton, New York

Fox K R 1997 (ed) The physical self: from motivation to well-being. Human Kinetics, Champaign, IL

Fox K R 2000 The effects of exercise on self-perceptions and self-esteem. In: Biddle S J H et al (eds) Physical activity and psychological well-being. Routledge, London

Fox K R, Corbin C B 1989 The physical self-perception profile – Development and preliminary validation. Journal of Sport & Exercise Psychology 11(4):408–430

Harter S 1996 Historical roots of contemporary issues involving the self-concept. In: Bracken B A (ed) Handbook of self-concept: developmental, social, and clinical considerations. Wiley, New York, p 1–37

Imrie R 1997 Rethinking the relationships between disability, rehabilitation, and society. Disability and Rehabilitation 19(7):263–271

James W 1892 Psychology: the briefer course. Henry Holt, New York

Kernis M H 1993 The roles of stability and level of self-esteem in psychological functioning. In: Baumeister R F (ed) Self-esteem: the puzzle of low self-regard. Plenum Press, New York, p 167–182

Lavigne J V, Faierroutman J 1992 Psychological adjustment to pediatric physical disorders – a meta-analytic review. Journal of Pediatric Psychology 17(2):133–157

Leary M R 1995 Self-presentation: impression management and interpersonal behavior. Brown & Benchmark, Dubuque, IO

Llewellyn A, Chung M C 1997 The self-esteem of children with physical disabilities – problems and dilemmas of research. Journal of Developmental and Physical Disabilities 9(3):265–275

Marcia J 1980 Identity in adolescence. In: Adelson J (ed) Handbook of adolescent psychology. Wiley, New York, p 159–187

Markus H, Wurf E 1987 The dynamic self-concept: a social psychological perspective. Annual Review of Psychology 38:299–337

Marsh H W 1992 Self-description questionnaire II: manual. Publication Unit, Faculty of Education, University of Western Sydney, Sydney

Marsh H W, Richards G E, Johnson S et al 1994 Physical self-description questionnaire: psychometric properties and a multi-trait multi-method analysis of relations to existing instruments. Journal of Sport & Exercise Psychology 16(3):270–305

Murphy G 1947 Personality: a biosocial approach to origins and structure. Harper and Row, New York

Roberts J E, Monroe S M 1994 A multidimensional model of self-esteem in depression. Clinical Psychology Review 14(3):161–181

Rogers C R 1951 Client-centered therapy. Houghton Mifflin, Boston, MA

Sherrill C 1997 Disability, identity, and involvement in sport and exercise. In: Fox K R (ed) The physical self: from motivation to well-being. Human Kinetics, Champaign, IL, p 257–286

Sonstroem R J 1984 Exercise and self-esteem. Exercise and Sports Sciences Reviews 12:123–155

Sonstroem R J 1997 Physical activity and self-esteem. In: Morgan W P (ed) Physical activity and mental health. Taylor and Francis, Washington DC, p 124–143

Sonstroem R J, Potts S A 1996 Life adjustment correlates of physical self-concepts. Medicine and Science in Sports and Exercise 28(5):619–625

Sonstroem R J, Harlow L L, Josephs L 1994 Exercise and self-esteem: validity of model expansion and exercise associations. Journal of Sport & Exercise Psychology 16(1):29–42

Spence J C, Poon P 1997 The effect of physical activity on self-concept: a meta-analysis. Alberta Center for Well-being: Research Update 4(3)

Stryker S 1987 Identity theory: developments and extensions. In: Yardley K, Holness T (eds) Self and identity. Wiley, New York, p 89–103

US Department of Health and Human Services 1999 Mental health: a report of the Surgeon General. Superintendent of documents, Pittsburgh, PA

van der Vliet P, Knapen J, Onghena P et al 2002 Assessment of physical self-perceptions in normal Flemish adults versus depressed psychiatric patients. Personality and Individual Differences 32:855–863

Wichstrom L 1998 Self-concept development during adolescence: do American truths hold for Norwegians? In: Skoe E, Von der Lippe A (eds) Personality development in adolescence: a cross-national and life-span perspective. Routledge, London

Wylie R C 1989 Measures of self-concept. University of Nebraska, Lincoln, NB

7 Physical activity and mental health

Nanette Mutrie and Guy Faulkner

Introduction

The role of exercise in improving mental health is a growing area of research interest. In an analysis of research trends in two international sport and exercise psychology journals during the 1990s, the topic of 'exercise and mental health' had increased in frequency by 400% from the late 1980s to the early 1990s (Biddle 1997). Following a summary of current consensus in this field, we will focus specifically on the possible mechanisms underpinning the relationship between exercise and mental health. We will then discuss some factors that might restrain greater consideration of exercise as a clinical adjunct before noting some practical considerations for those who might consider using physical activity to promote mental health.

Current consensus

The existing evidence suggests four main functions of physical activity for impacting mental health (Fox et al 2000):

1. to prevent mental health problems
2. to improve the psychological well-being of the general public
3. to improve the quality of life for people with mental health problems
4. as treatment or therapy for existing mental illness.

Physical activity for prevention

Reviews agree that lower instances of mental health problems are found among people who regularly participate in physical activity (Biddle et al 2000a). Mutrie (2000) reports four longitudinal studies that examined the effect of regular physical activity on the incidence of depression at follow-up several years later. In all four studies, people who were more active at baseline reported a lower incidence of depression at follow-up. These studies suggest a relative risk of 1.7 for the inactive individuals reporting depression at a later date. Mutrie concludes that current evidence indicates that physical activity has a protective effect against the development of depression. In contrast, evidence from the Nottingham Longitudinal Study does not provide strong evidence that increase in physical activity reliably promotes improvements in psychological well-being in the elderly (Morgan & Bath 1998). When the focus of attention turns to a broader notion of physical activity and other leisure activities (Dupuis & Smale 1995, Morgan et al 1991) the relationship between physical activity and depression becomes ambiguous, although validated measures of physical activity were not used in these studies. Further prospective epidemiological research is required before we can conclude that participation in regular exercise directly reduces the risk of mental health problems.

Based on Taylor's (2000) conclusion that aerobically fit individuals generally have a reduced physiological response to psychosocial stressors, exercise appears to offer a degree of protection from anxiety. Furthermore, exercise might help people become more resilient to stress (Salmon 2001). More research is required to investigate the extent that physical activity might be effective in preventing the onset of other types of mental health problems.

Physical activity to improve well-being in the general population

Participation in physical activity and exercise is consistently associated with positive affect and mood (Biddle 2000). This relationship has been confirmed in large epidemiological surveys and experimental studies. It would appear that exercise does 'make you feel good', and this phenomenon is supported by the finding that single bouts of exercise have a small to moderate effect on state anxiety whereas a period of exercise training can also reduce trait anxiety (Taylor 2000). Small but significant improvements in cognitive functioning in older adults have also been reported as a result of exercise participation (Boutcher 2000). For example, in a meta-analysis of fitness and cognitive performance studies, Etnier et al (1997) found a significant but small effect size (ES) for adults aged 60–90 years (ES = 0.19). Measurement difficulties have hindered research in this area.

Improvements in self-esteem and physical self-perceptions are further benefits that can be experienced by the general population through exercise participation. Fox (2000a) concluded that exercise promotes physical self-worth and other important physical self-perceptions, such as improved body image. For some people, in some situations, this generalizes to improvements in global self-esteem. Further discussion of the relationship between exercise and the physical self is provided in Chapter 8. Current consensus clearly supports an association between physical activity and numerous domains of mental health in the general population.

Physical activity for quality of life and coping with mental disorders

Preliminary evidence also suggests that regular physical activity improves positive aspects of mental health (such as psychological dimensions of quality of life and emotional well-being) in people with mental disorders. Specifically, positive psychological effects from physical activity in clinical populations have been reported even among those individuals who experience no objective diagnostic improvement and where complete remission may be unrealistic. For example, there is a potential role for exercise in the treatment of schizophrenia. Faulkner & Biddle (1999) concluded that exercise might alleviate the secondary symptoms of schizophrenia, such as depression, low self-esteem and social withdrawal. For some people, exercise might also be a useful coping strategy for the positive symptoms of schizophrenia, such as auditory hallucinations.

Finally, exercise might improve quality of life through the physical health benefits of exercise. For example, depression and anxiety are significantly prevalent causes of physical illness and mortality throughout the world (American Psychiatric Association 1994). Depressed individuals are more likely than others to develop cardiovascular disease and die of all-causes (Dinan 1999, Musselman et al 1998). In older adults 'depression and poor physical function are mutually reinforcing, causing a progressive downward spiral in the physical and psychological health of older persons' (Penninx et al 1998, p. 1725). Biddle & Faulkner (in press) suggested that, because of its impact on functional capacity, the potential of physical activity having an antidepressant effect for an elderly population far outweighs the possibility that it might not. Epidemiological surveys continually demonstrate the existence of an excess of physical morbidity and premature mortality in both treated and untreated populations of the mentally ill (e.g. Brugha et al 1989). For example, many people with chronic schizophrenia experience obesity, which is often associated with antipsychotic medication (Wetterling 2001). For all conditions, exercise might counteract the side-effects of medication and improve the general health of individuals with mental health problems.

Physical activity as intervention

Physical activity is emerging as an effective intervention or adjunct for existing mental health problems in clinical populations. Currently, the strongest evidence concerns the use of physical activity as a treatment for depression and a recent review found support for a causal link between physical activity participation and decreased depression (Mutrie 2000). Two recent meta-analyses report effects sizes of 0.72 (Craft & Landers 1998) and 1.1 (Lawlor & Hopker 2001) for exercise compared to no treatment for depression, and both meta-analyses show a comparable effect for exercise in comparison to other psychotherapeutic interventions. However, the importance of these large effects has been questioned on the basis of methodological weaknesses in existing research and lack of evidence for clinical outcomes (Lawlor & Hopker 2001). Furthermore, other reviewers using similar criteria have been less convinced of a causal relationship (Landers & Arent 2001, O'Neal et al 2000), but all researchers call for further research in the belief that there is an important relationship between exercise and depression that deserves further exploration.

In terms of anxiety, evidence supports the existence of a positive effect through physical activity participation for both trait and state anxiety (Taylor 2000). Although Taylor concluded that exercise has a low to moderate anxiety-reducing effect, he noted that the strongest effects were found in randomized controlled trials. At present, little evidence exists concerning the effects of physical activity on other mental health disorders, although it has been reported that exercise is effective in treating panic disorders (O'Connor et al 2000) and the symptoms of certain psychoses such as schizophrenia (Faulkner & Biddle 1999). Limited research also suggests that exercise may be a useful adjunctive strategy for drug and alcohol rehabilitation (see Chapter 20).

Summary   In conclusion, the recently published National Physical Activity and Mental Health Consensus Statements offer compelling evidence as to the positive relationship between physical activity and mental health (Biddle et al 2000a). Growing awareness of the importance of physical activity to physical and mental health should encourage the development of physical activity opportunities for individuals with mental health problems or for those at increased risk of developing mental health problems. At the same time, it is necessary to highlight the lack of strong research designs within the existing literature (see Biddle et al 2000b) and the uncertainty concerning the mechanisms underpinning such mental health benefits.

Mechanisms   The field of psychosomatic medicine has clearly established the idea that how we think and feel will affect the functioning of the body. What we do with our bodies can also affect how we think and feel but this somatopsychic approach is less well established or understood. In fact, there is considerable agreement that the underlying mechanisms that relate to the positive effects from exercise on mental health are not yet known (Biddle & Mutrie 2001, O'Neal et al 2000, Plante 1993). Several possible mechanisms, including biochemical changes such as increased levels of neurotransmitters such as endorphins or serotonin as a result of exercise, and psychological changes such as an increased sense of mastery, have been proposed (Petruzzello et al 1991).

La Forge (1995) has provided one of the best reviews of the possible mechanisms because he started from a standpoint of integrating the possible mechanisms rather than describing them as separate processes. This integration occurs via neural connections and to accept La Forge's model one has to accept the philosophical position that all emotions have a neurological explanation.

Table 7.1 shows the mechanisms that La Forge has integrated. This table provides a brief summary and commentary on these hypotheses. La Forge (1995) points out that all of the mechanisms in Table 7.1 overlap in terms of structure and function and in terms of neuroanatomic pathways. The integrated model that he proposes accepts

Table 7.1 *Mechanisms for exercise-associated mood changes reviewed by La Forge (1995)*

Name of hypothesis	Indicative reference	Major principles	Comments
Opponent-process theory	Solomon (1980)	Processes that oppose the heightened state of arousal brought about by exercise seek to return the body's systems to homeostasis. These opponent processes get stronger through training and thus can cause relaxation and anxiety reduction after exercise in trained individuals	Very difficult to obtain empirical evidence as many processes could potentially oppose. Thus linked hypothetically to all the other processes mentioned
Opioids	Schwarz & Kindermann (1992)	Opioids (e.g. endorphins, enkephalins, dynorphins) are associated with increased mood and decreased pain sensations. Exercise increases plasma levels of opioids and thus opioids could be responsible for postexercise mood enhancement. This system is linked to the cardiovascular, respiratory, reproductive and immune systems	It is not clear if the plasma levels reflect the central nervous system levels of opioids and research investigating the exercise and mood link has been equivocal
Monoamines	Chaouloff (1997)	Monoamines (dopamine, noradrenaline, (norepinephrine), adrenaline (epinephrine), serotonin) are involved in depression and anxiety. Much antidepressant medication is aimed at increasing the amounts of these amines. Exercise can also stimulate production	Most of the exercise research is animal based but since medications have extensive human research it is a very plausible hypothesis
Neocortical activation	Kubitz & Landers (1993)	Incoming signals from muscles, etc. during movement stimulate areas of the cortex responsible for mood. In addition, exercise might cause a shift to right hemisphere processing. Links to the concept of exercising to find 'optimal' levels of arousal	Methods have been inconsistent and often no mood or anxiety measure has been taken. Associating mood states with activity in specific brain regions is not an exact science at present

Table 7.1 *Cont'd*

Name of hypothesis	Indicative reference	Major principles	Comments
Thermogenic changes	Petruzzello et al (1991)	Increased core temperature decreases muscle tension and has been hypothesized to reduce anxiety. Certain types of exercise will increase core temperature	Very little support for this hypothesis has emerged from the literature. Given the body's ability to maintain core temperature against hostile environments, this does seem an unlikely explanation but the *process* of maintaining temperature might link to the opioids or to cortical activity
Hypothalamic–pituitary–adrenal (HPA) axis changes	Peronnet & Szabo (1993)	The HPA axis is the framework for mind–body communication. It plays a role in depression, eating disorders and stress response. Stress hormones are released by this axis in response to physical (exercise) and mental stress. High levels of stress hormones are associated with negative moods. Training decreases the amount of stress hormones released; overtraining increases the levels of stress hormones	The mechanisms that elicit responses by the HPA axis to exercise stress and to psychosocial stress are probably different and need to be better understood before this hypothesis can be advanced

this overlap and suggests that it is the integration that must be studied rather than the isolated mechanisms. This leads to the need for inter-disciplinary research to employ the latest imaging technologies to enhance understanding of what happens in the exerciser's brain.

What is particularly appealing in this integrated model is that, in terms of mental illness, exercise can be seen to play the same role as some antidepressant drugs but at the same time it could have more widespread (and potentially beneficial) effects. This is seen most clearly in the monoamine pathway. Landers & Arent (2001) describe how commonly prescribed antidepressants (such as Prozac), act by prevent-ing the reuptake of serotonin by neurons in the brain, thus allowing more of that monoamine to act. Higher levels of serotonin are related to heightened nervous system activity whereas lower levels are associ-ated with low levels of nervous system activity that would normally be seen in the lethargic behaviour of people with depression. Animal stud-ies show that serotonin discharge increases with motor activity and slows with sleep and disappears altogether with rapid eye movement (REM) sleep. Landers & Arent (2001) showed the integrated potential of exercise by explaining that exercisers probably have better sleep pat-terns than non-exercisers because they get to sleep faster, sleep longer but have less REM sleep, thus increasing the amount of serotonin avail-able. Exercise might therefore act to increase serotonin levels and pre-vent periods of sleep with no serotonin discharge. The notion of integration goes even further than that because the perceptions of sleeping well and feeling good after exercise could encourage more activity and thus more serotonin discharge.

However, some of the plausible explanations of why exercise can make people 'feel good' are not yet accounted for in this model. One notable exception is that of how exercise can provide a sense of mas-tery and control. For example, one theory of depression suggests that depression is a result of feeling that there is no action that can be taken to alleviate a problem. This feeling of helplessness is learned over a period of time and from a variety of situations, and results in the per-son having an external locus of control (Abramson et al 1978). It has been suggested that exercise can play a role in helping the person who is suffering in this way to gain control in one area of life, namely the physical self. In addition, if the exercise is programmed correctly, the sense of achievement and progression from week to week builds on this sense of control and could even provide a sense of mastery (Greist et al 1981). Self-esteem enhancement has therefore featured as a poten-tial explanation of how exercise can alleviate depression and anxiety (Ossip-Klein et al 1989).

La Forge's integrated model, as it stands, does not account for the neurobiology of achievement or self-esteem enhancement, but it could. New technologies such at PET scans and MRI will soon be able to show us which areas of the brain are activated when we are exercising and when we sense achievement and such pathways will probably link to those already identified by La Forge.

There is another drawback to the integrated model. It is built from examples of exercise related research that have almost exclusively focused on aerobic exercise and mostly acute exercise sessions rather than chronic exercise programmes. In terms of both anxiety and depression, Martinsen et al (1989a,b) have shown that both aerobic and non-aerobic exercise can have a positive effect. Only 'opponent process theory' and perhaps 'neocortical activation' (see Table 7.1) could account for non-aerobic exercise having positive psychological effects. However, La Forge does suggest there is a need to study other types and intensities of exercise.

Determining the mechanisms for the psychological effects of exercise for depression and other mental illness is a huge challenge for scientists. It would appear that much of the knowledge has to be developed in animal models until such times as we have the technology required to study humans during exercise. Brain imaging (MRI) is one possible technology that could advance our understanding of these mechanisms and there is now a real possibility that the human nervous systems can be explored by this technique during exercise. It is clear that the answer to this complex question will not be found in exercise laboratories alone.

La Forge (1995, p. 28) provided this sensible guide to future practice:

The mechanism is likely an extraordinary synergy of biological transactions, including genetic, environmental, and acute and adaptive neurobiological processes. Inevitably, the final answers will emerge from a similar synergy of researchers and theoreticians from exercise science, cognitive science and neurobiology.

Collaborative research is encouraged by many research councils. Those of us at the 'coal face' of dealing with people with mental health problems, or undertaking research about the effects of exercise, must seek-out and convince scientists who work in laboratory settings to work with us to determine the causal pathways that provide a feel-good effect from physical activity and exercise. However, although we are far from having the answer to this question, we should not stop recommending exercise as a potential therapeutic intervention. If we take the example of electroconvulsive treatment (ECT), which is still used in some situations in the UK, the fact that the mechanisms by which it has its effect are not well understood has not meant that it is not used. As MacLeod (1998, p. 566) said 'There is a debate about whether ECT is effective and even those who advocate its effectiveness would not claim to know how it works'. Similarly, despite the acceptance and widespread use of certain antipsychotic medications, for example, the biochemical basis for action for some drugs has not been clearly identified (Gerlach & Peacock 1995). Finally, within psychotherapy,

Llewelyn & Hardy (2001, p. 2) describe the question of mechanisms as the 'dodo bird' verdict. 'That is, we know psychotherapy is effective, but we also know that different apparently contradictory theoretical approaches are approximately equally effective in outcome, but very different in content'.

Why is exercise not used more in treating mental health problems?

Despite a developing evidence-base, exercise is rarely used as a form of treatment for mental health problems such as depression (Fox 2000b, Hutchinson et al 1999, Tkachuk & Martin 1999). In the US, there 'has been very little support on the system or program levels for the development and implementation of strategies and services aimed at improving the physical well-being of persons with psychiatric disabilities' (Hutchinson et al 1999, p. 356). Hale (1997) failed to mention exercise at all in discussing the treatment of depression in the UK. Neither the American College of Sports Medicine (ACSM; Pate et al 1995) guidelines nor many of the available international public policy documents on physical activity make specific recommendations concerning exercise and mental health (Scully et al 1998).

Fox (1999, 2000b) outlines a number of suggestions as to why the evidence for the mental health benefits of exercise has not been widely translated into mental health service practice:

■ Most research has been conducted within the exercise and sports sciences, which are themselves emerging disciplines.
■ The area remains poorly funded and is not seen as a serious area of medical or health research.
■ Lack of recognition of evidence-based research principles. Attention has been on academic rather than service outcomes. For example, studies have rarely addressed the cost-effectiveness of treatments or used intention-to-treat analyses. Criteria for randomized controlled trials are rarely satisfied (e.g. Lawlor & Hopker 2001).
■ The difficulties in moving from description to prescription in relation to mental health given the individual nature of benefit.

These factors are compounded by the lack of an established infrastructure for the translating of research into practice in exercise-related psychology (Gauvin & Spence 1995), which is exacerbated by the different goals, accountabilities and reward structures held by academic groups and practitioners (King et al 1998). It is also important to consider that changes in practice do not necessarily occur solely on the basis of an individual's evaluation of the scientific studies or even consensus statements (Bero et al 1998, Rogers 1995). There might be more subtle, conceptual barriers to a wider consideration of exercise as an adjunct treatment.

Such a possibility could be linked to the compatibility between the recommendation of exercise with existing roles and beliefs held by professionals working with people who have mental health problems. The consideration of exercise, or the need for physical activity, is not particularly prominent within the common models used to understand and formulate interventions for clinical conditions, such as depression. Furthermore, dualistic tendencies might continue to render any sense of the body 'absent'. In a survey of US psychotherapists' use of exercise, McEntee & Halgin (1996, p. 55) concluded that 'many therapists simply do not see their work as pertaining to the body' and that 'topics such as exercise are viewed as unimportant by some mental health workers who fail to appreciate the relationship between physical and psychological health' (McEntee & Halgin 1996, p. 58). They suggest this might be due to increased specialization in the health fields. Whereas greater connections are made between various health behaviours in general, many physicians and psychologists retain a narrow scope of specialization, failing to appreciate the interrelationship between the body and mind. As Baerveldt & Voestermans (1996, p. 693) suggest, 'the body as such is hardly a subject matter for psychology. Psychology is a science "buried in thought"'.

More controversially, Martinsen & Stephens (1994) first speculated that in the field of psychiatry, the status of exercise intervention was low. They suggested that this was partly due to exercise interventions being so 'simple'. Therapists who spend years learning a therapeutic technique are resistant to the concept that possibly analogous results could be achieved through exercise. In a qualitative survey of directors of clinical psychology training programmes in the UK, Faulkner & Biddle (2001) found perceived simplicity to be a recurring theme. Specifically, this concerned issues of legitimacy and deprofessionalization if exercise was used as a specific adjunct rather than as a general 'normalizing' activity. First, exercise might be seen as a frivolous activity when reflecting on the complexity of factors that could underpin the severe depression being experienced by a client. Second, anyone could recommend exercise! Consequently, it might not be seen as a profession-specific form of intervention. Given the possible incompatibility of exercise with common conceptual models that tend to ignore the body, the perception that exercise is not 'psychological' enough could be a final factor that results in an inconsistent consideration of exercise.

If exercise is to become more common as an adjunctive treatment then it might be important to frame 'exercise' more explicitly within existing practice (Faulkner & Biddle 2001). For example, there could still be the need to dispel common misperceptions regarding exercise. First thoughts regarding 'exercise' probably infer vigorous physical activity with specified parameters of intensity, duration and frequency. Although more research is necessary, less strenuous forms of activity such as walking might be sufficient to demonstrate significant treatment effects (Tkachuk & Martin 1999). Greater activity, which can possibly be accumulated throughout the day (Blair & Connelly 1994) can be promoted and fits easily into notions of activity scheduling in which many health professionals are already involved. Whereas activity scheduling can be useful for providing structure, the physical activity itself has been supported by a growing body of evidence in providing mental health benefits.

Second, cognitive–behavioural therapy (CBT) is becoming a common treatment modality for many mental health concerns, and indeed CBT techniques are increasingly being used to assist exercise initiation and maintenance. We would argue that exercise is itself an excellent behavioural modification, which can indeed influence cognitions. There is unambiguous evidence that becoming physically active changes people's perceptions of their physical self and identity in a positive way (see Chapter 6). Such changes can also generalize to global self-esteem and other markers of well-being. Both CBT and activity scheduling can involve structured exercise or habitual physical activity. Importantly, exercise can now be reconceptualized to, and by, clinicians as a process through which therapeutic goals can be reached rather than as a seemingly atheoretical therapy in itself. That is, it becomes compatible with existing practice. It could also reduce any concerns as to the perceived simplicity of the intervention. Physical activity is a demanding, complex behaviour with poor adherence rates (Laitakari & Miilunpalo 1998). Given the general difficulty in getting people active, health professionals might be an important resource for helping people do so in the future.

Practical considerations

Physiotherapists, occupational therapists and exercise specialists working with people with mental health problems have a number of considerations to make. First of all, the fitness levels of these people is likely to be very low. A review of recent activity history is essential to understand how to help the person become more active and, if resources allow, assessment of fitness might also be desirable. Creating a graduated programme, which is tailored to each person's needs, is important. The key elements are reinforcing success and providing variety. Using goal setting to increase the length of activity and reinforcing successful completion of early goals could assist motivation. Asking each individual to notice whether energy levels rise or fall immediately after exercise might also assist in overcoming lethargy and understanding that exercise can be used to boost energy levels. This is similar to certain aspects of behavioural activation therapy (Jacobson et al 2001). A clear long-term goal is for each person to become an independent exerciser. Loughlan & Mutrie (1995) have provided guidelines on how to counsel people into regular activity and these guidelines can easily be applied. Those who do not have clinical qualifications must also know the boundaries of their work with people with a mental health problem and know when certain topics of discussion should be stopped and when referral to other professionals is required. O'Neal & colleagues (2000) have provided an excellent set of recommendations for supervising exercise training for persons with depression, which is well worth consulting.

Exercise and drug therapy

There is another challenge for exercise programming for this particular group in the potential interaction of exercise and drug therapy. One of the common drug therapies is beta-blockade. Beta-blockers will attenuate heart rate response and thus exercise intensity is best introduced to each individual via rating of perceived exertion. This procedure focuses on how much effort exercisers perceive and it requires the use of a rating of perceived exertion scale. After some training, exercisers can judge the intensity of the workout without use of heart rates. For aerobic training an effort rating between 12 and 15 on the Borg 6–20 scale (Borg 1998) is normally recommended.

Neuroleptics, tricyclic antidepressants (TCAs) and monoamine oxidase inhibiting (MOAI) antidepressant medications can cause drowsiness and orthostatic hypotension as side-effects. Getting individuals motivated to exercise and teaching them how to avoid sudden movements that will make them feel dizzy are therefore additional challenges. Although the newer antidepressants (serotonin reuptake inhibitors; SSRIs) have fewer side-effects than TCAs or MAOIs, only moderate intensity exercise should be recommended because vigorous exercise for those on SSRI could lead to premature fatigue (Wilson & Maughan 1992). Some antipsychotic medications cause dehydration and frequent drinking of water before and during exercise will be necessary.

Martinsen & Stanghelle (1997) provided one of the few commentaries on the topic of the interaction of drug therapy and physical activity. Although noting that this is an area that requires further research, Martinsen speaks from the experience of a psychiatrist who has introduced exercise to the treatment programmes of many people with mental illhealth. Martinsen & Stanghelle noted that the side-effects of various drug therapies do bother these individuals but that they can still continue to exercise and that 'no serious complication to the combination of physical exercise and psychotropic medication has been published' (Martinsen & Stanghelle 1997, p. 90). Given that many people will have low initial fitness levels, and that drowsiness and fatigue are side-effects of many frequently used prescribed drugs, it is clear that a very gradual approach to exercise is the best initial course of action. This approach might lead to short sessions of 5 min several times in the day rather than the traditional 'exercise session'. It is important that these potential interactions of drugs and exercise are considered as part of the exercise programme, and should be discussed with the medical team.

Conclusions

The body of evidence supporting the relationship between exercise and mental health is growing. Increasing physical activity levels in the general population could have an impact on positive mental health and should be encouraged. Of course, the real difficulty is helping people start and independently maintain regular physical activity. With almost two-thirds of the UK population failing to meet the minimum recommendations for activity, of accumulating 30 min of moderate intensity activity on most days of the week, there is a huge public health challenge in promoting activity.

For those who are sceptical about the use of exercise in treatment of mental illnesses there are perhaps three potential concerns. The first is that it might not work. To this viewpoint we would counter that the potential benefit of advocating the use of exercise as part of a treatment package far outweighs the potential risk that no effect will occur. The second is that we do not know why it works. We have argued above that this should not in itself stop us from recommending exercise as part of a treatment package. The third potential concern of the sceptic is that there could be a harmful effect. However, there have been no negative outcomes reported in the literature. There are some potential negative side-effects, such as the risk of injury from exercise or the chance that a person could become dependent on exercise, but these, we would argue, are minor in comparison to many accepted side-effects from drug therapies. In addition, there are a host of potential physical health benefits from regular activity, which include reduced risk of dying prematurely from any cause and from heart disease; reduced risk of developing diabetes, colon cancer and high blood pressure; and promoting weight control, healthy bones, muscles and joints. Therefore we see the use of exercise as a 'win–win' situation and hope that many more therapists will begin using exercise and physical activity as part of their routine treatment packages.

Summary

- The evidence links physical activity to improvements in psychological well-being and in quality of life, and as a therapeutic intervention for people with existing mental health problems.

- Getting people started in exercise programmes and keeping them there is difficult.

- Low initial fitness levels, drowsiness and fatigue are side-effects of many frequently used prescribed drugs, indicating a very gradual approach to exercise as the initial course of action.

- Health benefits from regular physical activity far outweigh the potential risk of injury, indicating that exercise and physical activity should be included in all routine treatments.

References

Abramson L Y, Seligman M E P, Teasdale J D 1978 Learned helplessness in humans: critique and reformulation. Journal of Abnormal Psychology 87:49–74

American Psychiatric Association 1994 Diagnostic and statistic manual of mental disorders, 4th edn. CAPA, Washington DC

Baerveldt C, Voestermans P 1996 The body as a self-ing device. Theory and Psychology 6:693–713

Bero L A, Grilli R, Grimshaw J M et al 1998 Closing the gap between research and practice: an overview of systematic reviews of interventions to promote the implementation of research findings. British Medical Journal 317:465–468

Biddle S J H 1997 Current trends in sport and exercise psychology research. The Psychologist: Bulletin of the British Psychological Society 10:63–69

Biddle S J H 2000 Emotion, mood and physical activity. In: Biddle S J H, Fox K R, Boutcher S H (eds) Physical activity and psychological well-being. Routledge, London, p 63–87

Biddle S J H, Faulkner G 2002 Psychological and social benefits of physical activity. In: Chan K M (ed) Active aging. Lippincott Williams & Wilkins Asia Ltd, Hong Kong p 89–164

Biddle S J H, Mutrie N 2001 Psychology of physical activity: determinants, well-being and interventions. Routledge, London

Biddle S J H, Fox K R, Boutcher S H (eds) 2000a Physical activity and psychological well-being. Routledge, London

Biddle S J H, Fox K R, Boutcher S H, Faulkner G 2000b The way forward for physical activity and the promotion of psychological well-being. In: Biddle S J H, Fox K R, Boutcher S H (eds) Physical activity and psychological well-being. Routledge, London, p 154–168

Blair S N, Connelly J C 1994 How much physical activity should we do? The case for moderate amounts and intensities of physical activity. In: Killoran A J, Fentem P, Caspersen C (eds) Moving on: international perspectives on promoting physical activity. Health Education Authority, London, p 18–34

Borg G 1998 Borg's perceived exertion and pain scales. Human Kinetics, Champaign, IL

Boutcher S H 2000 Cognitive performance, fitness, and aging. In: Biddle S J H, Fox K R, Boutcher S H (eds) Physical activity and psychological well-being. Routledge, London, p 118–129

Brugha T S, Wing J K, Smith B L 1989 Physical health of the long term mentally ill in the community: is there unmet need? British Journal of Psychiatry 155:777–781

Chaouloff F 1997 The serotonin hypothesis. In: Morgan W P (ed) Physical activity and mental health. Taylor and Francis, Washington DC, p 179–198

Craft L L, Landers D M 1998 The effect of exercise on clinical depression and depression resulting from mental illness: a meta-analysis. Journal of Sport and Exercise Psychology 20:339–357

Dinan T G 1999 The physical consequences of depressive illness. British Medical Journal 318:826–827

Dupuis S L, Smale B J A 1995 An examination of the relationship between psychological well-being and depression and leisure activity participation among older adults. Society and Leisure 18:67–92

Etnier J L, Salazar W, Landers D M et al 1997 The influence of physical fitness and exercise upon cognitive functioning: a meta-analysis. Journal of Sport and Exercise Psychology 19:249–277

Faulkner G, Biddle S 1999 Exercise as an adjunct treatment for schizophrenia: a review of the literature. Journal of Mental Health 8:441–457

Faulkner G, Biddle S J H 2001 Exercise as therapy: it's just not psychology! Journal of Sports Sciences 19:433–444

Fox K R 1999 The influence of physical activity on mental well-being. Public Health Nutrition 2:411–418

Fox K R 2000a The effects of exercise on self-perceptions and self-esteem. In: Biddle S J H, Fox K R, Boutcher S H (eds) Physical activity and psychological well-being. Routledge, London, p 88–117

Fox K R 2000b Physical activity and mental health promotion: the natural partnership. International Journal of Mental Health Promotion 2:4–12

Fox K R, Boutcher S H, Faulkner G, Biddle S J H 2000 The case for exercise in the promotion of mental health and psychological well-being. In: Biddle S J H, Fox K R, Boutcher S H (eds) Physical activity and psychological well-being. Routledge, London, p 1–9

Gauvin L, Spence J C 1995 Psychological research on exercise and fitness: current research trends and future challenges. The Sport Psychologist 9:434–448

Gerlach J, Peacock L 1995 New antipsychotics: the present status. International Journal of Clinical Psychopharmacology 10:39–48

Greist J H, Klein M H, Eischens R R et al 1981 Running through your mind. In: Sacks M H, Sacks M L (eds) Psychology of running. Human Kinetics, Champaign, IL, p 5–31

Hale A S 1997 ABC of mental health. Depression. British Medical Journal 315:43–46

Hutchinson D S, Skrinar G S, Cross C 1999 The role of improved physical fitness in rehabilitation and recovery. Psychiatric Rehabilitation Journal 22:355–359

Jacobson N S, Martell C R, Dimidjian S 2001 Behavioral activation treatment for depression: returning to contextual roots. Clinical Psychology 8:255

King L, Hawe P, Wise M 1998 Making dissemination a two-way process. Health Promotion International 13:237–244

Kubitz K A, Landers D M 1993 The effects of aerobic training on cardiovascular responses to mental stress: an examination of underlying mechanisms. Journal of Sport and Exercise Psychology 15:326–337

La Forge R 1995 Exercise-associated mood alterations: a review of interactive neurobiological mechanisms. Medicine, Exercise, Nutrition and Health 4:17–32

Laitakari J, Miilunpalo S 1998 How can physical activity be changed: basic concepts and general principles in the promotion of health related physical activity. Patient Education and Counseling 33:S47-S59

Landers D M, Arent S M 2001 Physical activity and mental health. In: Singer R N, Hausenblas H A, Janelle C M (eds) Handbook of sport psychology : John Wiley, New York, p 740–764

Lawlor D A, Hopker S W 2001 The effectiveness of exercise as an intervention in the management of depression: systematic review and meta-regression analysis of randomised controlled trials. British Medical Journal 322:1–8

Llewelyn S, Hardy G 2001 Process research in understanding and applying psychological therapies. British Journal of Clinical Psychology 40:1–21

Loughlan C, Mutrie N 1995 Conducting an exercise consultation: guidelines for health professionals. Journal of the Institute of Health Education 33:78–82

MacLeod A 1998 Therapeutic interventions. In: Eysenck M (ed) Psychology an integrated approach. Longman, Harlow, p 563–589

Martinsen E W, Stanghelle J K 1997 Drug therapy and physical activity. In: Morgan W P (ed) Physical activity and mental health. Taylor and Francis, Washington DC, p 81–90

Martinsen E W, Stephens T 1994 Exercise and mental health in clinical and free-living populations. In: Dishman R (ed) Advances in exercise adherence. Human Kinetics, Champaign, IL, p 55–72

Martinsen E W, Hoffart A, Solberg Ø 1989a Comparing aerobic and non-aerobic forms of exercise in the treatment of clinical depression: a randomized trial. Comprehensive Psychiatry 30:324–331

Martinsen E W, Hoffart A, Solberg Ø 1989b Aerobic and non-aerobic forms of exercise in the treatment of anxiety disorders. Stress Medicine, 5:115–120

McEntee D J, Halgin R P 1996 Therapists' attitudes about addressing the role of exercise in psychotherapy. Journal of Clinical Psychology 52:48–60

Morgan K, Bath P A 1998 Customary physical activity and psychological well-being: a longitudinal study. Age and Ageing 27(suppl 3):35–40

Morgan K, Dallosso H, Bassey E J et al 1991 Customary physical activity, psychological well-being, and successful ageing. Aging and Society 11:399–415

Musselman D L, Evans D L, Nemeroff C B 1998 The relationship of depression to cardiovascular disease. Archives of General Psychiatry 55:580–592

Mutrie N 2000 The relationship between physical activity and clinically defined depression. In: Biddle S J H, Fox K R, Boutcher S H (eds) Physical activity and psychological well-being. Routledge, London, p 46–62

O'Connor P J, Raglin J S, Martinsen E W 2000 Physical activity, anxiety and anxiety disorders. International Journal of Sport Psychology 31:136–155

O'Neal H A, Dunn A L, Martinsen E W 2000 Depression and exercise. International Journal of Sport Psychology 31: 110–135

Ossip-Klein D J, Doyne E J, Bowman E D et al 1989 Effects of running and weight lifting on self-concept in clinically depressed women. Journal of Consulting and Clinical Psychology 57:158–161

Pate R R, Pratt M, Blair S N 1995 Physical activity and public health: a recommendation from the Centers for Disease Control and Prevention and the ACSM. Journal of the American Medical Association 273:402–407

Penninx B W J H, Guralnik J M, Ferruci L et al 1998 Depressive symptoms and physical decline in community-dwelling older persons. Journal of the American Medical Association 279:1720–1726

Peronnet F, Szabo A 1993 Sympathetic response to psychosocial stressors in humans: linkage to physical exercise and training. In: Seraganian P (ed) Exercise psychology: the influence of physical exercise on psychological processes. John Wiley, New York, p 172–217

Petruzzello S J, Landers D M, Hatfield B D et al 1991 A meta-analysis on the anxiety-reducing effects of acute and chronic exercise: outcomes and mechanisms. Sports Medicine 11:143–182

Plante T G 1993 Aerobic exercise in prevention and treatment of psychopathology. In: Seraganian P (ed) Exercise psychology: the influence of physical exercise on psychological processes. John Wiley, New York, p 358–379

Rogers E M 1995 Diffusion of innovations, 4th edn. The Free Press, New York

Salmon P 2001 Effects of physical exercise on anxiety, depression, and sensitivity to stress: a unifying theory. Clinical Psychology Review 21: 33–61

Schwarz L, Kindermann W 1992 Changes in B-endorphin levels in response to aerobic and anaerobic exercise. Sports Medicine 13:25–36

Scully D, Kremer J, Meade M M et al 1998 Physical exercise and psychological well-being: a critical review. British Journal of Sports Medicine 32: 111–120

Solomon R L 1980 The opponent-process theory of acquired motivation. American Psychologist 35:691–712

Taylor A H 2000 Physical activity, anxiety, and stress. In: Biddle S J H, Fox K R, Boutcher S H (eds) Physical activity and psychological well-being. Routledge, London, p 10–45

Tkachuk G A, Martin G L 1999 Exercise therapy for patients with psychiatric disorders: research and clinical implications. Professional Psychology: Research and Practice 30:275–282

Wetterling T 2001 Bodyweight gain with atypical antipsychotics: a comparative review. Drug Safety 24:59–73

Wilson W M, Maughan R J 1992 Evidence for a possible role of 5-hydoxytryptamine in the genesis of fatigue in man: administration of paroxetine, a 5-HT re-uptake inhibitor, reduces the capacity to perform prolonged exercise. Experimental Physiology 77:921–924

8 Adoption of physical activity in hospital and community settings

Andrew Clyne

Introduction

This chapter is divided into two sections. First, some of the possibilities for a physical activity service within a local mental health service are described. This section gives a rationale for the provision of physical activity. The second section concentrates on the practicalities of delivering physical activity. The need to be safe is emphasized, as is the need to know, and to show, that the physical activity has led to a positive outcome.

There is evidence that physical activity is a popular service within mental health and that many service users find physical activity very helpful (National Schizophrenia Fellowship, MIND and MDF 2000). However, this popularity does not reduce the responsibility to have clear clinical reasoning to support the planning and provision of a physical activity service. The purpose of this chapter is to assist health professionals to decide the reasons for providing physical activity in their local mental health service and to enable them to translate the evidence, that physical activity can improve mental health, into good practice within hospital and community settings.

Definition of terms

Throughout the chapter the following terms will be used: 'exercise professional' is used to cover a member of staff without a health professional qualification but with an exercise background. In some services this person might be employed as a technical instructor. 'Health professional' is used to describe the occupational therapist, physiotherapist or other health professional involved. 'Physical activity' is used rather than 'exercise'. Physical activity includes both structured and unstructured activity, e.g. going to a gym is structured physical activity, walking is unstructured. Although it is recognized that in some services and in some settings 'patient' or 'client' is the term in use, 'service user' is used throughout this chapter. Examples from one mental health centre have been provided solely to show how the background recommendations can be translated into practice within a local mental health service.

The possibilities   Occupational therapists and physiotherapists should be comfortable promoting physical activity within a mental health service because physical activity can be effective at improving mental health (see Chapter 7). Physical activity is within core professional skills of physiotherapists and occupational therapists. The service user can and should, be involved in developing physical activity opportunities. Also, physical activity can be included in mental health promotion work to help prevent mental illness. The presence of a physical activity service contributes to a more holistic service, where patients can feel that their mental and physical health needs are being addressed. However almost 80% of service users failed to list 'improving mental health' as a reason for physical activity when filling in a preactivity questionnaire (Clyne 2000).

Physical activity is an area where there can be user involvement in planning, promotion, funding, staffing, giving and receiving training and reporting. Occupation including leisure is a core activity of occupational therapy and exercise is a core skill of physiotherapy; both professions should be comfortable with some involvement with physical activity. Service user involvement and social integration are discussed in Chapter 9.

Aims of a physical activity service   If the aim of the service is not clearly understood by patients and other staff then the major demand could be to entertain and to pass the time. There is a role for making life more pleasurable but the role of a health professional is questionable if all activities are chosen for their entertainment value. The following are the aims of a physical activity service in a mental health day centre:

- to assist you to do something positive, which will help you feel fitter and better
- to provide a service that has high standards of safety
- to use the best evidence in our work
- to provide an individualized service that is realistic to your ability, interests and lifestyle
- to try our best to make it fun.

Four case studies are presented to illustrate different interventions. Some of the identifying details within the case studies have been changed.

Hospital and community settings   Physical activity in the community should reflect local surroundings, facilities and culture. The advantages of getting out of a hospital to provide a service include increasing social presence, better facilities, wider choice of activity and the fact that the activity can be ongoing after discharge from hospital or mental health service.

Case study 1

The volleyball player

Anne was a 46-year-old woman who was admitted to hospital with depression. While in hospital she engaged with gym sessions. Her major goal for the future was to try volleyball. She enjoyed a session organized at the local sports centre and was surprised at how 'good' she was at volleyball. Staff encouraged her to phone MIND to find out details of their session. Her family was informed of her plans to play volleyball each Thursday and they encouraged her to attend regularly.

Case study 2

The runner

Brian was a 38-year-old man attending a community drug rehabilitation programme. The physiotherapist obtained clearance from his GP for vigorous physical activity because Brian had high blood pressure. A Coopers Walking Test was carried out with blood pressure monitored. Then a walking/running programme was planned. Brian was given a choice of some local races to set as a target and he chose a run of 10 kilometres. The physiotherapist spoke to Brian each week but did not go running with him. As the run approached Brian requested that the physiotherapist ran with him, offering support. They both completed the run together. The physiotherapist discharged Brian at this point. Brian ran a half-marathon (21 kilometres) later that summer.

Case study 3

The gym member

Colin was a 36-year-old man who was admitted to hospital with depression. His walking was affected by psychomotor retardation. The physiotherapist worked to help improve posture and movements. After 3 weeks, Colin was confident to attend the gym sessions. Two months later Colin (still an inpatient) attended the supported gym session in a local authority sports centre. He continued to attend after discharge and for the next 18 months. He stopped attending only when he joined a private health club nearer to his home.

Case study 4

The walker

David was a 52-year-old man who was admitted to hospital with depression. He attended a walking group each week. However, he did not engage in any other physical activity and he was not keen to plan any physical activity after discharge. Two years later he was readmitted with another depressive episode. He reported that after his first admission he had developed a habit of walking 7 kilometres every evening after work. He had started the walks with his wife. Occasionally a neighbour and a friend of his neighbour join them.

A hospital gym or dedicated exercise facility might be the most practical option when service users are restricted to staying on site, particularly when an individual is staying for a long time. However, if an individual is likely to stay in hospital for less than 2 months then the amount of physical activity is likely to be insufficient to achieve many of the mental health benefits that a longer stay might allow. The aim of physical activity, in this case, might be to facilitate physical activity after discharge. Facilitating continued physical activity often requires a service to access community facilities close to where the individual lives.

Community settings for physical activity are frequently accessed in some kind of healthy alliance with leisure services or the voluntary sector. Healthy alliances are described later in the chapter. The barriers to providing a service in the community include cost, staffing, transport and risk.

In studies of 'free-living populations' (Hillsdon et al 1995), walking has been found to have the highest adherence rates. Its advantages are that it is available 7 days a week, it is free and you need no special equipment, it is sociable – the service user's family and friends can all walk, it is a good excuse to get out of the ward, it is practical for unfit people and it is practical for most staff to promote and supervise.

Preactivity assessment

Many health professionals who will be referring people to physical activity will have limited knowledge of the effect of physical activity on mental health. Likewise, their level of knowledge of exercise safety might be low. A preactivity assessment can help establish levels of safety, motivation and clinical effectiveness. It should include screening and could also include a fitness test and a more detailed assessment.

Pre-exercise screening is increasingly common before many exercise and sporting activities. Many screening questionnaires are based on the Physical Activity Readiness Questionnaire (PAR-Q). The PAR-Q is a standard to be met before moderate and vigorous exercise. The American Heart Association (AHA) and the American College of Sports Medicine (ACSM) have produced a joint position statement describing the 'Revised PAR-Q' (Balady et al 1998). The Revised PAR-Q is primarily designed to establish the presence or absence of angina pectoris.

Part of the 'Fit To Begin' assessment also questions for symptoms of mental illness and side-effects of medication (Fig. 8.1).

The AHA/ACSM joint position statement (Balady 1998) includes a more detailed questionnaire – the 'Health/Fitness Facility Preparticipation Screening Questionnaire', which can be used to decide the response to 'high risk' individuals and to people who do not, or cannot, complete a questionnaire. All health professionals supporting physical activity should carry out regular preactivity risk screens for CHD and other 'physical' risks. They should also have access to, and be part of, the general risk assessment process. Other relevant topics for risk assessment include:

Fit To Begin Questionnaire

Please write in yes or no for each question.

Question	Yes/No
1. Has a Doctor ever told you that you have a heart condition?	
2. Have you developed chest pain at any time in the last month or have you ever had chest pain brought on by physical activity?	
3. Have you ever fainted, lost consciousness or fallen over due to dizziness?	
4. Do you have muscle stiffness, or a bone or joint problem?	
5. Have you ever taken medication for your blood pressure or a heart condition?	
6. Do you experience headaches or blurred vision?	
7. Have you ever been told that you may have epilepsy?	
8. Have you ever been told that you may have diabetes?	
9. Has your weight changed in the last 6 months?	
10. Do you get dizzy if you stand up quickly?	
11. Have you ever been told that you have high or low blood pressure?	
12. Do you have any problems with your balance?	
13. Have you ever had asthma, panic attacks or breathing difficulties?	
14. Are you aware of any other reason that would stop you exercising normally?	

How fit are you? (Indicate by making a mark on the line below).

Very Unfit								Very Fit	
1	2	3	4	5	6	7	8	9	10

Figure 8.1 *The "Fit to Begin" Questionnaire*

- violence
- self-harm, including suicide
- abuse
- absconding
- use of alcohol or illicit drugs.

Most NHS mental health trusts have a standardized risk screen. This should have been carried out with each service user prior to physical activity. Health professionals need to plan their response to a service user not being screened, or being screened but not having the necessary risk assessments carried out. Physical activity should be fun, and can even be cathartic, but that does not rule out the possibility of an incident occurring.

Fitness testing

Fitness testing helps demonstrate likely tolerance of physical activity; it can also increase adherence (Franklin 1988). Indirectly, it can provide evidence of changes in physical activity level; lastly, it can provide evidence of clinical effectiveness.

The ACSM guidelines for exercise prescription (ACSM 2001) describe a range of protocols that can be used for fitness tests. A range of fitness tests should be available in response to the perceived level of fitness and risk of coronary heart disease. Possible options include (ACSM 2001):

■ a 6-min submaximal bicycle ergometer test, for instance the Åstrand and Rhyming protocol
■ the Rockport 1-mile Walking Test
■ the Coopers 12-min Walking Test (or even the 6-min version)
■ referral for maximal test.

The publication *Exercise referral systems: a national quality assurance framework* (NHS 2001a) provides UK recommendations for when different types of fitness testing are indicated. One apparent difference between the UK and North America is less frequent use of a maximal fitness test in the UK. A maximal fitness test is required when vigorous exercise is planned and one or more of the following are present (NHS 2001a):

■ age factors (men over 45 years, women over 55 years)
■ two or more risk factors for coronary heart disease
■ known cardiac, pulmonary or metabolic disease.

There is likely to be an inequality between who, in theory, should be sent for a maximal fitness test and the availability of the test. If a maximal exercise test is indicated but not available for an individual then the health or exercise professional has two options. Either decline to offer supervised physical activity or limit the intensity of the physical activity to well below 12 on the Borg scales (Borg 1998).

The Borg scales (Table 8.1) are an estimate of exertion without the need to measure heart rate. The 6–20 scale is widely used and respected. The modified scale (0–10) is used less in research but is commonly used in leisure centres and non-research settings.

Assessing physical activity level

Sustained physical activity can be effective at improving or ameliorating anxiety, depression, self-esteem, cognitive functioning, psychological dysfunction, mood and emotion (Biddle et al 2000). However, measuring

Table 8.1 *Physical activity intensity guide (adapted from Balady et al 1998 and ACSM 2001)*

Intensity	% maximum heart rate	RPE (Borg scale) (6–20)	RPE (modified Borg scale) (0–10)
Light	30–49	9–10	2–3
Moderate	50–69	11–12	4–5
Vigorous	70–100	13–20	6–10+

RPE, relative physical exertion

physical activity levels is not as easy as estimating fitness. An accelerometer or step-counter can be worn but compliance might be questionable. Structured physical activity can be measured but much physical activity occurs out of the sight of staff. Physical activity can be elicited by recall, for instance the 7-day Physical Activity Recall (PAR; Dunn et al 1999). The difficulty in accurately measuring physical activity provides another reason to fitness-test service users. Physical activity levels, especially in individuals who start with low fitness, influence aerobic fitness levels (Kostka et al 2000). Assessing the service users's motivation is useful to 'individualize' the approach, and the assessment can be part of the outcome measurement (Hunt & Hillsdon 1996).

Assessing mental health

There is considerable difference between what measures of mental health are required for an intervention study and what is required to indicate clinical effectiveness. Occupational therapists or physiotherapists must not exceed their role and competency to assess mental state. Some brief, validated, more general assessments can be used by a wide range of health professionals with a wide range of individuals; for instance the HoNOS scales (College Research Unit 1996). A health professional committed to physical activity might also be comfortable assessing the physical dimensions of self-esteem, e.g. using the Physical Self-Perception Profile described by Marsh (1997). Although this is a more detailed assessment than, for example, the HoNOS scale, it measures 'the physical self'. This is distinctive and is more likely to be accepted as providing evidence of effect of a physical activity intervention.

Discharge

A discharge report can provide motivation to stay focused on the physical activity plan and the identified outcome of physical activity. A discharge report could include:

- the physical activity plan/record
- the fitness test
- assessments of intention to be physically active
- an assessment of mental health.

Outcome measurement

One of the guiding principles quoted in *Turning evidence into everyday practice* (Dunning et al 1998, p. 19) is that service outcome measures should 'focus on the process of implementation rather than on health outcomes'. Some examples of outcome measures are given in Box 8.1.

Box 8.1
Example of objectives from a mental health centre

- That 50% of all inpatients will engage with physical activity at least twice during their stay.
- That four or more physical activity sessions will be available to inpatients each week.
- That the percentage of inpatients achieving 180 min of moderate exercise, in 1 month, increases each year.

Motivation to be physically active

Franklin (1988) listed some 'programmatic' variables that influence adherence. The presence of all seven variables would indicate that the physical activity service provides very high levels of encouragement for adherence. The variables are:

1. instruction and encouragement
2. regular routine
3. freedom from injury
4. enjoyment, fun, variety
5. group camaraderie
6. progress testing and recording
7. spouse and peer approval.

Transport and cost

Providing free physical activity might be justifiable for inpatients but is unlikely to lead to sustained physical activity in outpatients. A local decision therefore needs to be taken about what to charge service users. Grants are rarely available directly to the NHS but are available to voluntary organizations. Cost as well as staffing is a good reason to provide community physical activity in partnership with other organizations. The decision about providing transport is similar to the decision about cost. The more that is provided free of charge, the greater the shock when the free transport stops. However, staff and a minibus outside your home are strong incentives to get up and out to the physical activity. One positive variable for physical activity is group camaraderie (Franklin 1988). Sharing lifts may indicate good group camaraderie.

Staff qualification

Encouraging someone to walk to the shops would not require a health professional to obtain additional qualifications but supervising a session using a climbing wall, or using an unsupervised gym, *would* require additional qualifications. A health professional without any exercise qualification should not be considered competent to teach weight lifting. Clearly, the more vigorous and more dangerous the activity, the greater the need for additional qualification. A professional qualification in occupational therapy or physiotherapy does not guarantee that the individual is an effective physical activity leader. One of the most influential variables that affects adherence to physical activity is 'instruction and encouragement' (Franklin 1988, p. 240). Technical Instructor is a grade that reflects a background and qualification as an exercise professional. Table 8.2 outlines some of the better-known qualifications available.

Promoting a physical activity service within a mental health service

Probably the most effective way to promote a physical activity service within a mental health service is to be associated with good quality work and positive outcomes. Other ways to win support are through:

Table 8.2 *Some widely recognized qualifications for physical instruction*

Purpose	Required qualification
For instructing people in the use of a multigym or weights	B.A.W.L.A Leaders award
For instruction of exercise in a range of structured physical activity	GNVQ Exercise and Health Levels 1 and 2 RSA Exercise to Music YMCA Fitness Instructor or Exercise to Music Awards
Additionally	Yoga, Tai Chi, EXTEND, plus awards in specific sports or activities

- education of staff
- having a high profile
- audit and activity measurement
- outcome measurement
- service user feedback
- links with other agencies, e.g. leisure services, local universities, user groups and other mental health agencies
- involving staff in the referral process
- annual report and newsletter.

Health promotion (healthy alliances)

Standard 1 of the Mental Health National Service Framework (NSF) relates to mental health promotion. The executive briefing (The Sainsbury Centre for Mental Health 2000) provides examples of how physical activity could be an activity to tackle social exclusion and promote mental well-being. A GP exercise referral scheme in Redbridge and Waltham Forest (in the UK) is described as being supported by good quality of evidence.

This exercise referral scheme is an example of a healthy alliance. Healthy alliances can be between health and leisure services, as well as the voluntary sector. The Health Education Authority (HEA) and Wessex Institute of Public Health (1995) described the benefits of healthy alliances under six 'indicators'.

1. Policy change: changing or creation of a 'health promoting' policy, for instance greater access to leisure services.
2. Service and environmental change: e.g. including mental health as referral criteria in an exercise referral scheme.
3. Skills development: a healthy alliance should increase the health professional's knowledge of physical activity opportunities and increase the exercise professional's knowledge of mental health.

4. Publicity: coverage needs to reach the intended audience. This could be people who do not usually engage with the mental health service.

5. Contact: likewise, healthy alliances can aim to maximize contact with people who are not usually mental health service users.

6. Knowledge, attitude and behaviour change: 'Healthy alliances have long been recognised as the best way to achieve real and lasting changes to improve the health of communities' (HEA and Wessex Institute of Public Health 1995).

Although the joint working can be initially time consuming, it can bring a longer lasting service and a higher profile for the service.

Summary

This chapter described some possibilities for a physical activity service. The responsibilities of the different health professionals influence the activities and style of service. Particular importance has been placed on why a physical activity service should be offered. The second part of this chapter discussed some of the practicalities of providing a service. The popularity of the service does not remove the need to be focused on what (and why) services are provided. Many service users will be unfit, at increased risk of coronary heart disease and be experiencing side-effects from medication. Safe practice therefore needs to be maintained. However, the benefit to mental health and the physical health advantages of exercise mean physical activity has much to offer the mental health service user.

A good physical activity service should have:

■ Publicized rationale for physical activity.

■ Screening and safety procedures.

■ Assessment and outcome measurement.

■ Healthy alliances.

■ Strong physical activity promotion.

References

ACSM 2001 Guidelines for exercise testing and prescription, 6th edn. Williams and Wilkins, Philadelphia

Balady G, Chaitman B, Driscoll D et al 1998 Recommendations for cardiovascular screening, staffing and emergency policies at health/fitness facilities. Joint position statement of the AHA/ACSM. Medicine and science in sport and exercise 30(6):1009–1018

Biddle J, Fox K, Boutcher S 2000 Physical activity and psychological well-being. Routledge, London

Borg G 1998 Borg's perceived exertion and pain scales. Human Kinetics, Champaign, IL

College Research Unit 1996 HoNOS: Health of the nation rating scales: raters' pack. Royal College of Psychiatrists, London

Clyne A 2000 Internal audit of 'Fit to begin' questionnaires. Sandalwood Court, Swindon

Dunn A, Marcus B, Kampert J et al 1999 Comparisons of lifestyle and structured interventions to increase physical activity and cardiorespiratory fitness. Journal of the American Medical Association 281:327–334.

Dunning M, Abi-Aad G, Gilbert D et al 1998 Turning evidence into everyday practice. The King's Fund, London, p 19

Franklin B 1988 Program factors that influence exercise adherence: practical adherence skills for the clinical staff. In: Dishman R (ed) Exercise adherence: its impact on public health. Human Kinetics, Champaign, IL, p 237–258

Hillsdon M, Thorogood M, Anstiss T, Morris J 1995 Randomised controlled trials of physical activity promotion in free living populations – a review. Journal of Epidemiology and Community Health 49:448–453

Hunt P, Hillsdon M 1996 Changing eating and exercise behaviour: a handbook for professionals. Blackwell Science, Oxford

HEA and Wessex Institute of Public Health 1995. Towards healthier alliances – a tool for planning, evaluating and developing healthy alliances. Health Education Authority, London

Kostka T, Rahmani A, Lacour J et al 2000 Quadriceps muscle function in relation to habitual physical activity and VO^2 max in men and women aged more than 65 years. Journal of Gerontology series A: Biological Sciences and Medical Sciences 55:481–488.

Marsh H 1997 The measurement of physical self-concept: a construct validation approach. In: Fox K (ed) The physical self: from motivation to well-being. Human Kinetics, Champaign, IL, p 27–58

National Schizophrenia Fellowship, MIND and MDF 2000 A question of choice – initial findings of a survey. Online. Available: www.nsf.org.uk/information/research

NHS 2001a Exercise referral systems: a national quality assurance framework. Department of Health, London

NHS 2001b NHS Beacon Handbook. Department of Health.

HYPERLINK http://www.nhsbeacons.org.uk/main.htm (accessed 9 July 2001)

The Sainsbury Centre for Mental Health 2000 An executive briefing on mental health promotion: implementing standard one of the national service framework. The Sainsbury Centre for Mental Health, London

Activity and social inclusion

Tina Everett and Colin Godfrey

Introduction

The aims of this chapter are to provide a brief insight as to how service provision for people with mental health problems has changed over the last hundred years.

Exercise provision within psychiatric institutions in the last century is contrasted with the problems of social isolation and sedentary lifestyles that have developed with the advent of community care. Recent government initiatives to increase the uptake of exercise, supported by the National Service Frameworks, provide opportunity to engage service users in community-based activities that will promote a healthier lifestyle and opportunities for social integration. The chapter outlines examples of this illustrated with the views from users of the service

Historical perspective

The asylums built in the nineteenth century for people with mental health problems generally had a very large hall for exercise and recreation, and outdoor 'airing courts' for walking. In the 1920s and 1930s, 90% of the patients at the asylum at Colney Heath lived in locked wards and were confined to hospital gardens for fresh air and exercise. It is reported that female patients were kept fit by a masseuse (but this could only have been for a few privileged women), and male patients by physical training classes and games. Both were supervised on long walks on paths constructed around the inside of the boundary wall – patients could sometimes cover up to 7 miles a day in this way (Hunter & Macalpine 1974). Prior to this, in the latter part of the nineteenth century, a passive form of hydrotherapy became a standard treatment in the asylums 'hot baths for melancholia, cold for mania, plunge or prolonged, sat in or poured over, vapour or wet' (Hunter & Macalpine 1974, p. 85).

Patients in the county asylums were kept occupied during the day either in workshops or doing suitable light work within the hospital. Most hospitals had their own farms and were self-sufficient in the supply of vegetables: 'potatoes, mangel-wurzel, turnips and cabbages!' (Hunter & Macalpine 1974, p. 39) for all their residents, who often numbered up to 2000. The situation in the county hospitals was perhaps better than in other institutions. In 1939, the then private Warneford hospital in Oxford was described as a place where patients were 'less occupied, less useful and more inclined to brood over their own inadequacies than in the nearby county hospital' (Jones 1960, p. 137).

The mid-1950s saw both the introduction of chlorpromazine and the beginning of the decline in total inpatient numbers, and from this period there was an increased range of occupational and industrial therapy, often led by nursing staff. These were now housed away from the wards to provide changes in scenery and staff. From the 1960s and 1970s, at differing rates around the UK, resettlement of long-stay residents into hostels and group homes became increasingly widespread.

With the advent of community care and the closure of the old asylums, many people previously confined to hospital for a variety of medical and social reasons were able to resume useful lives in the community. But for some with enduring mental illness, living alone or with their families, isolation has become a real problem. For them, and for patients still requiring long-term hospital care, social exclusion and societal attitudes have yet to be tackled. The British government is attempting to address these problems through the National Service Framework (see Chapter 3).

Government initiatives and local schemes

The national exercise referral scheme (DoH 2001) enables doctors to refer patients for prescribed exercise at their local leisure centre. Therapists can tap into this and can set up an agreement with local leisure centres to refer their own clients directly. This is proving a useful way of progressing people from the hospital gym setting to community facilities. However, it is not an easy option, and can take a great deal of networking and negotiation. In some areas, a member of the physiotherapy team takes a group at the local leisure centre and clients can progress from that to the exercise referral scheme when they feel confident enough to attend on their own. Some people with long-term mental health needs will always find this difficult, and the success of the scheme can depend in part on the attitudes of the leisure centre staff. See Chapter 8 for other examples of integrated service provision in the community.

In Oxfordshire, therapists have initiated mental health awareness seminars for leisure staff aiming to break down barriers and to confront fear and stigma. Service users are involved in the seminars, which have been very well received. A comment from the evaluation form submitted by a member of the leisure centre staff highlights the benefit of these shared sessions:

> *Listening to real-life cases is the key to future help towards mental health – these guys could really help others, they are the ones that have been there and are able to say what they have been through.*

A sample plan for a 'mental health awareness seminar' could include:

- Introduction.
- Ice-breaker, e.g. ask participants what ambition they have and what stops them achieving it.
- Brief explanation of the role of physiotherapy and occupational therapy in mental health.
- Brainstorm – what is mental illness, common names, labelling, etc?
- Service users speak about their experience of exercise.
- Workshop in small groups – discussion of sample case studies 'what would you do if...?'
- Way forward – feedback and questions.

The following is an extract from a service user's contribution to the seminar:

> *What are people looking for from the mentally healthy population? We are looking for the fear and disquiet to go, and we would like people to know the difference between a nutter and a mentally ill person. We don't want special treatment and we don't want sympathy, but we do want respect, understanding and knowledge.*
>
> *The free, supervised use of leisure centres is very much appreciated by mentally ill people. It is important for us to have exercise as a stress-buster. It is also important for us to get into a routine of doing things because this guards against isolation, idleness and torpor – which are easy things to slip into.*

Another example of innovative practice is a community gym in the North of England. This facility for people with mental health problems was awarded NHS beacon status in 2000. The original hospital-based service moved to a building in the town centre providing easy access and a very open referral system. Its most unique quality is that it provides opportunity for users to take part in the running of the gym and to have input into its planning, development and evaluation. A formal volunteer system provides users with a range of opportunities to gain work experience and qualifications (Truman & Raine 2001). The gym has been developed by a Community Trust physiotherapy department and is jointly financed by the Regional Mental Health Partnership Fund and the local health authority. Qualitative research has been carried out by a local university to evaluate the process of developing the gym and to explore user perspectives on their participation in the project (Truman & Raine 2001). Emphasis is placed on strengthening links with a range of community agencies and user involvement ensures the gym is flexible and responsive to user needs. By providing a volunteer scheme and training opportunities users gain more control in their lives (as is evidenced in the quote below from a service user), which is likely to increase their employment possibilities:

> *I'll see one of my friends. 'What have you been up to?' What can you say? 'I've just been sat at home all day'? I can say, 'I've been down to the gym'. It sounds a lot better.*

A programme based on the multigym is neither a suitable, nor preferable, form of exercise for all clients and the physiotherapist can help each individual in their choice of recreational exercise. The Countryside Agency (2000) along with the British Heart Foundation has set up a scheme entitled 'Walking the way to health', funded by the National Lottery and Kia cars. It aims to train local people to lead walks for health in their own locality and could provide an opportunity for service users to participate as they regain their independence. Free or reduced rate swimming sessions are also often provided for disadvantaged groups. Service users can also support each other in buddy schemes at the local pool.

Extending the boundaries

Further innovative practice is found in a Mental Healthcare Trust's 'Activities Development Service'. The service works with isolated and non-progressing individuals with enduring mental health problems through challenging outdoor activities. Referrals are accepted from any health professionals for inpatients, and through the community mental health teams for outpatients. The service users are, or often have been, resident for long periods on an acute admission ward, or are living in hospital or social services accommodation.

The nurse in charge of this service works as part of the physiotherapy team and has supervisory qualifications in rock climbing and general outdoor pursuits. The nurse aims to establish positive therapeutic relationships with service users, particularly those who find it difficult to engage or be engaged by conventional therapeutic regimes. Team building and enjoyment of health-promoting activity leads to an increase in motivation, self-confidence, independence and sociability. The Activities Development Nurse is both facilitator and participant, working to a flexible timetable and not limited by standard hours or fixed sites. No patients are discharged from this service so a network has evolved of users and staff with a positive shared experience. Regular evening and weekend sporting groups for badminton and football have been established, as well as a series of annual events. These include a 2-week coast-to-coast walk, a 5-day coast-to-coast (C2C) mountain bike ride, a series of local day-long walks and some overnight visits to North Wales. Abseiling and rock climbing are on offer both locally and in North Wales. Each activity demands a positive application of mind and body and engenders a true feeling of achievement in taking part. The activities also enhance social integration and give powerful positive messages both to the local community and to the wider mental health fraternity. Risk assessment is a key part of this therapeutic role. Activities must be pitched at the user's perceived ability or perceived potential ability, and a continuous assessment of the participant in a holistic (mental, physical and psychological) sense is essential. Benefits of this approach are given in this user's quote:

I had a terrible experience in hospital. I was sent to two medium secure units for violence in response to auditory hallucinations. When I think back to those many years of treatment there is one event that changed my life: joining nurses and other patients on a 190-mile coast-to-coast walk. I found it particularly difficult as I am overweight and not very fit. The first few days were the worst. They involved very rugged terrain and I needed a good head for heights. During the walk the best moment was finishing 24 miles in a day. The worst moment was climbing up a rock-face waterfall – don't look down. The walk improved my self-esteem, now I feel much more confident. I got to know my fellow walkers very well. Our experience drew us together as friends. I know I can't change the past. All I can do is take each day as it comes, much like on the walk and make the most of it. I gained a new outlook on life. I am glad I met the challenge but I would never do it again. Once is enough.

(Mackay & Bowery 1998)

The continuous evolving of the network has led to service users becoming part of the activities development team, with Trust honorary contracts for work done by users to fund raise or provide logistic support such as driving. Some users are taking a full part in evaluative research, supported by the local university. This qualitative research project is investigating:

- physical and mental health of users
- social integration
- sense of well-being
- admission rates
- prescription of psychotropic medication
- development of positive relationships with statutory mental health services.

Summary

- Community care has brought freedom and autonomy to many people who were previously confined to the large asylums.

- Problems of isolation and social exclusion still exist and are being tackled in a few innovative schemes around the UK.

- Nationally, the 'Exercise referral scheme' and 'Walking the way to health' are providing exercise opportunities at reduced cost in many areas.

- There are still barriers of inequality and stigma to be overcome.

- The National Service Framework is providing opportunity and an obligation to listen to users of mental health services and to make radical changes.

- Physiotherapists and occupational therapists in partnership with their clients can be pioneers in this field.

References

DoH 2001 Exercise referral systems: a national quality assurance framework. Department of Health, London

Hunter R, Macalpine I 1974 Psychiatry for the poor. W Dawson & Sons, Folkstone, UK

Jones K 1960 Mental health and social policy. Routledge & Kegan-Paul, New York

Mackay G, Bowery C 1998 Side view... there's nothing like a coast-to-coast walk to mark mental health day and test your mettle. Nursing Times 94(40):7–13

The Countryside Agency 2000 Walking the way to health. The Countryside Agency, Cheltenham, UK

Truman C, Raine P 2001 User participation, mental health and exercise: learning from the experiences of Barrow community gym. Department of Applied Social Science, Lancaster University

10 Cognitive–behavioural therapy in physiotherapy and occupational therapy

Edward A S Duncan

Introduction

Cognitive–behavioural therapy (CBT) is the term given to a specific psychological approach to conceptualizing and treating clients' difficulties. An emphasis upon implementing evidence-based interventions has assisted its rapid development since the 1980s. CBT, in one form or other, is often the mode of psychological intervention cited as having the greatest evidence-base for effective intervention with a variety of disorders, including anxiety, depression and psychotic disorders (Department of Health 2001). More recently, evidence has emerged supporting the use of CBT with various other conditions such as chronic pain (Strong 1998) and chronic fatigue syndrome (Prins et al 2001).

As CBT has been found to be effective within an increasing range of conditions, so too has the interest of physiotherapists and occupational therapists grown in this treatment approach. Although CBT is non-profession specific, it is important that both occupational therapists and physiotherapists thoroughly understand the approach, so as to incorporate the principles effectively within their working practice. It is equally important for such professionals to have an awareness of the limitations of their core professional skills and to acknowledge situations in which they are not competent to utilize a cognitive–behavioural approach.

This chapter gives a general introduction to cognitive–behavioural therapy. The evidence for the efficacy of the approach within both professions will then be illustrated. The text purposively omits detailed description of the various therapeutic techniques related to CBT: the cognitive–behavioural approach is guided more fundamentally by its tenets than by the techniques utilized. Focus upon techniques has led to a highly prescriptive understanding of the cognitive–behavioural approach to intervention. Such techniques are described in greater detail in other texts and the interested reader is recommended to follow-up the references at the end of this chapter. Cognitive–behavioural interventions take place in both an individual and group format. The information given in this chapter is of relevance to both settings.

Historical developments

Cognitive–behavioural therapy, as it is understood today, is the result of a series of theoretical and clinical developments. The behavioural component of therapy, strongly influenced by the evolutionary perspective of health, can be traced to the beginning of the twentieth century, when the principles gained from animal behaviour research were applied to human beings (Hawton et al 1996). The cognitive component of the approach claims even more historical roots, linking itself with the Roman emperor Epictetus who wrote in the Enchiridion, 'Men are disturbed, not by things, but of the view they take of them' (Beck et al 1979). A comprehensive examination of the historical development of the model can be found in Hawton et al (1996).

Cognitive therapy

Although the first cognitive approach to therapy was developed by Meichenbaum (1975), it is the work of Aaron T. Beck that has become synonymous with the term 'cognitive therapy'.

Aaron Beck (born in 1921) developed cognitive therapy through an examination of the links between the environment, the person and his or her emotion and motivation. Surprisingly, Beck, a psychiatrist, did not come from a foundation in behaviourism; instead, his roots are in the psychoanalytical perspective. Commencing his career, Beck trained in psychoanalytical theory and practice. Despite an initial hesitancy regarding the nature of psychoanalytical theory, he soon commenced a research project aimed at proving the efficacy of the approach in relation to depression, in a bid to convert the doubtful. It is in the findings of this research, which highlighted discrepancies in the psychoanalytical approach, that the origins of cognitive therapy can be found. A fuller account of Beck's life and work can be found in his biography (Weishaar 1993).

Tenets of cognitive therapy

Although several developments have taken place within cognitive therapy since its inception, the general assumptions surrounding its practice remain:

- *Perception and experiencing in general are active processes which involve both inspective and introspective data.*
- *The patient's cognitions represent a synthesis of internal and external stimuli.*
- *How a person appraises a situation is generally evident in his cognitions (thoughts and visual images).*
- *These cognitions constitute the persons 'stream of consciousness' or phenomenal field, which reflects the person's configuration of themself, their world, past and future.*
- *Alterations in the content of the persons underlying cognitive structures affect his or her affective state and behavioural pattern.*
- *Through psychological therapy, a patient can become aware of his cognitive distortions.*
- *Correction of these faulty dysfunctional constructs can lead to clinical improvement.*

(Beck et al 1979)

Cognitive–behavioural therapy (CBT)

The term 'cognitive–behavioural therapy' is now commonly given to interventions that encompass the above tenets of therapy. Increasingly, therapists utilize a combination of behavioural and cognitive components within their therapeutic practice.

Characteristics of cognitive–behavioural therapy

Whereas the fundamental paradigm of CBT, as described above, provides the basis to the approach, the structure and processes of therapy are also characteristic and distinguish it from other psychotherapeutic approaches:

- *Present focused.* With a few notable exceptions, mainly in the field of personality disorders, the majority of CBT is centred on the 'here and now'. Historic information (e.g. about the client's childhood) is of interest only in gaining an understanding of the person. The focus of therapy is on current cognitions, behaviours and emotions.
- *Time limited.* In treating anxiety and depression, for which the approach was originally developed, CBT was typically considered as a 12-session approach. Today, as therapists tackle more complex dysfunctions, such as personality disorders and psychosis, this guide is becoming less rigid. The time-limited philosophy to intervention, however, still stands as a guiding principle.
- *Collaborative.* The relationship between therapist and client is central to the process of CBT. Beck et al (1979) describes this relationship as a 'collaborative empiricism' in which both the therapist and the client work together as a team and aim to develop a shared understanding of the client's problems.
- *Problem focused.* Clients who present themselves, or are referred for therapy, often have multiple and complex problems. Therapists might initially draw a problem list with the client, outlining the various problems the client has. Together, they will then decide upon a problem priority list, thus providing a focus for intervention. Although the list is developed in a collaborative manner, there might be occasions in which the therapist addresses some areas of concern (e.g. suicidality) before moving to other areas.

The therapist–client relationship

A collaborative relationship is central to the therapeutic process. The utilization of therapeutic techniques, in a toolbox fashion, has led to the perception of CBT as lacking in due attention to the client as an individual. This danger has been recognized since the inception of the approach:

> *A word of caution is in order. Cognitive and behavioural techniques often seem deceptively simple. Consequently, the neophyte therapist may become 'gimmick orientated' to the point of ignoring the human aspect of the therapist–patient interaction.*

(Beck et al 1979)

Thus, since its inception, the development of a positive, collaborative therapeutic relationship has been recognized as a fundamental component of the cognitive–behavioural approach.

Desirable therapist characteristics are described as the ability to exhibit warmth, accurate empathy and genuineness (Beck et al 1979). Regarding the therapist–client relationship, Beck et al (1979) outline its basis in trust, rapport and collaboration.

Structure of therapy

The following structure is often considered to be the 'classic' course of CBT. This was developed from its original conceptualization as a therapeutic intervention designed to address the affective disorders (e.g. anxiety and depression). As the spectrum of disorders addressed by CBT has increased, so too has the flexibility of the original structure.

Initially, sessions are held weekly. Towards the end of the agreed number of sessions, the therapist and client might agree to meet on a less frequent basis (e.g. fortnightly). This has the added benefit of lessening any dependence on the therapist, that might have developed during the course of the intervention. The duration of each session is normally between 45 and 60 minutes.

Assessment

The assessment process allows the therapist to gain information relating to the client's problems and develop the basis for a therapeutic relationship. This can be achieved through a variety of methods including, interview, questionnaires, observational techniques and self-monitoring (Wells 1997). The information gained is used in the development of the individual's case formulation. This cognitive conceptualization of the client's problems is presented to the client as a method of explaining the therapist's perspective. It is important to note, however, that the formulation is presented as a working hypothesis and the therapist should ask the client for his or her feedback on its perceived accuracy. In this manner, the formulation becomes a collaborative effort to understand the client's problems and will often be referred to and refined throughout the course of therapy. The client's problem formulation often forms an initial component of another aspect of the therapeutic process, socialization.

Socialization

'Socialisation refers to "selling" the approach and providing a basic mental set for understanding the nature of treatment' (Wells 1997). Clients who enter the therapeutic process but do not engage with the fundamental tenets of the cognitive–behavioural approach are unlikely to engage meaningfully in the therapeutic process. Socialization can occur in a variety of manners. Further to the case formulation, the therapist could provide written material about the approach, as well as examples and demonstrations of the links between cognition and behaviour and emotion.

Intervention

The therapist will draw upon a wide range of therapeutic interventions/ techniques to assist the client to alter the cognitive/behavioural/-

environmental variables that are causing the individual to experience distress or dysfunction. CBT texts for specific disorders have been widely developed and outline these interventions in detail. As sessions progress, the focus might move from the immediate cognitive factors causing the difficulties to more schema-driven concepts. Schemas are the maintaining beliefs from which an individual forms unhelpful cognitions. The process of schematic change in clients is a complex and lengthy therapeutic process, which is beyond the scope of this chapter (Beck & Freeman 1990, Young 1999).

Concluding therapy

Throughout the whole process of therapy, the therapist should aim towards the development of the clients as 'his or her own therapist'. This empowering process, which is ongoing throughout therapy, is designed to assist clients to recognize the triggers that initiated their problems and to develop effective strategies for dealing with them. This focus on 'relapse prevention' is a fundamental component of the therapeutic process.

Session content

Each session follows a core programme. Both client and therapist can add to this collaboratively at the beginning of each session:

1. Recap of previous session and the completion of baseline assessment measures.
2. Agenda setting. The therapist and client both agree on the subjects to be discussed during the session.
3. Feedback from homework. Following each session, the client and therapist agree upon the 'homework' or task that the client will complete between the therapy sessions. These tasks, which can be very varied, are all aimed at gathering further information or reinforcing the content of the therapy sessions. This is viewed as a vital component of the therapeutic process.
4. Implementation of interventions. These can be either cognitive or behavioural in nature, and the reader is referred to the referenced texts for a detailed explanation of their function and practice.
5. Provision of new homework tasks.
6. Feedback. The therapist will always seek feedback from the client on the session and conclude with a synopsis of the session.

It is important to outline the above structure in an introductory text such as this chapter, although it could lead to misunderstandings that the cognitive–behavioural approach is overly rigid and systematized. Beck himself has described effective therapy sessions as akin to a good conversation. In 1990, Beck (cited in Salkovskis 1996) was asked for his vision for the future of CBT. He replied:

> *I hope in 10 years it no longer exists as a school of therapy [he hoped that]...what we call cognitive therapy (conceptualizations and treatment plans informed by research, collaboration and guided*

discovery) will be taken for granted as the basics of all therapy, just as Carl Rogers's principles of warmth, empathy and genuine regard for patients were adopted as necessary basics for all therapy relationships.

Clinical applications

This section will review the utilization of the cognitive–behavioural approach in occupational therapy and physiotherapy practice and outline emerging key themes. The literature reviewed in this section should not be considered as a comprehensive review of the topic area.

Occupational therapy

Cognitive–behavioural approaches within occupational therapy can be traced back as early as 1969 (Braund & Moore 1969). Taylor (1988) firmly grounds the cognitive–behavioural approach within an occupational performance context and highlights the benefits to occupational therapists as follows:

- The approach is based on theories already familiar to occupational therapists and is readily incorporated into practice.
- The methods of assessment utilized are also familiar to therapists.
- The flexibility of the approach is attractive to the client group occupational therapists often work with.
- The approach lends itself to scientific investigation.

It would appear that occupational therapists find the utilization of a cognitive–behavioural approach valuable. Indeed, the approach has been utilized by occupational therapists for a variety of reasons including anxiety management, problem solving (Keable 1997, Meeson 1998, Prior 1998a,b), skill enhancement (Gilbert & Strong 1994), and anger management (O'Neill 1999, Taylor 1988), amongst others.

The use of the cognitive–behavioural approach by occupational therapists has been criticized for blurring of the role of occupational therapists and being symptomatic of a loss of professional identity. Such a stance is perhaps more reflective of early developments within the cognitive–behavioural approach, but is certainly unsustainable within the current collaborative approach outlined above. Figure 10.1 outlines the naturally shared nature of occupational therapy and CBT.

Activities

Activities form an excellent basis for utilizing the cognitive–behavioural approach:

- During an activity, occupational therapists are ideally suited to monitoring the client's thought processes and challenging any unhelpful automatic thoughts that might arise (Gardiner 1997). Such interventions facilitate an in vivo approach to therapy: the therapist can work with patients, in real time, to assist them in challenging their cognitions and behaviour and to help develop positive coping strategies for functioning.

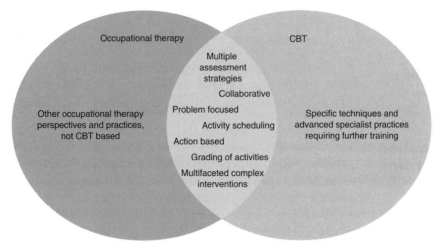

Figure 10.1   *The relationship of cognitive–behavioural therapy (CBT) to occupational therapy*

■ An activity being carried out by both client and therapist can create a safe environment in which a client is able to discuss experiences that he or she is finding distressing or unhelpful. Clinical experience has illustrated how the traditional didactic interview can be too stressful for disturbed clients. The utilization of activity often provides an environment in which clients feel safe and can actively engage in therapeutic interventions to optimal benefit.

Research into these aspects of the cognitive–behavioural approach by occupational therapists is sadly lacking.

Physiotherapy

Research within physiotherapy and mental health remains an underdeveloped area of the profession. The cognitive–behavioural approach has, however, been used within several areas of practice by physiotherapists, which highlights its applicability to the profession.

The main area of practice in which physiotherapists utilize and publish their work on the cognitive–behavioural approach is with clients suffering from pain (Harding & Williams 1998, Hellsing & Linton 1989, Nicholas et al 1992, Taimela et al 2000). Interestingly, it would appear that physiotherapists within these studies have mostly utilized behavioural techniques such as relaxation (Hellsing & Linton 1989, Nicholas et al 1992, Taimela et al 2000). Other techniques utilized include biofeedback (Hellsing & Linton 1989) and more cognitively based techniques such as developing coping strategies (Nicholas et al 1992). It could be that physiotherapists find the practical aspect of behavioural techniques more in keeping with their physical approach to therapy.

Physiotherapy has also developed the use of the cognitive–behavioural approach in a health promotion environment. In a publication entitled *Glad to be yourself*, Payne (1989) outlined a health promotion project, facilitated by a physiotherapist, which focused upon health education, relaxation, stress relief, physical health and disease promotion.

Physiotherapists utilize cognitive–behavioural interventions in a variety of settings. To date, little has been published regarding the use of the approach by physiotherapists working in mental health environments. This is an area that would benefit from further research and dissemination.

Skills required for practising CBT

For occupational therapy and physiotherapy, the utilization of cognitive–behavioural interventions falls within the shared and specialist skill level (Duncan 1999). Undergraduate education within occupational therapy and physiotherapy varies nationally in its coverage of the cognitive–behavioural approach. It is difficult, therefore, to define clearly where each professional will be competent and to develop a list of shared cognitive and behavioural skills. It is vital that professionals recognize the limitations of their knowledge and skill and practise within these, with appropriate supervision. Failure to do so is negligent and a breach of one's ethical code of conduct.

Any professional who wishes to practice cognitive–behavioural therapy as a form of psychotherapy must recognize that this requires a specialist level of skill and should undertake further training and become an accredited practitioner in this area. The British Association of Behavioural and Cognitive Psychotherapy (BABCP) is the recognized interdisciplinary national body of cognitive–behavioural psychotherapy, through which most cognitive–behavioural specialists are accredited.[1]

Summary

- CBT has been found to be effective in the treatment of anxiety, depression and psychotic disorders.

- Cognitive–behavioural interventions can take place in both an individual and group format.

- CBT, as it is understood today, is the result of a series of theoretical and clinical developments and its efficacy is well supported by research.

- Physiotherapists and occupational therapists need to acknowledge situations in which they are, and in which they are not, competent to implement a cognitive–behavioural approach.

- Cognitive–behavioural interventions fall within the shared and specialist skill level of both physiotherapists and occupational therapists. However, there is a need for research to support the effectiveness of this approach when utilized by these professional groups.

---

1   The BABCP can be contacted at www.babcp.org

References

Beck A T, Freeman A (eds) 1990 Cognitive therapy of personality disorders. The Guilford Press, New York

Beck A T, Rush A J, Shaw B F, Emery G 1979 Cognitive therapy of depression. The Guilford Press, New York

Braund J L, Moore R J 1969 The use of behaviour therapy in occupational therapy with psychiatric patients. Australian Occupational Therapy Journal 16(3):27–32

Department of Health 2001 Treatment choice in psychological therapies and counselling. DoH, London

Duncan E A S 1999 Occupational therapy in mental health: it is time to recognise that it has come of age. British Journal of Occupational Therapy 62(11):521–522

Gardiner M 1997 Cognitive approaches. In: Creek J (ed) Occupational therapy and mental health. Churchill Livingstone, Edinburgh

Harding V R, Williams A de C 1998 Activities training: integrating behavioural and cognitive methods with physiotherapy in pain management. Journal of Occupational Rehabilitation 8(1):47–60

Hawton K, Salkovskis P, Kirk J, Clark D M (eds) 1996 Cognitive behaviour therapy for psychiatric problems: a practical guide. Oxford University Press, Oxford

Hellsing A, Linton S 1989 Chronic headache treatment in an occupational setting: a pilot study. Physiotherapy Practice 5:3–8

Keable D 1997 The management of anxiety: a guide for therapists. Churchill Livingstone, Edinburgh

Meeson B 1998 Occupational therapy in community mental health, part 1: intervention choice. British Journal of Occupational Therapy 61(1): 7–12

Meichenbaum D A 1975 A self-instructional approach to stress management: a proposal for stress inoculation training. In: Spielberger C, Sarason I (eds) Stress and anxiety, vol 2. Wiley, New York

Nicholas M K, Wilson P H, Goyen J 1992 A comparison of cognitive–behavioural group treatment and an alternative non-psychological treatment for chronic low back pain. Pain 48(3): 339–347

O'Neill H 1999 Managing anger. Whurr, London

Payne R 1989 Glad to be yourself: a practical course of practical relaxation and health education talks. Physiotherapy 75(1):8–9

Prins J B, Bleijenberg G, Bazelmans E et al 2001 Cognitive behaviour therapy for chronic fatigue syndrome: a multicentre randomised controlled trial. Lancet 357:841–847

Prior S 1998a Determining the effectiveness of a short term anxiety management course. British Journal of Occupational Therapy 61(5): 207–213

Prior S 1998b Anxiety management: results of a follow-up study. British Journal of Occupational Therapy 61(6):284–285

Salkovskis P M (ed) 1996 Frontiers of cognitive therapy. The Guilford Press, New York

Strong J 1998 Incorporating cognitive–behavioural therapy with occupational therapy: a comparative study with patients with low back pain. Journal of Occupational Rehabilitation 8(1):61–71

Taimela S, Takala E, Asklf T et al 2000 Active treatment of chronic neck pain: a prospective randomized intervention. Spine 25(8):1021–1027

Taylor E 1988 Anger intervention. American Journal of Occupational Therapy 42(3):147–155

Weishaar M 1993 Aaron T. Beck. Sage Publications Ltd, London

Wells A 1997 Cognitive therapy for anxiety disorders: a practical manual and conceptual guide. Wiley, Chichester, UK

Young J E 1999 Cognitive therapy for personality disorders: a schema-focused approach (Practitioner's Resource Series). Professional Resource Exchange, New York

11 Stress and mental health

Mick Skelly

Introduction

The purpose of this chapter is to discuss the issue of stress, both causes and effects, in relation to mental health problems. The causes of stress include chemical, physical, social and personal/psychological elements. The neurochemical systems involved include the monoamines, the opiate peptides and in particular cortisol (Walker & Diforio 1997, Wessely et al 1998).

Defining stress

Historically, stress has been defined largely in psychological terms, as a product of perception or cognitive evaluation (Cassidy, 1999). According to Rose (1994), 'the psychophysiological response to challenge' becomes negative when it exceeds the individual's coping resources/abilities. However, a slightly different perspective is offered via research into epidemiology regarding both general health issues and mental health (Wilkinson 1998). This perspective suggests that some factors act directly upon the physiology of the individual and require no psychological mediation (Goldberg & Huxley 1992). Stress can generally be defined as a form of stimulation that places a demand on one or more body systems, thus including a psychological dimension, particularly in higher mammals. If such stimulation acts as a stressor, it will produce (Freund & McGuire 1995, p. 77–82):

- increased blood pressure, increased central and decreased peripheral circulation
- the release of sugars and fats into the circulation
- suppression of the immune system.

Eustress and distress

Stress can be divided into eustress and distress:

- *Eustress* is that level of demand that promotes a level of performance from a dimension of individual potential up to the maximum possible. A track athlete breaking a world record is an obvious example of the peak of eustress in an individual.
- *Distress* is that level of demand that requires a level of performance beyond the potential of the individual. A person trying to lift a weight

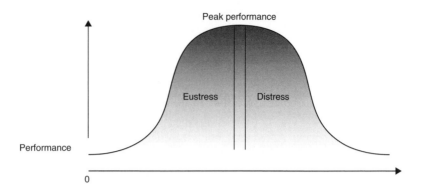

Figure 11.1 *Stress performance curve*

that is too heavy for them, or the same track athlete whose performance deteriorates because of overtraining, are examples of distress.

In the 1970s Hans Selye (Cunningham 1998) produced the stress–performance curve to illustrate this idea (Fig. 11.1). An increasing demand produces an increasing performance until the demand becomes too great and performance decreases. Even a relatively low level of demand has the potential to move the individual from eustress to distress if it continues for long enough.

Both evolutionary theory and ethological studies support the idea that our stress system has evolved to deal with a particular lifestyle (Stevens & Price 1996). This lifestyle was that of our ancestors – the hunter-gatherers – the lifestyle that characterizes almost all of human history. Hunter-gatherers lived in 'aggressively egalitarian' communities, worked a 3–4-hour day and spent the rest of their time on useful handicrafts, playing and socializing (Wilkinson 2000); 99% of life was fairly predictable, with some controlled physical demands due to hunting, and most time was spent in productive, sociable 'leisure' activities. Stress for hunter-gatherers was usually a time-limited crisis that required immediate action, not a lifestyle. Stress for hunter-gatherers took place in the context of a close-knit and supportive community.

Our stress system does not seem well designed to cope with the kinds of stresses that group living now imposes, known as 'social stressors', especially when competition and hierarchialism are predominant group dynamics (Wilkinson 2000). In a sense, this concept is the cornerstone of social interaction/social learning explanations of schizophrenia (Bateson 1973). The general consensus appears to be that the human stress system seems ideally designed to deal with short-term crises that the individual can do something about to resolve swiftly and when the individual is living within an environment that meets his or her 'archetypal needs' (Stevens & Price 1996). What our stress system appears not to be designed to deal with are lots of persistent minor 'hassles' that the individual cannot sort out and which are not entirely under the individual's control because they are intrinsic to the contemporary social environment.

To understand the damage stress can do we need to understand something about the neurochemistry of stress. As the stressful event begins to happen the brain reacts by releasing adrenocorticotrophic stimulating hormone (ACTH), which travels through the circulatory system to the adrenal cortex on the top of each kidney, causing the release of the hormone adrenaline. Another hormone – cortisol – is also released into the circulation and has an effect on every cell in the body (see Fig 11.2). The monoamine system in the brain is affected, increasing the respiratory and heart rates, largely via changes in the levels of noradrenaline. Attention/concentration are affected via dopamine whereas decreasing calmness/increasing anxiety results from serotonin suppression. There is an increased sensitivity to pain, probably mainly via serotonin/noradrenaline–opiate–peptide system interactions. As the brain also functions as a gland (Rose 1999), communicating with the rest of the body via the circulation as well as through the nervous system, these further neurochemical changes will also produce effects down to the cellular level. The body goes into 'fight or flight' mode, with increased sensitivity and increased preparedness for the rapid use of energy, mainly via glycogen (the carbohydrate stores within the body, but there also appears to be a minor release of fatty acids into the circulatory system, although this might have other roles related to coping with short-term stress). Awareness is also increased and reactions are speeded up. With short-term stress, once the stressful situation has been coped with, the physiology of the body rapidly returns to normal.

What causes distress in one person can produce eustress in another. It is all a matter of how life has prepared the individual, physiologically and psychologically, plus the environmental circumstances, particularly the individual's perceived ability to cope and perceived social support. All these factors determine 'hardiness' or vulnerability (Cassidy 1999).

It will be useful at this point to consider first the causes of (di)stress and then some further aspects of the effects of long-term stress.

Causes of stress

Roughly speaking, the causes of stress can be placed into one of four categories:

1. chemical stressors
2. physical stressors
3. social stressors
4. psychological stressors.

Chemical stressors

These include any and all chemicals taken into the body via the digestive or respiratory systems, or via the skin. Some of these chemicals are so toxic to everyone that they can produce massive damage, even death; metals such as lead and mercury fall into this category. Most chemical stressors are more subtle and insidious, undermining one or more body systems or increasing the risk of disease; cigarettes are a

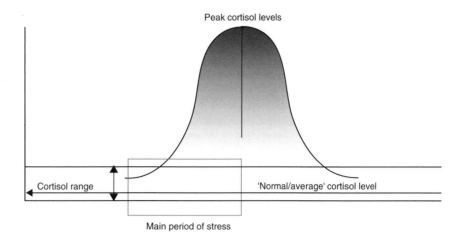

Figure 11.2 *Normal stress response*

prime example of this kind of chemical stressor. The tars in cigarettes massively increase the risk of all cancers and the nicotine causes the heart to beat faster and the arteries to contract, both raising the blood pressure and having a negative effect on the peripheral circulation. This latter effect is thought to be one of the reasons why smoking is highly correlated with low back pain (Deyo & Bass 1989).

Alcohol is a chemical stressor that directly weakens the muscles (including the heart), raises blood pressure and, in combination with nicotine, is thought to contribute to atherosclerosis. Women are more vulnerable to alcohol and there might be gender differences regarding other drugs (Pease & Pease 2001; see also Chapter 20).

Individuals who are sensitive to caffeine might be more likely to suffer from mental health problems. Caffeine is a powerful dopamine agonist that produces a rapid and massive short-term rise in dopamine levels, this might be particularly significant in schizophrenia (Hamera et al 1995). The diathesis–stress paradigm predicts that some individuals will be more susceptible than others to these effects. Throughout life, chemical stressors can affect the individual's ability to cope with other potential causes of distress.

Physical stressors

Physical stressors are those that have a direct physical impact on the individual. For most people, these forms of stress are usually due to 'load' demands placed upon the body in working environments. People have to be fit enough and conditioned specifically to deal with the kinds of physical stressors they face in their everyday working lives and their leisure activities; this is known as fitness for function. It includes endurance and cardiovascular fitness, strength, power, flexibility, and coordination/reaction times. A reasonable level of physical fitness, just making the effort to exercise regularly, is also associated with higher self-esteem, lower risk of mental health problems and greater physical health (Fox et al 2000). See Chapters 7 and 8 for full discussion of the effects of exercise on mental health. In short, a physically fit person feels more able to deal with psychological and social stressors, as well as more capable of dealing with physical stressors (Taylor 2000). This can be explained partly by the effect that regular exercise has on the chemistry of the body. Exercise appears to help to balance out the neurochemistry in a positive way; possibly by centralizing cortisol within its 'normal' range, raising serotonin levels (Chaouloff 1989) and modulating the other two monoamines, dopamine and noradrenaline (Dishman 1994). This is useful, because rises in noradrenaline associated with psychological and social stressors raise the levels of low density lipoprotein (LDL) in the blood and contribute to coronary heart disease (CHD). (Even when on the same fat intake, high-status individuals have higher levels of 'good' cholesterol, high density lipoproteins (HDL) and lower levels of LDL than low-status individuals.) This action of noradrenaline is one of the reasons why long-term stress is probably a contributory factor in CHD.

Social stressors

People usually think of coping with stress as being entirely 'within' a particular individual, regarding the way they think, feel and react to the world around them. In this context, not coping can be regarded as indicating a 'weakness' or inadequacy. People often do not want to admit that their performance, or their physical/mental health, is being affected by stress for this reason. The most important causes of stress are social. 'These social stressors cannot be dealt with without adverse effects on the health and behaviour of the individual' (Sparkes 1997, p. 88).

Social stressors such as differentials in wealth and status can act to suppress the immune system and make people more vulnerable to any disease or medical condition (Wilkinson 2000). Poverty, isolation and physical disability are associated with depression, especially in older people (Eastwood 1994). In the UK, women from social classes 1 and 2 live, on average, 8 years longer than men from social classes 4 and 5. More important than the mortality rates, however, are the morbidity rates. Men from social classes 4 and 5 not only die sooner but are ill and disabled through illhealth far more frequently and for longer than men in other social classes (Gordon et al 2001). Stress has a more devastating effect on male manual workers than any other sector of the population. Young men from this sector of the population are around four times more likely to commit suicide than anyone else. People with a perceived inadequacy of income, one indicator of financially related social stress, are three times more likely to develop low back pain than people who are satisfied with their income (Papageorgiou et al 1997). 'In the developed world, it is not the richest countries which have the best health, but the most egalitarian'. (Wilkinson 1998, p. 3). Wilkinson concludes that more egalitarian societies ensure that the maximum number of people can live safe, healthy lives.

Rose (1999) cites work on animal studies that suggests that environmental stressors have an impact that is more important or decisive than genetics in determining neural structure, the neurophysiology of the individual, and the individual's ability to function in any dimension. Long-term stress appears to profoundly affect the potential for intelligence and, therefore, for emotional self-control and intelligent behaviour (Aldridge 2001). It might also affect physical capabilities through effects on the control of movement by the nervous system. These 'distress simplified' nervous systems are more vulnerable to injury caused by trauma, chemical neurotoxins such as alcohol and disease, and 'normal' changes due to ageing (Eastwood 1994). This lends some support to a neurodevelopmental model of schizophrenia (Bentall 1999).

Psychological stressors

These are often regarded as related to the personality of the individual, i.e. some types of personalities are more likely to suffer from stress than others. Here personality is defined as (Maddi 1989, p. 8):

> *A stable set of tendencies and characteristics that determine those commonalities and differences in people's psychological behaviour (thoughts, feelings, and actions) that have continuity in time and that may not be easily understood as the sole result of the social and biological pressures of the moment.*

Using this definition, it can be seen that personality is linked to beliefs about the way the world really is, what type of person the individual believes him- or herself to be and beliefs about how other people should behave or are behaving. Beliefs are largely determined by the conceptual currency of a particular culture plus the individual's experience of the reality of life (the 'phenomic' world). Personality traits are not consistent because they can be reduced or exacerbated by environmental factors (Cassidy 1999). Even the most exacting personality tests have poor behavioural predictive validity, and behaviour is more likely to be driven by contingency than by trait (Dawes 1994). Gender might also influence perception and behaviour (Pease & Pease 2001).

Individuals have a tendency to hold 'irrational beliefs' regarding relationships between themselves and others, which help to determine their concept of themselves. These so-called irrational beliefs are usually thought to be logical constructs based upon social and/or familial 'myths' about the world and the way the world works (Cunningham 1998). People experiencing stress as a result of a dissonance between such a 'myth', their experience of the world and/or their fundamental psychological needs are described as being in a 'double bind' (Sue et al 1997). This interpretation of the meaning of the behaviour of others helps to create both our concept of the world and our concept of our self (Smail 1984).

A key factor to acknowledge, accept and take responsibility for dealing with, is manipulation. It is an inevitable fact of the human condition that we manipulate others and that others manipulate us.

This is often done as a 'transaction', with the other person trying to play either an obviously dominating (parental) role or being more subtly manipulative in the 'child' role (Berne 1968, see Fig. 11.3). Transactional analysis (TA), is the concept that all human interactions can be conceptualized as transactions in which individuals take on parental, adult, or child roles. Parent–child interactions emphasize the authority of the former and the dependence of the latter with the transaction being related to power differentials and inequality. Power can be obtained via manipulation either from an authoritarian or a dependent stance. The person in the dependent or child-like role has the options of 'good' or 'recalcitrant' child as a means of manipulating the parent into being 'nurturing' or 'critical'. Although there may be a need to adopt a parent or child role at times, TA holds that good relationships are generally characterized by equal and honest adult-to-adult transactions.

In transactional analysis, the idea is that the ideal quality of communication, for most of the time, is adult-to-adult (Berne 1968.) This is a useful model from which to generate a strategy for dealing with interpersonal stress.

Another, less scientific but older model, of Chinese origin, is the Yin/Yang model. In this model, the individual observes to see if the other person is being hard and aggressive (Yang) or soft and yielding (Yin) towards them. The Chinese idea is that the first person complements the second person, for example by being 'soft'/Yin when the other person is being 'hard'/Yang. This originally physical idea becomes a metaphor for all human interactions.

These are all useful perspectives for the individual to actively interpret another's behaviour in order to respond in the most appropriate way – the best way for them and, hopefully, for the other person too. They are also useful structures for 'self-consciousness' plus understanding the situation to enable informed behaviour. This is referred to as 'right awareness' in the Buddhist 'eight-fold path', perhaps one of the earliest cognitive–behavioural manifestos! (DeSilva 1984).

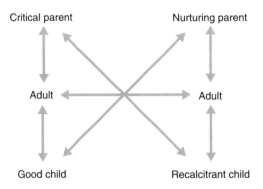

Figure 11.3
Transactional analysis (TA)

A further facet of psychological stress comprises the beliefs that the individual has learned to have about themselves. These are often learnt by listening to the opinions of others (plus by interpreting/misinterpreting the meanings of the behaviour of others), particularly of 'significant others', the most significant of which are parents, other close family and close friends. These 'things' we come to know about ourselves might or might not conform to what we are actually like. People's beliefs about themselves and what they are actually doing to themselves and/or others might or might not have anything to do with their habitual behaviours (Laing 1967). These individual beliefs are constructed within the context of larger stories, or 'meta-narratives', about the 'self' in the world, such as 'the myth of normality' (Smail 1984). In actuality, it might be that much of people's behaviour tends to be contingent, designed to get them through an immediate situation with the least effort, least physical risk or least risk of social criticism and/or attract some kind of social reward at the same time if at all possible (Crooks & Stein 1991).

As a rule, individuals who have negative beliefs regarding themselves, their abilities and the world in general, tend to be the least likely to cope with anything and the most likely to succumb to stress (Gatchel 1996). It is possible that these beliefs are influenced by an altered neurophysiology produced by long-term stress. New information and new skills, a different way of thinking and feeling about things, especially those that put the individual more in control of his or her life, can act as a form of environmental change. The key issues appear to be:

- *Control*: the individual's sense that he or she has control over the environment and over his or her life – that choices and responsibilities exist, particularly the responsibility to face the consequences of whatever choices the individual has made.
- *Safety*: the sense that the environment, although challenging, is a safe one in which to take risks and to make the occasional mistake, because things always turn out well in the end. An environment that is full of supportive social contacts – a social environment that also has clear boundaries, as much for the 'social space' as for the physical space.
- *Stimulation*: the sense that the environment is full of interesting potential, things to investigate and 'play' with or work on. Things that challenge the individual and which, if they choose, will stretch the person to the (safe) limit. An environment where there are individuals who will be challenging and who will also be supportive in helping each other to develop their potential to the full, if that is what each person chooses.

Managing stress

Using ideas from this chapter, it should now be possible to begin to create a general, individualized, plan for dealing with the stressors that are likely to undermine mental health. The individual should be informed and supported in his or her choices (not led or pushed) and should be in control of the plan and of the timescale, and supported in realizing it. It might be useful for the individual to ask the following questions:

- What are the sources of stress in my life? In particular what are the sources of social stress?
- What are the effects of stress upon my performance, both at work and in the rest of my life?
- What are the effects of stress on my health?
- What are the areas in my life where I need to make changes?
- What do these changes need to be? (What behavioural changes do I need to make at home and at work? What structural changes need to be made at work and at home?)
- Who do I need to help me through these changes?
- What further knowledge will I need?
- What skills am I likely to need?

Ten possible stress management areas emerging from this process are:

1. Strategy for financial security.
2. Strategy for social status.
3. Diet plan – general dietary strategy (see Holford & Cass 2001, Holford & Pfeiffer 1996, Walford & Walford 1994).
4. Physical well-being via regular exercise for:
   - muscular endurance/cardiovascular fitness
   - strength with muscular endurance
   - flexibility with muscle balance and avoiding hypermobility
   - coordination/reaction times.
5. Structural/physical/safety factors at work.
6. Interpersonal factors at work:
   - team working: effectiveness and efficiency
   - assertiveness and individual interactions.
7. Physical home environment.
8. Interpersonal home environment: appropriate support rather than more stress.
9. Intellectually challenging hobbies/activities.
10. Engaging in strategies for relaxation (see Payne (2000) for instructions on relaxation techniques).

Conclusions

All mental health problems are strongly influenced, if not caused, by 'distress'. Stressors come in four major forms or dimensions, the most important of which, in relation to mental health, appear to be social stressors (Goldberg & Huxley 1992). The other dimensions of stress are chemical, physical and psychological. In actuality, it is most likely that factors from all four dimensions will be at work on the individual.

From the neurochemical perspective, in particular, mental health problems do not conform to discrete diagnostic categories but exist on neurochemical and neural constellation continua and are likely to be responsive to variations on a single theme of intervention for this reason. This concept has explanatory power in terms of the apparent general effectiveness of cognitive–behavioural approaches (Roth & Fonagy 1996) and provides a theoretical basis for the use of 'stress management programmes', including exercise and relaxation, in the care pathways for most, if not all, individuals with mental health problems.

This ensures a fundamental role for physiotherapists and occupational therapists in the overall management of mental health problems. It also means a fundamental need for therapists to consider the impact that stress, from any source, is having upon the people they work with in institutional or community settings.

Summary

- Stress can generally be defined as a form of stimulation that places a demand on one or more body systems. It thus includes a psychological dimension, particularly in higher mammals.

- Stress can be divided into eustress and distress.

- Both evolutionary theory and ethological studies support the idea that our stress system has evolved to deal with a particular lifestyle.

- Stress can be triggered by chemical, physical, social and psychological stressors.

- All mental health problems are strongly influenced, if not caused, by 'distress'.

- The neurochemical changes and psychosocial triggers associated with stress provide a theoretical basis for the use of exercise and relaxation, in the care pathways for most, if not all, individuals with mental health problems.

References

Aldridge S 2001 Seeing red and feeling blue. A new understanding of mood and emotion, 1st edn. Arrow Books, The Random House Group Ltd, London

Bateson G 1973 Steps to an ecology of mind. Paladin, Frogmore, St Albans, p 173–198, 242–249

Bentall J 1999 Why there will never be a convincing theory of schizophrenia. In: Rose N (ed) From brains to consciousness. Penguin, Harmondsworth, UK

Berne E 1968 Games people play. The psychology of human relationships. Penguin, Harmondsworth, UK

Cassidy T 1999 Stress, cognition and health, 1st edn. Routledge, London

Chaouloff F 1989 Physical exercise and brain monoamines: a review. Acta Physiologica Scandinavica 137:1–13

Crooks R L, Stein J 1991 Psychology, science, behaviour, and life, 2nd edn. Harcourt Brace Jovanovich, Holt, Rinehart and Winston, Orlando

Cunningham J B 1998 The stress management source book: everything you need to know. Lowell House Extension Press, NTC/ Contemporary Publishing Group, Lincolnwood, Illinois

Dawes R M 1994 House of cards. Psychology and psychotherapy built on myth. Free Press, a division of Simon and Schuster, New York

DeSilva P 1984 Buddhism and behaviour modification. Behaviour Research Therapy 22(6):661–678

Deyo R A, Bass J E 1989 Lifestyle and low-back pain – the influence of smoking and obesity. Spine 14(5):501–506

Dishman R K (ed) 1994 Advances in exercise adherence, 1st edn. Human Kinetics, Champaign, IL

Eastwood R 1994 Epidemiology in the study of functional psychiatric disorders of the elderly. In: Chiu E, Ames D (eds) Functional psychiatric disorders of the elderly. Cambridge University Press, Cambridge, p 31–44

Fox K R, Boutcher S H, Faulkner G E, Biddle S J H 2000 The case of exercise in the promotion mental health and psychological well-being. In: Biddle S J H, Fox K R, Boutcher S H (eds) Physical activity and psychological well-being. Routledge, London

Freund P E S, McGuire M B 1995 Health, illness, and the social body. A critical sociology, 2nd edn. Prentice Hall, Englewood Cliffs, New Jersey, p 71–141

Gatchel R J 1996 The biopsychosocial model. In: Gatchel R J, Turk D C (eds) Psychological approaches to pain management. A practitioners handbook. Guilford Press, New York, p 33–52

Goldberg D, Huxley P 1992 Common mental disorders. A bio-social model. Routledge, London, p 83–113

Gordon D, Adelman L, Ashworth K et al 2001 Poverty and social exclusion in Britain. Joseph Rowntree Foundation, York

Hamera E, Schneider J K, DeViney S 1995 Alcohol, cannabis, nicotine and caffeine use and symptom distress in schizophrenia. Journal of Nervous and Mental Disease 183(9):559–565

Holford P, Cass H 2001 Natural highs. Piatkus, London

Holford P, Pfeiffer C 1996 Mental health and illness. The nutrition connection. Ion Press, London

Laing R D 1967 The obvious. In: Cooper D (ed) The dialectics of liberation. Pelican, London

Maddi S R 1989. Personality theories. A comparative analysis, 5th edn. Brooks/Cole, Pacific Grove, California, p 8

Papageorgiou A C, Macfarlane G J, Thomas E et al 1997 Psychosocial factors in the workplace – do they predict new episodes of low back pain? Evidence from the South Manchester back pain study. Spine 22(10):1137–1142

Parker G 1992 Counting care: numbers and types of informal carers. In: Twigg J (ed) Carers research and practice. HMSO, London, p 6–29

Payne R 2000 Relaxation techniques, 2nd edn. Churchill Livingstone, Edinburgh

Pease A, Pease B 2001 Why men don't listen and women can't read maps. Orion Books, London

Rose N D B (ed) 1994 Essential psychiatry. Blackwell Scientific Publications, Oxford

Rose S (ed) 1999 From brains to consciousness? Essays on the new sciences of the mind, 1st edn. Penguin, Harmondsworth, UK, p 1–52

Roth A, Fonagy P 1996 What works for whom? A critical review of psychotherapy research. Guilford Press, New York

Smail D 1984 Illusion and reality. The meaning of anxiety, 1st edn. Dent & Sons Ltd, London

Sparkes A C 1997 Reflections on the socially constructed physical self. In: Fox K R (ed) The physical self from motivation to well-being. Human Kinetics, Champaign, IL, p 111–139

Stevens A, Price J 1996 Evolutionary psychiatry. A new beginning. Routledge, London

Sue D, Sue E, Sue S 1997 Understanding abnormal behaviour, 5th edn. Houghton Mifflin, Boston, New York

Taylor A H 2000 Physical activity, anxiety and stress. In: Biddle S J H, Fox K R, Boutcher S H (eds) Physical activity and psychological well-being. Routledge, London

Walford R L, Walford L 1994 The anti-aging plan. Strategies and recipes for extending your healthy years. Four Walls Eight Windows/Turnaround, London

Walker E F, Diforio D 1997 Schizophrenia: a neural diasthesis-stress model. Psychological Review 104(4):667–685

Wessely S, Hotopf M, Sharpe M 1998 Chronic fatigue and its syndromes, 1st edn. Oxford University Press, Oxford, p 250–276

Wilkinson R G 1998 Unhealthy societies. The afflictions of inequality, 1st edn. Routledge, London, p 73–109, 175–192

Wilkinson R G 2000 Mind the gap. Published in the series 'Darwinism Today'. Wiedenfeldt and Nicholson, London

Further reading

Goffman E 1961 Asylums. Doubleday, Garden City, NY

Newnes C, Holmes G, Dunn C 1999 This is madness: a critical look at psychiatry and the future of mental health services. PCCS Books Ltd, Ross-on-Wye, Herefordshire

Newnes C, Holmes G, Dunn C 2001 This is madness: too critical perspectives on mental health services. PCCS Books Ltd, Ross-on-Wye, Herefordshire

Smail D 2001 The nature of unhappiness. Robinson, an imprint of Constable and Robinson, London

12 Chronic pain

Derek Jones and Denis Martin

Introduction

Therapists are involved in the care of people with chronic pain in all clinical settings, including mental health. Successful care of the person with chronic pain depends on the establishment of a two-way working relationship between the patient and therapist to promote active self-management. Thus the therapist must have a sympathetic understanding of the effects of chronic pain on the individual and, within this context, the role of his or her social environment. If the therapist's knowledge, attitudes and beliefs about chronic pain are not appropriate then successful management is at risk. It is hoped that this chapter will help the reader by presenting an overview of current thinking about pain to stimulate discussion of how the knowledge can translate into better practice. Readers should note that the focus of this chapter is on chronic non-malignant pain.

Definitions of pain

Although its very definition can spark heated debate among eminent scientists and clinicians who have devoted many years to its study, most agree that pain is multidimensional and that it is fundamentally a personal experience. This recognition is often seen as making the treatment, management and assessment of pain difficult. A more realistic view is that awareness of its multidimensionality and fundamental subjectivity makes possible its appropriate treatment/management and assessment.

The International Association for the Study of Pain (Merskey & Bogduk 1994, p. 210) has defined pain as:

> *An unpleasant sensory and emotional experience associated with actual or potential tissue damage, or described in terms of such damage.*

Definitions of what constitutes *chronic* pain vary, but its key features are that it persists beyond the normal time of healing and can be constant or intermittent. The timescale beyond which acute pain becomes chronic is open to debate. Some authors classify pain lasting more than 3 months as chronic; others choose 6 months. To an extent, these cut-off points are arbitrary as, for any one individual, the point at which pain begins to have long-term consequences will vary depending on the interaction of biological, psychological and social factors. Chronic pain is often associated with chronic conditions such as joint disease, where there is identifiable tissue damage. However, it is now recognized that pain mechanisms and neural pathways can undergo changes in the way they function and that chronic pain can also be experienced in the absence of tissue damage.

Before outlining the assessment and management of chronic pain, it is useful to look at the way in which pain has traditionally been viewed, as vestiges of this linger on in both professionals and patients.

Historical perspective

In the not too distant past, and in thankfully shrinking pockets of the present, pain has been viewed as a direct linear response to tissue damage – an idea that can be traced back to René Descartes (Fig. 12.1).

Although compact, this simplistic thinking in terms of a one-to-one relationship between pain and tissue damage has failed clinicians and pain sufferers alike. The complex relationship between tissue damage and the pain experience might be something you have encountered. You might recollect the toothache that kept you awake all night only to 'disappear' during a busy day at work and then reappear in the evening. Now, clearly the pathology underlying the toothache has not gone away, so how do we explain the disappearance of the pain? Underlying current thinking about pain is the recognition that there is not always a direct correlation between tissue damage and the pain experienced. People with apparently horrendous injuries can feel no or little pain and people with no apparent tissue damage can be in excruciating agony. Increasing understanding of the neural mechanisms underlying pain provides an explanation for this strange occurrence.

Current thinking

Consider the following statement written by Hanson & Gerber (1990, p 57):

The foundation for self-management is the biopsychosocial model of pain. We suggest that more effective control over chronic pain

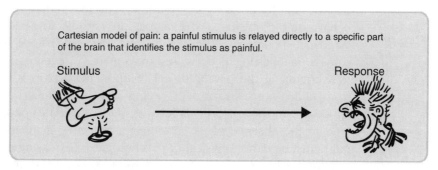

Cartesian model of pain: a painful stimulus is relayed directly to a specific part of the brain that identifies the stimulus as painful.

Stimulus   Response

Figure 12.1 *Cartesian model of pain.*

requires a thorough and accurate understanding of the nature of pain. Dualistic notions that consider pain as either entirely physical or psychological must be abandoned. All pain involves a combination of biological or physiological factors, psychological factors (mental, emotional and behavioural) and social–environmental factors.

These factors will now be explored in more detail.

Biological factors

Pain clearly has sensory discriminative components, and this involves the transmission of signals through pathways in the nervous system. In recent years there have been major advances in the understanding of the biological dimensions of pain. Much work has been done to describe psychoneurobiological mechanisms to link stress with chronic pain. The role of cortisol has been given prominence in this mechanism (Van Houdenhove 2000). By way of careful neurophysiological and neuroanatomical research, it is possible to map out relatively well-defined pathways by which pain perception can occur and through which the effects of pain can be mediated (Fields 1999, Treede et al 1999). The role of the structures within the spinal cord has been clearly and cleverly described and functional nuclear magnetic resonance imaging can now demonstrate activity in different anatomical and functional areas of the brain as the person is thought to be experiencing pain (Casey & Bushnell 2000).

Philosophically, the Cartesian mind–body duality is no longer popular, and research has made great strides in closing the gap in favour of a more integrated explanation. The Neuromatrix Theory has been developed to bring together the multitude of influences in pain (Melzack 1999). This comprehensive model builds on the gate control theory and is more inclusive of neuroplasticity and environmental factors. The phenomenon of pain, however, extends beyond a full neurophysiological explanation. Pain is inextricably linked with psychological theories of the mind, changes in behaviour and cognitive processing.

Psychological factors

Chronic pain is more than a sensation. It is a perception that has an emotional overlay. Psychological factors are now prominent in discussions of chronic pain and they form a focus for many forms of intervention. The understanding of these components takes place within a cognitive–behavioural framework and chronic pain has been associated with behavioural problems. For example, in chronic low-back pain, fear-avoidance behaviour describes an excessive, misplaced fear of tissue damage manifesting as decreased movement (Vlaeyen & Linton 2000).

Recognizing the psychological component of pain is very different from falling into the trap of seeing any unexplained pain as 'psychogenic'. In the past, this label was often applied to people who had pain in the absence of tissue damage, reflecting a dualistic view that pain must be either physical or psychological. Increasing understanding of neural mechanisms has led to the rejection of this term and it should be noted that 'psychogenic pain' is not included in DSM IV (McCaffery & Pasero 1999). In some cases, chronic pain *can* be indicative of psychopathology. However, diagnostic labels with clearly defined criteria (such as hypochondriasis) exist to cover such circumstances.

Social/ environmental factors

Of course the individual with chronic pain does not exist within a vacuum. The pain experience takes place within a social context and this social context influences the individual's understanding of pain. The pain experience is framed within a cultural context and affected by the wider society in terms of the response of health, welfare and employment services (Bendelow & Williams 1995). It has been well documented that social and economic inequalities are linked with poor health in general and chronic pain is no exception (Elliott et al 1999). Chronic pain has been discussed as '. . . a phenomenon of industrialised societies . . .' and, as such, treatment must be targeted at '. . . the social structure and physical environment in which the individual works and plays' (Loeser 2000). The importance of socioeconomic factors has been overlooked in many health problems and, again, chronic pain is no exception. Whether this is by neglect or design is obvious to some or a point for long debate for others. Interestingly, in recognition of the importance of social factors, some commentators go so far as to discuss pain in terms of a biosocial model.

Because it is clear that a biomedical explanation is insufficient to explain chronic pain, the biopsychosocial model has gained acceptance as a framework for viewing the multidimensional nature of pain. As a result, issues of function and quality of life have gained prominence in chronic pain – one of the reasons why occupational therapists and physiotherapists are seen to be key agents of rehabilitation.

Assessment of pain and its effects

Optimum management of the person suffering from pain depends on knowing as much as is necessary about the person and the condition – assessment of pain and its effects. The recent Clinical Standards Advisory Group report *Services for patients with pain* (CSAG 1999) recommends the 'regular use of assessment and outcome tools' in managing chronic pain. In response to this report, the Pain Management Programmes Special Interest Group of the Pain Society has attempted to establish a consensus on assessment/outcome measures (Johnson 2001).

Unfortunately for the person with chronic pain, attempts at systematic assessment of pain and its effects are usually scant and chaotic, when they happen at all. Clinicians from all disciplines tend to rely on their expert opinion when deciding on the extent or nature of pain. In doing so there is a fairly systematic underestimation of patients' distress. A more systematic approach using valid, reliable and practical measurement tools might help.

The most common measurement tool is the simple visual analogue scale (VAS) marked with such descriptors as 'no pain' at one end and 'worst pain possible' at the other. The scale is attractive because it is relatively easy to score and has been credited, albeit arguably, as showing validity and reliability. Validity and reliability have been tested mainly under controlled experimental conditions. In clinical assessment, however, the apparent simplicity of the VAS has been shown to mask a complex amount and type of information contained within the score obtained (Williams et al 2000). Because this complex information is not easily extracted from the VAS score in clinical practice, multidimensional assessment is advocated. The number of dimensions of chronic pain and their definition is arguable but probably not far off the mark is the suggestion that chronic pain has seven dimensions (Morley et al 1999) described in Box 12.1.

Each of the seven dimensions can be measured to some extent. Some measures have been developed by specific professions and relate to their role, other measures are more generic. Regardless of the type of measure used, it should have demonstrated reliability and validity and it should be practical within the given clinical context. There is a received wisdom that measurement is often driven by the available tools rather than the other way about. Stannard (2001) has reminded us that when the only tool you have is a hammer everything can look nail shaped. Patients should not be put through batteries of assessments just for the sake of collecting data. The exercise must have a purpose: outcome measure, diagnosis, treatment/referral allocation. An enlightened case for good practice is that assessment should measure what is important not just what is possible.

A primary consideration in assessment of pain and its effects, especially in the clinical situation, is the need to gather complex information through parsimonious measurement. Worthy of special mention within this context is the patient-generated index (Ruta et al 1994). This has a special appeal in that it combines practicality with a subtle statistical sophistication. The patient indicates aspects of the condition that he or she would like to improve and these are then listed, weighted for impor-

Box 12.1

Seven dimensions of chronic pain (Morley et al 1999)

1. Pain experience: described by subjective reports of intensity and unpleasantness.
2. Mood/affect, e.g. depression.
3. Cognitive coping strategies: both negative and positive.
4. Biological activity and physical capacity.
5. Activity level and behaviour: these can signal the presence of pain.
6. Social role functioning, e.g. the effect on relationships at work and at home.
7. Use of healthcare systems, e.g. number of medical consultations.

tance and combined to give an overall score. The overall score can be used to group findings with other patients for statistical analysis.

With measurements of pain and its effects, the information will always be grey as opposed to black and white. Thus, the user of the information must be aware of its limitations and must use it appropriately. For the clinician, this requires using the information in conjunction with clinical experience and expert judgement. In other words, to be of real value the information needs intelligent processing. For a more detailed exploration of assessment of pain and its effects, the reader is referred to Peat (2000) and Watson & Parker (2000).

Pain management

Pain management takes place in a number different contexts: it can take place in inpatient, outpatient or community settings; it can be offered by individual professionals with relevant knowledge and expertise, or by multi- or interdisciplinary teams working in specialist programmes.

The IASP (1994) has suggested a core curriculum for professionals involved in pain management and has listed the roles of occupational therapy and physiotherapy (Table 12.1). It is important to note that there is a powerful ongoing lobby to replace the passive components of physiotherapy with active rehabilitation management strategies incorporating aspects of cognitive–behavioural therapy. Evidence supports a hands-off approach, not a hands-on or physical-modality based intervention. As discussed below, the delineation between the two professions is blurred: this is a conceptual problem for the professions rather than a practical problem for the patients. For more information on pain management see the list of further reading at the end of the chapter.

The next section of this chapter focuses on what goes on in pain management programmes; therapists working in other contexts need to adapt the principles to suit their setting.

Pain management programmes

Increasingly the focus of pain management is the interdisciplinary pain management programme. Occupational and physiotherapists have been identified as core members of the pain management team (Pain Society 1997). Although these programmes are still relatively limited in terms of availability their efficacy is well supported by research.

Cognitive–behavioural therapy

A cognitive–behavioural approach underpins the way in which pain management programmes operate. This reflects the understanding that the pain experience is mediated as much as by what people feel and believe about their pain as by the nature of biological response to tissue damage. This approach is based on the assumption that:

■ People do not passively react to sensory data – they process it actively.
■ Thoughts influence emotions and physiological responses and act as an impetus to behaviour – these thoughts are, in turn, influenced by environmental factors.

Table 12.1 *Roles of occupational therapy and physical therapy (IASP 1994)*

Therapy	Assessment	Aims	Intervention strategies
Occupational therapy	Assessment of the impact of pain on occupational performance in the areas of: ■ self-care ■ paid and unpaid work ■ interests and leisure pursuits, customary habits and routine ■ family relationships ■ psychosocial and environmental factors aggravating pain in the home and workplace	■ To increase self-esteem ■ To restore self efficacy ■ To promote optimal occupational function despite pain	These might include: ■ assistive devices and adaptive equipment, purposeful and productive occupations/activities ■ vocational rehabilitation or work hardening to improve endurance and work skills and re-establish roles, habits and routines of everyday life ■ education about pain ■ supportive individual, family or group counselling (utilized as needed)
Physiotherapy	Assessment of factors that contribute to pain, the pain–activity cycle and overall function, including: ■ primary and secondary chemical factors (infection/inflammation) ■ biomechanical factors (stress/strain) ■ behavioural factors	■ To modify the effect of primary and secondary contributors to pain ■ To promote tissue healing ■ To reduce the factors that might lead to the recurrence of pain and dysfunction	These might include: ■ education ■ exercise ■ manual therapy ■ movement facilitation techniques ■ application of electro-/physical agents based on thermal/ mechanical/electrical/ phototherapeutic modalities

- Behaviour is influenced by individual and environmental factors.
- Individuals can learn more adaptive ways of thinking, feeling and behaving.
- Individuals should be active collaborative agents in bringing about change (Turk & Meichenbaum 1994).

This approach has been broadly supported by research, although it is true to say that which part of programmes work for which patients is still unclear (Guzman et al 2001, Morley et al 1999).

Occupational therapists are likely to have been introduced to cognitive–behavioural therapy (CBT) as part of their undergraduate programme, and to have observed it in practice during fieldwork in mental health. Increasingly, physiotherapy students are also being given grounding in CBT (see Chapter 10). Although therapists will therefore be able to use this approach, it is important that they practise within the limits of their competency. Support and supervision can be obtained from therapists who have gained an additional qualification in cognitive-behavioural therapy, or from clinical psychologists.

Intervention strategies

Pain management programmes typically use a set of key interventions. The Pain Society (1997) has recommended the following elements be included in accredited pain management programmes:

- physical reconditioning
- posture and body mechanics training
- applied relaxation techniques
- information and education about pain and pain management
- medication review and advice
- psychological assessment and intervention
- gradual return to activities of daily living.

The interdisciplinary nature of programmes means that, in well-established and experienced teams, there might be a great deal of role overlap between team members. Such teams must avoid interprofessional 'turf wars' over who should do what, while at the same time recognizing the value of the diverse perspectives provided by professionals from different backgrounds. Ultimately, the important point is that the professional delivering the service is appropriately skilled and qualified. In addition, all professionals can gain from regular support and supervision.

Conclusion

Pain is a multidimensional phenomenon and the management of chronic pain is increasingly focused on recognizing the psychosocial dimension. Occupational therapists and physiotherapists need to understand the neural mechanisms underlying the pain experience. Note should be taken of the relevant professional specialist interest groups (National Occupational Therapy Pain Association and Physiotherapy Pain Association) and the guidelines they have produced for therapists working in this area.

Summary

- The focus of this chapter is on chronic non-malignant pain.

- Occupational therapists and physiotherapists work with patients with chronic pain in different clinical settings, including mental health.

- Pain can be defined as an unpleasant sensory and emotional experience associated with actual or potential tissue damage, or described in terms of such damage.

- Pain is multidimensional and fundamentally a personal experience.

- Current thinking about pain suggests that there is not always a direct correlation between tissue damage and the pain experienced.

- Pain management programmes are interdisciplinary in nature and are based on set recommendations acknowledged by the Pain Society.

- Psychosocial dimensions are recognized as being key determinants in the management of chronic pain.

References

Bendelow W A, Williams S J 1995 Transcending the dualisms: towards a sociology of pain. Sociology of Health and Illness 17(2):139–165

Casey K L, Bushnell M C (eds) 2000 Pain imaging progress in pain research and management (18). IASP Press, Seattle, WA

CSAG 1999 Services for patients with pain. The Stationery Office, London

Elliott A M, Smith B H, Penny K I et al 1999 The epidemiology of chronic pain in the community. Lancet 354(9186):1248–1252

Fields H L 1999 Pain: an unpleasant topic. Pain suppl 6:S61–S69.

Guzman J, Esmail R, Karjalainen K et al 2001 Multidisciplinary rehabilitation for chronic low back pain: a systematic review. British Medical Journal 322:1511–1516

Hanson R W, Gerber K E 1990 Coping with chronic pain. Guilford Press, New York

IASP ad hoc sub-committee for occupational therapy and physical therapy curriculum 1994 Pain curriculum for students in occupational therapy or physical therapy. IASP Newsletter Nov/Dec:3–8

Johnson T 2001 Pain management programmes outcome consensus meeting. The Pain Society Newsletter 1(13):8

Loeser J D 2000 The future: will pain be abolished or just pain management specialists? Clinical Updates: International Association for the Study of Pain 8(6):1–4

McCaffery M, Pasero C 1999 Pain: clinical manual, 2nd edn. Mosby, St Louis

Melzack R 1999 From the gate to the matrix. Pain Suppl 6:S121–S126.

Merskey H, Bogduk N (eds) 1994 Classification of chronic pain: descriptions of chronic pain syndromes and definitions of pain terms, 2nd edn. IASP Press, Seattle, WA

Morley S, Eccleston C, Williams A 1999 Systematic review and meta-analysis of randomized controlled trials of cognitive behaviour therapy and behaviour therapy for chronic pain in adults, excluding headache. Pain 80(1,2): 1–14.

Pain Society 1997 Desirable criteria for pain management programmes. Pain Society, London

Peat G 2000 Evaluation of outcome. In: Main C, Spanswick C S (eds) Pain management: an interdisciplinary approach. Churchill Livingstone, Edinburgh

Ruta D A, Garrat A M, Leng M et al 1994 A new approach to the measurement of quality of life:

the patient generated index. Medical Care 32(11): 1109–1126

Stannard C 2001 Editorial. The Pain Society Newsletter 1(13)

Treede R-D, Kenshalo D R, Gracely R H, Jones A K P 1999 The cortical representation of pain. Pain 79 (2–3):105–111

Turk D C, Meichenbaum D 1994 A cognitive—behavioural approach to pain management. In: Wall P D, Melzack R (eds) Textbook of pain, 3rd edn. Churchill Livingstone, Edinburgh

Van Houdenhove B 2000 Psychosocial stress and chronic pain. European Journal of Pain 4(3):225–228

Vlaeyen J W S, Linton S J 2000 Fear-avoidance and its consequences in chronic musculoskeletal pain: a state of the art. Pain 85(3):317–332

Watson P, Parker H 2000 Assessment of pain, disability and physical function in pain management. In: Main C, Spanswick C S (eds) Pain management: an interdisciplinary approach. Churchill Livingstone, Edinburgh

Williams A, Davies H, Chadbury Y 2000 Simple pain rating scales hide complex idiosyncratic meanings. Pain 85(3):457–463

Further reading

Gifford L (ed) 1998 Topical issues in pain. Vol 1. Whiplash: science and management. Fear avoidance beliefs and behaviour. CNS Press, Falmouth

Gifford L (ed) 2000 Topical issues in pain. Vol 2. Biopsychosocial assessment and management. Relationships and pain. CNS Press, Falmouth

Melzack R, Wall P D 1983 The challenge of pain. Penguin, London

O'Hara P 1996 Pain management for health professionals. Chapman Hall, London

Strong J 1996 Chronic pain: the occupational therapists perspective. Churchill Livingstone, Edinburgh

Wells P E, Frampton V, Bowscher D 1994 Pain management by physiotherapy, 2nd edn. Butterworth Heinemann, Oxford

Helpful websites

INPUT Pain Management Unit, St Thomas' Hospital, London, UK

http://www.inputpainunit.org/index.html

Physiotherapy Pain Association
http://www.ppaonline.co.uk

The International Association for the Study of Pain
http://www.iasp-pain.org

The Oxford Pain Internet Site
http://www.jr2.ox.ac.uk/bandolier/painres/PRintro.html

The Pain Society (The British and Irish Chapter of the IASP)
http://www.painsociety.org

Useful addresses

National Occupational Therapy Pain Association
Sue Tambor (Membership Secretary), Occupational Therapist, Pain Management Programme, Tom Rudd Unit, Moorgreen Hospital, Botley Road, Southampton SO30 3JB

Physiotherapy Pain Association
Sue Mickleburgh (Membership Secretary), 9 Lowen Way, Threemilestone, Truro, Cornwall TR3 6TR

13 Aggression and mental disorder

Emma Williams

Introduction

The focus of this chapter is on understanding and managing aggressive behaviour in mental health settings. There are many misconceptions regarding the link between aggression and mental disorder. The media has reinforced popular beliefs that people with a mental disorder are violent and dangerous. In reality, few acts of extreme violence are committed by this population. There are approximately 600–700 homicides in England and Wales per year, of these less than 20 are committed by people with a history of mental disorder; less than 10 homicides each year are committed by people with a primary diagnosis of schizophrenia (Geddes 1999).

The belief that mental disorder causes aggressive behaviour is also largely a misconception. A recent survey found that the major predictors of criminal and violent recidivism were the same for mentally disordered offenders as for non-disordered offenders. Criminal history variables were the best predictors, whereas clinical variables showed the smallest prediction (Bonta et al 1998).

Aggressive behaviour by people with mental disorders occurs mainly within psychiatric hospitals. This is partly because violent behaviour often leads to hospitalization. It is estimated that between one in ten to one in three admissions are preceded by violence (Crichton 1995). Approximately 10% of psychiatric inpatients commit assaults against staff; NHS staff were three times more likely to suffer injury than industrial workers, mainly due to assault (Health Services Advisory Committee 1987).

Understanding aggressive behaviour

Aggression can be defined as any form of behaviour directed towards the goal of harming or injuring another living being or object. It does not occur spontaneously (except in rare cases associated with organic brain damage) but commonly arises from interrelated factors associated with: (1) the individual; (2) the interaction; and (3) the situation. Therefore, in attempting to predict and manage aggressive behaviour, individual, interactional and situational factors should be considered.

Individual factors that could increase a person's likelihood of behaving aggressively might include poor ability to cope with stress, current life events, previous life experiences, personal victimization or traumatization and cultural and attitudinal variables. In regard to the interaction, the single most important factor is the individual's perception of the interaction. Aggression is driven by underlying thoughts and feelings; most commonly those associated with anger. Anger is an emotional state experienced as the impulse to behave in order to protect, defend or attack in response to a threat or a challenge. For the initiation of anger the individual must experience a perceived fear or threat, such as an insult, verbal abuse, frustration, annoyance or unfairness. Thus it is not the trigger itself that causes anger but the way in which the person thinks about the interaction. The individual factors specific to a person described above, such as current life stressors, affect their degree of sensitivity to the trigger. Emotions such as fear, hurt and jealousy generate further negative thoughts, which in turn can lead to aggressive behaviour.

The situational context in which the behaviour takes place also influences the likelihood of aggression. Henderson (1986) conducted an analysis from self-reports of offenders about the types of situation in which they were violent. This produced four general situations in which violence was most likely to occur: (1) violence in conjunction with crime; (2) in a family context; (3) in clubs and bars; and (4) in institutions. Situational vulnerability is the increased likelihood of behaving aggressively towards others in a given situation. It has been proposed that seven circumstances are likely to have particular situational vulnerability in inpatient mental health settings. These are: physical contact, limit setting, problems of communication, changes/readjustments, specific persons, high-risk contact and drugs/stimulants (Bjørkly et al 1996).

Risk Reduction and managing aggression

Mental health professionals commonly encounter people who are personally vulnerable to aggressive behaviour because of their individual experiences, are sensitive to potentially conflictual interactions and who are in situations that might increase their likelihood of behaving aggressively. It is important, therefore, to be mindful of reducing the risk of aggression when interacting with these people. Davies (1989) describes four potentially counterproductive attitudes that could provoke confrontational responses:

1. overly rigid and controlling attitudes
2. not showing any fear response despite an escalating incident
3. not responding or problem-solving in a potentially conflictual situation
4. not referring the person on if a successful therapeutic relationship is not established.

Davies proposed that professionals should be aware of their attitudes towards individuals and should cognitively rehearse a range of potential 'aggressive behaviour' scenarios and their management.

Guidelines to reduce the likelihood of aggressive behaviour

- Show warmth, respect and understanding.
- Get to know the person. Ensure that you have as much information as possible about him or her, including the nature and outcome of any previous incidents of aggressive behaviour.
- Communicate effectively with your colleagues, and those from other agencies, about individual people; keep yourself and others up to date.
- Ensure colleagues know where you are and who you are with.
- Schedule potentially difficult people for times when others are around and when you function at your best.
- If at all possible, avoid making people wait beyond the appointment time and allocate sufficient therapeutic time to engage them fully, so they feel valued and the session worthwhile.
- Conduct a non-clinical risk assessment of all areas where service users have access, to include, for example, access to potential weapons (I was recently shown to an interview room in a secure unit in which pool balls and cues were stored!). Health and safety guidance is often helpful in identifying potentially hazardous situations.
- Develop departmental contingency plans for a range of eventualities, including potential 'hostage' situations.
- Arrange your office/therapeutic rooms to allow a free exit path for yourself and the person you are seeing.
- If an individual has a known anger-control problem, address this openly by questions such as 'How would I know if you were getting angry?' and 'What particular things make you angry?' Discuss and agree contingency plans with them, e.g. identification of a 'bolt hole' for them to go to for a short time if they start to feel agitated during the session.

If preventive measures are not possible or are unsuccessful, and you are confronted with an agitated person, the following three-step process could be followed:

1. Try to reduce the person's anger. This can be done by showing empathy, paraphrasing the content of what is being said, and acknowledging the person's feelings.
2. Problem-solve. Attempt to clarify exactly what the problem is, generate possible solutions and discuss these together.
3. Act. Help the individual put into practice whatever was decided at stage 2.

Formal training in managing aggressive behaviour is becoming widely available for NHS staff. Various short courses have been developed from the Home-Office-approved Control and Restraint training that was originally organized for the Prison Service and Special Hospitals. Control and Restraint is based on the premise that aggressive clients should be physically controlled only as a last resort. Control and

Box 13.1
*Defusing an
aggressive situation
(Cembrowicz & Ritter
1994, Davies 1989)*

General points to consider when attempting to defuse a situation
include:
- not 'taking sides' but trying to find a solution
- 'depersonalizing' the problem
- giving the person physical space
- being aware of non-verbal behaviour and trying to retain a
  normal pattern of eye contact (and, if standing, angling
  yourself rather than standing directly in front of someone).

Restraint courses, usually of 5 days duration, focus on teaching non-physical and physical interventions in the management of aggression and in preventing physical injury to both parties. Specific modules teach staff how to restrain a person as part of a team using a recognized series of techniques.

'Breakaway' techniques can be taught over 1 or 2 days, and are particularly valuable for ancillary staff and non-ward based staff; these are essentially 'escape' techniques.

Use and abuse of touch

As outlined above, physical contact can be considered to increase some people's situational vulnerability to aggression. Touch, whether it is used instrumentally (as when guiding a person's actions), expressively (as in placing a hand on a shoulder in friendship) or therapeutically (e.g. massage) can be experienced by the recipient as pleasurable, irritating, welcome or aversive. What might be intended as reassurance could be misinterpreted as a sexual advance – clear verbal communication and establishing of therapeutic boundaries is important to ensure that the person wants to be touched and that the touch is interpreted correctly.

People with anger-control problems are often sensitive to perceived invasion of their personal space and can feel threatened by direct touch or by interactions in which they do not feel in control. Particular attention should therefore be paid to establishing safe and agreed therapeutic boundaries before using touch in therapy. Touch, in the form of massage, is an ancient form of treatment used by many societies, including the Chinese, Egyptians and Greeks. Massage can be used as a relaxation technique, often combined with other forms of relaxation. People with high levels of tension and anxiety symptoms can be helped to relax by massage, which works directly on the parasympathetic nervous system to produce a reversal of the physiological symptoms of arousal. This can be particularly beneficial for those with aggression problems who often have high levels of tension and physical arousal (Poon 1995).

Support, supervision and debriefing for everyone involved

The recent national audit (National Audit of the Management of Violence in Mental Health Settings 2000) found that of 3609 people who work on, use or visit psychiatric wards, one-third of service users and visitors reported that they had experienced violence. Seventy-two per cent reported that they had not been given advice on what to do and 47% said that they did not know how to summon help. With regard to staff training, development and supervision, 34% of staff had not had any training that was directly related to the management of violence in the past 5 years and 52% of staff reported they were receiving regular supervision. The National Audit recommends that Mental Health Services should develop coherent strategies for dealing with the aftermath of violent incidents. These should take account of the needs of service users as well as staff.

As part of routine support and supervision for staff, specific attention should be given to the sequelae of working with potentially aggressive people. Staff and service users assaulted in mental health settings experience similar effects to those assaulted in the community and should expect similar consideration and access to professional support.

The personal effect of witnessing or being the victim of aggression depends on a combination of factors, including the seriousness of the incident, the injuries sustained, the victim's personality, the responses of colleagues and social networks. Psychological consequences can include stress reactions, such as increased startle response, hypervigilence, tension, irritability and phobic anxiety, as well as generalized anxiety, depression, guilt, loss of confidence, anger, decreased concentration, 'burnout' and post-traumatic stress disorder. Physical sequelae include insomnia, nightmares, appetite disturbance, lethargy and headaches. Behavioural effects such as increased alcohol and cigarette consumption, avoidance of patient contact, social withdrawal, loss of interest and involvement in work are common (Mezey & Shepherd 1994).

Timely and appropriate support and debriefing can reduce the likelihood of developing such symptoms. Critical incident debriefing is a widely used and recognized process to ensure that the victims and witnesses of traumatic experiences receive optimum support.

Critical incident debriefing is a three-stage process: first, an informal meeting is held as soon as possible after the event to support the individuals involved. This is normally led by a senior member of staff and should be prioritized and attended by all associated staff. The second

Box 13.2
Critical incident debriefing

The goals are to:
- reassure the person that their reactions are normal, e.g. feeling helpless, shocked, humiliated, outraged
- promote the cohesiveness of the healthcare team
- anticipate and deal with immediate, medium and longer-term emotions and responses
- reduce tension and stress
- provide immediate and continuing support.

stage is a more formalized private meeting of approximately 2 hours, 1 or 2 days after the event. Again, as many of the staff team as possible should attend. The focus is on members talking about the event, their feelings and any coping and non-coping responses. Educational material can be presented, peer support encouraged and opportunities for further help or necessary intervention and action, e.g. reporting to police, discussed. The third stage is a follow-up group meeting, the format and timing of which are agreed at the second stage (Cembrowicz & Ritter 1994).

Similar support and debriefing should be organized for service users. Often, users have experienced traumas and assaults prior to admission and should rightly expect to find a place of safety and care in hospital. Many will be experiencing symptoms of anxiety, depression and stress, and these can be increased significantly by experiencing or witnessing aggressive behaviour. Even apparently minor assaults can result in significant and prolonged responses; the incident might trigger emotions associated with past experiences or cause unresolved personal conflicts to emerge.

Conclusion

Working with people with aggressive behaviour problems can be very rewarding – forming a good therapeutic relationship and helping such people to change, to feel more in control of themselves and less disadvantaged by their difficulties. Although people with mental health needs *can* be aggressive and occasionally violent, the nature and frequency of this violence is often overestimated. In mental health settings the risk of aggressive behaviour can be greatly reduced by focusing on the individual's specific vulnerabilities, the interaction and the situational context. Appropriate training in physical and non-physical techniques and strategies to manage aggression can ensure that the likelihood of such incidents is minimized, and that mental health settings are safer for all.

Summary

- The chapter focuses on challenging misconceptions associated with aggression and mental disorder.

- Guidance is presented for the containment and management of aggressive behaviour in mental health settings.

- Beliefs that aggression is associated with mental health needs are unfounded, with fewer than 10 homicides each year being committed by people with a primary diagnosis of schizophrenia.

- Aggression rarely occurs spontaneously and most commonly arises from interrelated factors associated with the individual, the interaction, and the situation.

- Guidelines to reduce the occurrence of aggressive behaviour are presented.

■ Formal training in managing aggressive behaviour is becoming widely available for NHS staff.

■ Recommendations from the National Audit highlight the need for mental health services to develop coherent strategies for dealing with the aftermath of violent incidents.

■ Forming a good therapeutic relationship with, and enabling people with problems of aggression to feel more in control can be very rewarding.

References

Bjørkly S, Havik O E, Løberg T 1996 The interrater reliability of the scale for the prediction of aggression and dangerousness in psychotic patients. Criminal Justice and Behaviour 23(3): 440–454

Bonta J, Law M, Hanson K 1998 The prediction of criminal and violent recidivism among mentally disordered offenders: a meta-analysis. Psychological Bulletin 123(2):123–142

Cembrowicz S, Ritter S 1994 Attacks on doctors and nurses. In: Shepherd J (ed) Violence in health care: a practical guide to coping with violence and caring for victims. Oxford University Press, Oxford, p 13–41

Crichton J 1995 A review of psychiatric inpatient violence. In: Crichton J (ed) Psychiatric patient violence: risk and response. Duckworth, London, p 9–23

Davies W 1989 The prevention of assault on professional helpers. In: Howells K, Hollin C R (eds) Clinical approaches to violence. John Wiley, Chichester, UK, p 311–328

Geddes J 1999 Suicide and homicide by people with mental illness. British Medical Journal 318: 1225–1226.

Health Services Advisory Committee 1987 Violence to staff in the health service. HMSO, London

Henderson M 1986 An empirical typology of violent incidents reported by prison inmates with convictions for violence. Aggressive Behaviour 12: 21–32

Mezey G, Shepherd J 1994 Effects of assault on health-care professions. In: Shepherd J (ed) Violence in health care: a practical guide to coping with violence and caring for victims. Oxford University Press, Oxford, p 1–11

National Audit of the Management of Violence in Mental Health Settings 2000 The multi-centre audit team. College Research Unit, London

Poon K 1995 Touch and handling. In: Everett T, Dennis M, Ricketts E (eds) Physiotherapy in mental health: a practical approach. Butterworth-Heinemann, London, p 91–101

14 Enabling occupation

Jennifer Creek

Jennifer Creek

Introduction

The word 'occupation' is usually taken to mean employment, or the main productive activity in which a person spends time. It often contributes to the individual's sense of identity, and one of the first questions we ask a new acquaintance is 'What do you do?' meaning 'What is your main job?'. The answer to this question would be something like 'I'm a doctor' or 'I work for social services' or 'I mend clocks'.

However, 'occupation' also has a range of other meanings, including holding a physical position (as in the occupation of university buildings by protesting students), and holding a social position (as in having the same occupation, i.e. job, for over 30 years) (Caulton 1993). An occupation is not usually a brief or temporary event but generally implies activities that take place over time. For example, a physiotherapy student who does a summer job stacking shelves in the local supermarket is more likely to think of his or her occupation as physiotherapist or student than as shelf stacker. The concept of occupation also suggests active commitment to, and engagement in, what is being done rather than a passive acceptance of events. To be occupied is to be busy and engrossed (Caulton 1993).

This chapter offers definitions of occupation, occupational form and occupational performance, and the related concepts of activity and skill. It discusses the importance of occupation in organizing human life, creating meaning, supporting self-esteem and maintaining health. The effects on the individual of occupational dysfunction are illustrated by a case study. The same case study is then used to illustrate two models for practice based on the concept of occupational performance: the personal adaptation through occupation model and the person–environment occupational performance model.

Defining occupation and activity

Taking the concepts of activity, identity, time and engagement, we can define occupation as a number of activities that can be grouped together under a name and that form a part of the individual's personal and social identity. Occupations organize the time and effort a person

153

spends on activities throughout life. For example, fly fishing, occupational therapy, parenting, youth work and boxing are all occupations. Occupations are commonly classified as self-care, productivity and leisure, although these are artificial divisions. For example, cooking could be productive work for a housewife, self-care for a student and leisure for someone entertaining friends to dinner.

The word 'activity' is sometimes used synonymously with 'occupation' but it can be helpful to differentiate the two terms. Hagedorn (2000) saw occupations and activities in a hierarchical relationship, with our occupations determining the activities that we do. For example, I am a mother (occupation) therefore I listen to my daughter's piano practice (activity), make fashionable clothes for her (activity) and frequently cook chips (activity). Hagedorn (2000, p. 307) defined activity as 'a series of linked episodes of task performance which takes place on a specific occasion, during a finite period, for a particular reason'.

Skills   To carry out the range of activities that make up our daily occupations, we need to develop skills. A skill is 'a specific ability or integrated set of abilities...learnt and practised to a standard required for the effective performance of a task' (Hagedorn 2001, p. 161).

Skills can be classified into three main groups (Reed & Sanderson 1992):

1. Sensorimotor skills, including sensory skills, perceptual skills, visual sense, motor skills and neuromuscular skills.
2. Cognitive skills, including arousal, orientation, attention, recognition, memory, reality testing, association, categorization, concept formation, sequencing, problem-solving, judgement, learning and time management.
3. Psychosocial skills, including psychological (intrapersonal) skills, such as self-concept and affect, and social skills.

The wider the range of skills a person has, and the greater the level of competence in them, the more activities he or she will be able to perform satisfactorily and the more occupations will be open to him or her.

Occupational form and performance   All human activity occurs within a social context that influences both the occupations that we choose or are given and the ways in which we enact them. We learn what constitutes an appropriate range of occupations, and the standards of performance that are expected of us, within a particular physical and social environment. The rules that society lays down for acceptable occupational performance have been called the 'occupational form':

> *An* occupational form *is an objective set of circumstances, independent of and external to a person. The individual's occupational performance (the doing)*

can be understood only in terms of the environmental context in which the performance takes place (that is, only in terms of the occupational form).

(Nelson 1988, p. 633)

Occupational form consists of the materials, physical environment, human context and temporal context in which the occupation is performed, as well as the values, norms, sanctions, symbols, rules and guidelines governing that performance. For example, chess has an occupational form independent of anyone playing the game.

Occupational performance is the doing of the occupation, the active behaviour of the individual within the context of the occupational form, for example, playing a game of chess. Each person will carry out an occupation differently, even within the same environment, as a result of their individual skills, level of competence, values, goals and interests.

Occupational dysfunction

Occupational performance equates to the ability to function within a social, cultural and physical environment. Function is dependent on the interaction between environmental supports and barriers, the individual's skills and the individual's occupational demands (Baum & Edwards 1995).

To understand the effects on the individual of not being able to carry out a normal range of occupations, we need to be aware of the purposes that occupation serves for each person.

The functions of occupation

We have already considered how occupations guide the activities that we carry out in our daily lives. They are the framework that allows us to structure our time in a healthy and purposeful way. 'Man learns to organize time and he does it in terms of *doing* things...we might call it the ingestion and digestion and proper use...of *time* with its succession of *opportunities*' (Meyer 1977, p. 642).

Occupations not only structure our time but also give meaning to our lives. We make sense of the human and non-human world by acting within and upon it through the medium of activity. In turn, our experiences of activity shape the meanings that we give to people, places and events. Further, our sense of who we are, our identity, is created by the things that we do:

Doing *is a process of investigating, trying out, and gaining experience of one's capacities for experiencing, responding, managing, creating, and controlling. It is through such action that an individual comes to know the potential and limitations of self and the environment and achieves a sense of competence and intrinsic worth.*

(Fidler & Fidler 1978, p. 306)

Wilcock (1998), an Australian writer, suggested that occupation has an even more fundamental purpose to human existence. It is an innate behaviour and 'an evolutionary mechanism for the maintenance and promotion of health' (Wilcock 1998, p. 1). The two most important functions of occupation are survival and health. Survival occupations include those that provide for the essential needs of the person, such as food, water and shelter. Occupations that maintain or promote health are those that exercise physical, mental and social capacities, keeping them in balance. Devoting too much time to one aspect of the self at the expense of others is likely to lead to illhealth, for example, eating too much and not taking enough exercise has been linked with a range of diseases such as heart disease and arthritis.

The effects of occupation on health were demonstrated by the well elderly study, a randomized, controlled trial of the effectiveness of occupational therapy in preventing illhealth among 361 well, elderly people. The study demonstrated that participants in two activity groups gained significant benefits across various measures of health, function and quality of life over participants in the non-activity control group (Clark et al 1997).

The effects of occupational dysfunction

Occupational performance can be disrupted, temporarily or permanently, by developmental delay, disease, injury or environmental constraints. A single case study is used here to illustrate the effects of occupational dysfunction on an individual's life. Parallels with this case can be drawn across all the social and ethnic diversity of human occupational experience.

Case Study: Sue

Sue is a single woman in her early 50s. She had hyperthyroidism in her teens, necessitating several periods in hospital with severe restriction of physical activity. Since then, she has felt guilty if she is not as active as her contemporaries.

In 1977, Sue was ill for several months with swollen glands and fatigue. This was eventually diagnosed as sarcoidosis. A second episode occurred in 1982, when Sue had problems with her breathing and was treated with steroids for 7 years. During this time, she gave up many of her more physically demanding activities, such as weight training, and concentrated her limited energy on work. She became more interested in intellectual activity and moved to an academic job. Her intellectual ability became an important source of self-esteem and satisfaction.

A third episode of sarcoidosis occurred in 1996, affecting Sue's breathing and her eyesight. The fatigue became more extreme and Sue took medical retirement at the age of 48. Her health continued to deteriorate so that her activity levels remained low, even after she gave up work. This led to her becoming socially isolated and depressed, for which she was treated with antidepressant medication.

At this time, Sue was living in a large Victorian house with her four cats. She was confined to the house for much of the time, unable even to come downstairs on bad days. She put on a lot of

Continued

Case Study: Sue
Continued

weight, which made her breathing more laboured. Her concentration was so poor that she was unable to read.

In January 2000, Sue had a heart attack. Unfortunately, she was not able to manage a cardiac rehabilitation programme because her breathing was not strong enough to cope with the exercise. She was not offered pulmonary rehabilitation.

Over the course of the next year, Sue continued to have problems with fatigue and difficulty with breathing but her concentration improved and she registered to do a PhD. With the help of friends, she took on an allotment where she was able to take gentle exercise at her own pace.

This case study illustrates the effects of illness and disability on occupational performance. As Sue's physical limitations led to a reduction in certain occupations, she attempted to salvage her identity and self-esteem by turning to more intellectual pursuits. When these were affected by her illness, she became depressed. Her world changed from the busy life of an active, working, independent woman to days of isolation and inactivity. As she became well enough to take up some of her former occupations, and found new ones, her quality of life and her mood improved.

Models for enabling occupational performance

The process of enabling occupational performance has been described as:

Using interventions to improve the occupational performance of persons who lack the ability to perform an action or activity considered necessary for their everyday lives. This is accomplished through a joint effort of the person and the clinician, where the person's problems, strengths, and assets are identified; followed by therapeutic interventions, educational strategies, access to resources, and environmental adaptations, so the person can accomplish his or her goals.

(Law & Baum 1994, quoted in Baum & Edwards 1995, p. 1019–1020)

To assist people to adapt, access resources and learn or relearn skills to a level of competence that will support their necessary and chosen occupations, the therapist can use a model for practice. A model for practice is 'a set of theories applicable in a particular field of practice that provides an explanation of clinical phenomena and suggests the type of intervention the therapist should make' (Creek & Feaver 1993, p. 5).

Several models for enabling occupational performance have been developed (Hagedorn 2000). All of them describe how people maintain themselves in the world by engaging in a balanced range of occupations. Two of these models are described here.

Personal adaptation through occupation model (Reed & Sanderson 1992)

People are conceptualized as living in three, overlapping worlds: (1) the personal, psychobiological environment (the body); (2) the physical,

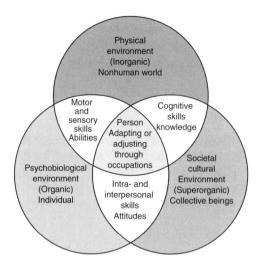

Figure 14.1
Conceptional model of occupational therapy (Adapted from Reed & Sanderson 1992, with permission)

non-human environment; and (3) the sociocultural human environment (Fig. 14.1). Each person is changed by, and adapts to, changes in any of these three environments by using occupations. Occupations are supported by four types of skills and abilities: motor and sensory, cognitive, intrapersonal and interpersonal.

All the occupations a person undertakes are determined by the environment and are developed to meet needs. People adapt or adjust to their circumstances by using occupations either to change themselves or to change the environment, therefore, the degree to which a person is able to adapt depends on the occupations he or she is able to perform. Change in an individual's occupations is affected by change in the environment, in individual skills and in adaptive potential.

There are three levels of intervention. The first is to teach the normal way of carrying out a task; for example, after some graded exercise, Sue is able to walk upstairs to bed. The second is to teach an alternative way of carrying out the task; for example, Sue is able to walk upstairs to bed if she rests every few steps. The third is to adapt the environment; for example, a stair lift is fitted so that Sue does not have to walk upstairs.

With the model as an organizing framework for the assumptions and theories underpinning practice, intervention takes place in a logical process:

- The therapist gathers data about the client's past and present performance skills and functional ability to determine whether an intervention is indicated.
- The therapist and client analyse and identify the occupations that will be most useful to the client.
- The therapist analyses the skills needed to perform specific occupations.

- The therapist evaluates the client's performance to identify problems in skill development and acquisition.
- The therapist predicts problems with occupational performance based on analysis of skills deficits.
- The therapist and client agree on a hierarchy of goals to be attained through intervention.
- The therapist and client design a programme of intervention through which the client is enabled to learn or relearn skills.
- The therapist and client work together to integrate the skills needed to perform occupations.
- The client is assisted to adapt to the environment through the use of selected occupations.
- The therapist might assist the sociocultural environment to adapt to the client through the use of selected occupations.
- The client's progress is measured against baseline performance and the stated goals.
- When goals have been attained, or the therapist or client judge that no further progress can be made, the client is discharged with recommendations for support and assistance.

Person–environment occupational performance model (Christiansen & Baum 1997)

This model is based on the belief that people are intrinsically motivated to explore their world and develop skills to adapt successfully to it. Adaptation is the process by which individuals meet the challenges of daily living by using the resources (personal, social and material) available to them. Through their occupations, people develop their identity and derive a sense of fulfilment so that they come to an understanding of who they are and their place in the world.

The three components of the model describe what people do in their daily lives, what motivates them to act and how their occupational performance is influenced by a combination of personal characteristics and circumstances (Fig. 14.2). The latter are called 'performance enablers' because they support the occupational performance of the individual. They include intrinsic enablers (such as cognition) and extrinsic enablers (such as environmental demands).

The goal of intervention is to enable people to develop or use resources that will support their necessary and chosen occupations. For example, to carry out the occupations that will enable her to survive and be happy, Sue needs to improve her physical fitness (personal resource) and organize her house so that she can carry out domestic activities with the minimum of effort (material resource). She buys in help with housework and house maintenance (social resource). If she wants to have an evening out, she has learned to manage her time (personal resource) so that she can rest for a day or so either side of the

Figure 14.2
Person–environment occupational performance model (reprinted from Christiansen & Baum 1997, with permission from SLACK Incorporated)

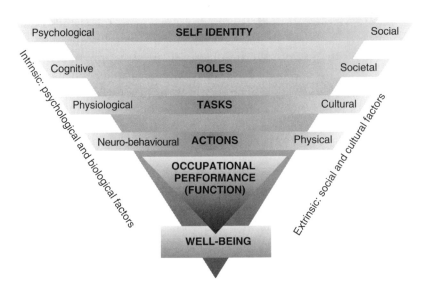

outing. She has kept her car (material resource) so that she can get about more easily, but she shares the use of it and the costs with a neighbour (social resource).

The process of intervention is client-centred and includes:

- Referral.
- Initial assessment – this involves identifying the intrinsic and extrinsic factors that support and limit activities. It includes assets as well as deficits.
- Determination of needs – a list of goals is developed by the therapist and client.
- Intervention plan – this will include both interventions to restore skills and re-engagement in meaningful occupations. The therapist and client agree on which parts of the plan will be given priority.
- Intervention and formative assessment – the major intervention categories used by occupational therapists are: occupation, education and training, sensory and neuromuscular remediation, modification of the physical environment and use of technological aids and devices.
- Summative assessment.
- Termination of treatment.

Conclusion   Occupations form the fundamental framework of human life. If they are disrupted, the individual will encounter problems in all aspects of living. It is the job of the therapist to assist people to lead the lives they want, or expect, to lead, despite disorder or disease, so that they are able to participate fully in their social world.

Summary

- The concept of occupation and its part in human life was explored.

- The chapter discussed how occupations are made up of activities that, in turn, are supported by skills.

- Some of the functions of occupation for individuals and the effects of occupational dysfunction were considered.

- Two practice models used for enabling occupation were reviewed.

References

Baum C M, Edwards D 1995 Position paper. Occupational performance: occupational therapy's definition of function. American Journal of Occupational Therapy 49(10):1019–1020

Caulton R 1993 Occupation and healing. Occupation 1(1):6–17

Christiansen C, Baum C 1997 Occupational therapy: enabling function and well-being, 2nd edn. Slack, New Jersey

Clark F, Azen S P, Zemke R et al 1997 Occupational therapy for independent-living older adults. Journal of the American Medical Association 278(16):1321–1326

Creek J, Feaver S 1993 Models for practice in occupational therapy: Part 1, defining terms. British Journal of Occupational Therapy 56(1):4–6

Fidler G S, Fidler J W 1978 Doing and becoming: purposeful action and self-actualization. American Journal of Occupational Therapy 32(5):305–310

Hagedorn R 2000 Tools for practice in occupational therapy: a structured approach to core skills and processes. Churchill Livingstone, Edinburgh

Hagedorn R 2001 Foundations for practice in occupational therapy, 3rd edn. Churchill Livingstone, Edinburgh

Meyer A 1977 The philosophy of occupation therapy. American Journal of Occupational Therapy 31(10):639–642

Nelson D L 1988 Occupation: form and performance. American Journal of Occupational Therapy 42(10):633–641

Reed K L, Sanderson S N 1992 Concepts of occupational therapy, 3rd edn. Williams & Wilkins, Baltimore

Wilcock A 1998 A theory of occupation and health. In: Creek J (ed) Occupational therapy: new perspectives. Whurr, London

Occupation: a view from users

Patsy Brodie and Shelagh Creegan

Introduction

This chapter considers how users of the service view occupation as a strategy to facilitate living with mental health needs. The narratives of several people are considered within the context of occupational therapy and their experience provides valuable insight into the importance of occupation as both a social expectation and as a therapeutic intervention contributing towards the process of recovery for people with mental health problems.

People with enduring mental health problems are prone to experience occupational deprivation, which can have a profound impact, both mentally and physically, on their lives. The erosion of the quality of life is often demonstrated by a basic lack of structure to the day, which has the effect of generating low self-esteem, a lack of motivation and general hopelessness, all of which exacerbate the original problem (Williams 1997).

Case study: Ian

> Ian is 58 years old, nearly 59. He has had a good work record, holding a number of senior positions as a computer programmer. Ian suffers from manic-depressive psychosis. After 4 or 5 years of poor mental health Ian's marriage crumbled. His self-esteem and self-confidence were at a low ebb. He felt lonely and alone. Ian's motivation to go to work and focus on everyday tasks waned. He left his job and became more and more despondent. In the depths of depression, Ian slashed his wrists and was admitted to a psychiatric hospital. Ian continues in his own words. 'Five or six years ago I thought about getting back to work. I dug out my old curriculum vitae (CV) and thought about what job I could do. I could drive a van or a minibus, be a warehouseman or stack supermarket shelves. I applied for lots of jobs like that. Potential employers looked at my CV. My last job had a salary of £28,000. I didn't want a job like my last one because of the stress. But now I was physically fit, I was keen, mental health was certainly good enough and I was chasing jobs to get back to work. Did employers want me? No. As soon as they saw 'mental health problem requiring inpatient treatment' on my CV that was it. It was very depressing.'

Case study: George

> George is aged 35 years and suffers from schizophrenia. He has had two admissions to hospital as a result of severe depression and suicidal ideation. He is an intelligent man. He has an honours degree in business studies and a postgraduate degree in marketing. His last job, which he lost due to poor mental health 5 years ago, was as a product design and development manager with a life assurance company. George is single and he lives alone. He has an uneasy relationship with his family. He has lost contact with his friends since becoming ill. 'When I was working,' he recalled, 'I used to play football with colleagues and stuff like that. I lost my job through illhealth and now I don't really have any hobbies. My social life has stopped.'

'Doing' has historically been a core principle of occupational therapy practice in mental health. The role of occupational therapists is to promote occupation as a route for people to find meaning in everyday pursuits and to gain an appreciation and enjoyment of life. The focus of this chapter is to examine the perceived benefits of engagement in occupation by relating the experiences of a small group of people with enduring mental health problems who make use of National Health Service (NHS) Occupational Therapy Services.

Generating motivation

Peter, a 47-year-old, single man related his experience of being in hospital and attendance at occupational therapy (OT):

> In the early days I used to attend the Occupational Therapy Department from the ward...OT then the ward...OT then the ward. I didn't speak to anybody, I didn't look at anybody. The OT staff were very good at channelling you and bringing you out. They helped me to develop a more settled existence. After I was out of hospital, for a while, I thought I was cured. That was when I started chasing jobs but when nothing came up I went down again and felt very bad. So I started attending OT again. That helped a lot as it gave me a routine and I proved to myself I could do things.

Peter suffers from severe anxiety and has a great lack of self-confidence. He constantly fears failure. He has a good relationship with his family but he is very dependent on his elderly mother. He has few other social contacts and he becomes very anxious and agitated if pressurized. He feels unable to cope with a job and has been unable to find work which he can commit to. He dislikes change. Through discussion, the OT staff found out that Peter had enjoyed woodwork and gardening in the past. His OT programme focused upon these activities as a means of achieving personal growth and self-confidence. Working within group settings promoted Peter's development and use of interpersonal and social skills. He revealed to staff a past love of fishing before going on to organize a fishing trip for a small group of people attending OT. Peter went as far as donating a winner's trophy.

Sense of purpose

Ian also attended OT as a day patient after his discharge from hospital. Like Peter, he chose woodwork as a work activity:

> *I attended OT from the ward and when I was discharged I just kept coming because I knew everybody. You actually make things that are really quite good. You can also chat to people who are in the same situation as yourself and share a bit of black humour. The woodwork instructor is great. He doesn't make you feel awkward or things like that. He is just one of the boys rather than a member of staff. You get a laugh and are part of something good and relaxed.*

Organization of time

The need to fill time in a meaningful way was a major concern for all the service users. Mark's experience was not untypical:

> *On the three days I attend OT I have a set time of when to go to sleep and when to get up. I get washed and have breakfast and get to OT on time. I enjoy doing woodwork. It gives me the enthusiasm to get up in the morning and so helps with how I feel. On the days I don't attend OT I don't really get up. I tend to lie in my bed. I just laze about and don't do anything. I get a bit bored.*

Mark is a 33-year-old, single man. He suffers from paranoid psychosis. He disclosed to OT staff that he felt idle, lonely and unable to engage in work activities because the paranoia he experienced made it difficult for him to be among people. Personal growth is a challenge that requires a safe and supportive environment. By demonstrating flexibility in determining his days and hours of attendance, Mark engaged with the OT department and learned to make a varied range of woodwork items. With encouragement, he joined OT staff at local craft fairs to sell the woodwork items to the general public. Being able to progress from a small group setting in the OT department to helping out at busy craft fairs was a source of great satisfaction and personal achievement for Mark. Like Ian and Peter before him, being involved in productive occupation and/or having the opportunity to socialize appeared to be a motivating force for Mark in terms of providing a sense of purpose and an organization of time.

Environmental influences

The environment also plays an important role in generating motivation. Peter described his need for something purposeful and meaningful to do that filled his time rather that staying at home where he seemed to have difficulty finding motivation. Peter becomes anxious and upset without a structured programme of activities. This manifests in various physical complaints and he tends to stay at home. This upsets his elderly mother. Having somewhere to go and something to do has enabled Peter to keep busy and occupied:

> *I like attending OT. Being outside and working in the garden gets me out the house. It is very easy to sit in the house and after a week or two you start thinking that you can't be bothered doing anything. But having OT makes you come out the house. It makes you do things.*

As a group, the users identified that a welcoming, friendly and sociable atmosphere, free from pressure, was an important element in motivating them to attend OT. 'I like coming here,' said Ian. 'I like the way you are treated. You get a laugh and make new friends.' Enjoying each others' company and having the opportunity to talk about problems and concerns improved the users' abilities to express their own needs and meet those of others. Ian explained, 'You make friends with people who have been in the same position as yourself. Things can be said or left unsaid because we all understand the experiences we have been through.'

Medication

Medication plays a central role in the management of people with mental health problems. This group of users accepted the role of medication in maintaining their well-being but expressed problems in the management of medication and finding a balance between controlling symptoms and living with debilitating side effects. 'We are all extremely grateful for medication' said Ian. 'We have discussed it many times. I am on antidepressants. That is the fourth lot I've been on and each time it gets better.'

The negative effects of medication related mainly to diminished motivation, tiredness and poor tolerance for activity. For Brian, a 46-year-old married man, being on medication made work a struggle and participating in predetermined programmes difficult. Previously, he had worked as a pre-caster with a local building firm. Following a motor cycle accident, with resultant nerve damage and shoulder pain, he had suffered from anxiety and panic attacks. 'I went down to the office to talk to someone about voluntary work. I was making a weekly commitment. At that stage I knew there were some weeks I couldn't get up. I am supposed to pick up a mini bus at 8.30 a.m. and I am still in bed. You can't commit and then let people down.'

Where are they now?

For the small group of people with enduring mental health problems who make use of NHS occupational therapy services, engagement in occupation gave them a sense of purpose and helped them to organize time. Being in a supportive environment that fostered choice and autonomy contributed to generating intrinsic motivation which they acknowledged that they either lacked or had previously lacked. Their personal testimonies of the power of occupation to generate motivation supported the belief that occupations can be used as therapeutic means to contribute towards the process of recovery of health and well-being of people with mental health problems.

Forced social involvement carries with it the risk of failure and usually involves emotional demand which can provoke relapse. However, active but task-orientated involvement in occupational therapy activities can increase the likelihood of social involvement and task attainment. For instance, Ian continues to attend the OT department three times per week. He accepts that paid employment is not an option for him now due to his age and the length of time he has been out of work. Ian is happy with his current programme: 'It keeps me going and helps me get on with other things like keeping the house and even going out for a pint occasionally. I have never been particularly sociable but I enjoy the company at OT and will make social chit-chat in the pub.' Ian says he is happy to be involved in small group discussions regarding service users' needs. Such interaction has proved to be a dynamic and potent therapeutic exercise. 'Work is important for people with mental health problems and I can share my experiences to help others in the future.'

George achieved his goal of returning to paid employment. He was successful in getting a part-time job dealing with enquiries at a local bank. 'I am thrilled to be starting work again. It is not at the same level as I was before but it is a start and there is the opportunity to progress on to other areas if things go well.' Three months have passed and George is still in his job. Moreover, he is optimistic about his chances of re-establishing a social life through the contacts he has made at his work.

Peter continues to suffer from severe anxiety but he has coped with a change of house. His self-confidence is better and he has extended his range of activities, now doing pottery and cooking when at OT. He has been able to go on holiday with a local fishing group. Peter says, 'I now know that having a routine helps me cope with other things. I feel a great weight off my mind when I know I can speak to staff and other patients about my various concerns. Going on holiday with others has helped me feel more normal.'

Mark has demonstrated competent basic work habits at OT. He has progressed to a stage where he is able to assemble the full range of woodwork items available in the OT department independently. He is accurate, safe and tidy in his work. Socially, Mark gets on well with most people. On the odd occasion, his paranoia leads to altercations with young women attending the department. However, he is able to resolve these difficulties with support from staff. Mark expressed an interest in therapeutic paid employment beyond the OT department setting. Contact was make with the Employment Disability Unit (EDU). The EDU secured a position as a handyman's assistant in a nursing home for a 12-week trial period. Mark completed 4 weeks of the placement before it was brought to an abrupt end:

At my work placement I was going to be building things, putting up partitions, knocking down walls, ripping up lino. I was good. I enjoyed it but I was pretty sad when it stopped. The nursing home said it did not have the funding or something. The staff said they did not need me anymore because the two guys who were looking after me were off doing other things. They were handymen as well but they were working elsewhere and they could not look after me. So I would just be in the nursing home on my own doing nothing. There were no jobs to do and no supervision.

Mark returned to the OT department. Latterly, he had been observed as becoming increasingly unsteady in his gait, with poor balance, although he did not fall. He subsequently suffered three small cerebrovascular accidents. After a spell in hospital, Mark again resumed attendance at OT. He has since learnt picture frame assembly and spends most of his time engaged in this activity. Although his poor balance can still cause him problems Mark feels it does not unduly affect his work performance. Socially, he is friendly towards visitors going as far as to engage them in social chit-chat. He also goes out of his way to welcome new people attending the department. Mark has come to realize that work does not necessarily have to be paid work. It can be paid work or voluntary work or just how he occupies his time in a constructive way to get him through the day.

Medication can have positive and negative effects on mental health. The users accepted that prolonged treatment with medication contributed to their well-being but at the cost of long-term side-effects including insidious weight gain and a reduction in energy levels. Deficit symptoms such as a lack of initiative and social unresponsiveness can be overcome, they felt, by engagement in meaningful occupations.

Brian progressed from undertaking simple woodwork tasks like sanding and painting to picture framing. He also learned to use a variety of tools and machinery and showed an interest in developing do-it-yourself (DIY) skills. Brian now feels he has something positive to offer his friends and family: 'I can do things at home like putting up shelves. I even laid someone's floor for them. I learned a lot when attending OT.' The freedom to choose both the frequency and the length of attendance, plus whether to engage in occupation or not, was an individual choice given to all attenders, including Brian: 'To have something to do without pressure, like attending OT is voluntary. You can take days off if you want. It is not the same as the pressure of work.' This autonomy appeared to be a key to generating motivation for Brian. Over the summer he made a time-limited commitment to look after his daughter's house and babysit for 3 months. His anxiety about making this commitment was lessened on learning that his place at OT would be kept open for him. The security of the knowledge enabled him to cope with this task successfully. He has since recommended attendance at OT: 'I am happy to get back to OT. Being away was okay but I need something practical to do.'

Conclusion

The uniqueness of the occupational therapy approach in mental health lies in the belief that service users have the ability to influence their own health through occupation. Their personal knowledge and experience of living with a mental health problem enables them to explain their lives, goals, plans and environments, to contribute to their OT programme, to make personal changes and changes in their environments and to evaluate the personal impact of OT mental health services. Occupational therapists' personal as well as professional knowledge and experience prepares them to: (1) enable service users to focus on their own experience so as to enhance their occupational performance within their environments; (2) advocate with and for service users; and (3) evaluate the process and outcome of service from the occupational therapist's perspective. Together, occupational therapists and service users actively seek to structure opportunities that promote real choice and autonomy commensurate with the service users' skills and experience. Ultimately, the balanced use of time in daily living activities, including meaningful occupation, is an indicator for service users and occupational therapists as to the state of their health.

Summary

- Meaningful occupation is a key element in the recovery process for service users.

- Components of the occupational therapy programme most valued by service users include flexible programming, a wide range of activities, unforced social interaction, and the promotion of real choice.

- The provision of a safe, supportive environment in which staff encourage independence and respect the needs of individuals are motivating factors for service users.

Acknowledgements

We would like to thank Audrey Cuthill, Secretary, and the small group of service users who utilize the NHS Occupational Therapy Service, without whose valuable contribution this chapter would not have been possible.

References

Williams N 1997 Temporal dysfunction: time is their enemy. Therapy Weekly 17th July:8

16 Mental health problems in children and adolescents

Part A: **THE CHILD IN THE CONTEXT OF CHILD AND ADOLESCENT MENTAL HEALTH SERVICES**

Jonquil Drinkwater, Nicola Connolly and Alice Farrington

Child and adolescent mental health problems are important because of the distress they cause to the child and, also, because if not addressed at this stage they can lead to a lifetime of difficulties. This chapter puts child and adolescent services into context and gives a brief outline of the types of assessment and treatment undertaken with children. There is then a review of how children are assessed and treated in the context of their families.

The child in the context of child and adolescent mental health services

Child and adolescent mental health services in the NHS are organized into four levels or 'tiers'. The first tier is primary care; the second tier involves referral to an individual trained in one of the mental health professions; the third tier involves referral to a multidisciplinary team; and the fourth is for complex cases including specialist provision in inpatient units.

The referral route into child and adolescent mental health services is often by the parent or young person going to his or her GP. Alternative referral routes are via other professionals such as health visitors and community paediatricians. Multidisciplinary teams vary in composition but can include a range of different professionals such as occupational therapists, clinical psychologists, family therapists, psychiatrists, psychiatric nurses, physiotherapists, dieticians, psychiatric social workers, play therapists, child psychotherapists and art therapists. These teams might refer more complex cases for inpatient assessment and treatment, or for more specialist services, such as neuropsychology.

Other agencies also work with children and adolescents with mental health problems, such as social services, youth offending teams, physical health services and education. This means that an important role of professionals who work with children and adolescents with mental health problems is liaison with other professionals and agencies.

Assessment and treatment approaches for children and adolescents with mental health problems

Assessing children

The purpose of the assessment is to gather information to develop a comprehensive understanding, or formulation, of the child's difficulties on which to base an effective treatment plan. It is important to gather information from different settings and from multiple sources, such as the child, family and teachers.

Most assessments begin by interviewing the child and the parents. The interview should gather a thorough account of the development and occurrence of symptoms and problem behaviours. The child's early development, progress in education and family and individual strengths and vulnerabilities are explored. Any mental health problems in the extended family, family lifecycle issues and marital problems are also investigated and a genogram will often be drafted (Fig. 16.1).

It can be useful to interview parents and children separately to gain an understanding of everyone's point of view and to allow any sensitive information to be shared in confidence. Clinicians have developed various techniques to illuminate the child's perspective, such as the 'bag of feelings', in which the child is asked to draw all their feelings and thoughts in a bag (Binney & Wright 1997), and the Family Relations Test (Bene & Anthony 1957) to explore the child's perception of family members. In addition, structured clinical interviews exist to aid psychiatrists in diag-

Figure 16.1
Example of a genogram

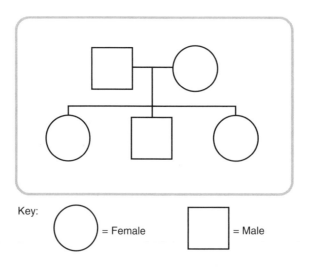

Key: ◯ = Female   ☐ = Male

nosing children and adolescents with a particular mental health difficulty (Angold et al 1995).

Observations of the child and family can support the information gathered through interview and can take place in various settings, such as the clinic, home and school. Clinicians can be watching for the degree of individuation between parents and child, responsivity of parents to the child's needs and the child's interactions with others. The type of play the child engages in can suggest developmental difficulties.

More formal assessments include psychometric tests. Common tests that measure the child's functioning across a variety of areas are the Bailey Scales of Infant Development for 1- to 42-month-olds (Bayley 1993) and the Wechsler Intelligence Scale for Children for 5- to 16-year-olds (Wechsler 1991). More detailed tests of functioning are completed by neuropsychologists. Questionnaires can be administered to explore the nature and severity of symptoms further. These can be for children to complete themselves, such as the Children's Depression Scale (Lang & Tisher 1983), or for parents to complete about their child, such as the Conners Questionnaire for Attention Deficit Hyperactivity Disorder (Conners 1997). In addition, clinicians can use questionnaires for parents to report about themselves, such as the Parenting Stress Index (Abidin 1995).

Assessing adolescents

Assessments of adolescents are similar in content to those for children, but adolescents are usually more able to report their own emotions and cognitions than younger children. This means that more of the assessment will be spent interviewing the adolescent individually. Indeed, adolescents might be more likely to give more accurate and detailed information without the presence of their parents. Nonetheless, it is usually still useful to interview parents, particularly for information about early development and to gain an understanding of parents' views of any difficulties.

Observation is used less often with adolescents than with children because adolescents are more able to describe their own and others' behaviour reliably. Formal assessments of functioning can be used, but should be age appropriate. Questionnaires that are appropriate for adolescents are used, such as the Depressive Experiences Questionnaire for adolescents (Blatt et al 1996).

Formulation

The multiple types of information from the various sources are pulled together into a comprehensive formulation within a developmental framework (see Connor & Fisher (1997) for a discussion of formulating child and adolescent problems). The planned treatment approach targets those parts of the system indicated by the formulation to be driving or maintaining the difficulties.

Treating children

Moving on to treatment issues, the treatment of preschool children tends to focus primarily on parents. Intervention might need to address parental mental health issues and commonly helps parents implement behavioural strategies. For example, Sadeh & Anders (1993) describe treatment of infant sleep problems, including behavioural work, challenging unhelpful maternal thinking patterns, such as 'my child will feel abandoned if I don't go up to him' and other maternal mental health issues, such as depression.

School-age children can be seen for treatment alone, using such treatments as play therapy (Axline 1989), counselling (Geldard & Geldard 1997), cognitive–behavioural therapy (Graham 1998), or psychopharmacology, such as Ritalin for attention deficit hyperactivity disorder (Taylor 1986). However, it is usually crucial to involve parents in treatment and there are several ways of doing this. The work might be done primarily with parents, for example, working on marital difficulties and parenting. Alternatively, parents could be invited to support individual work with the child and be encouraged to change any of their own behaviours that are unwittingly maintaining their child's problems. Finally, family therapy could be carried out to alter family interactional patterns.

Working with adolescents

Treatment of older adolescents is more likely to rely on individual work, reflecting the adolescent's greater verbal abilities and maturity. There is a clear evidence-base for using talking therapies with adolescents, such as cognitive–behavioural therapy (Wilkes et al 1994). The involvement of parents can again be to varying degrees, depending on the formulation of the problem. Treatment effectiveness can still be influenced by the support that parents show for treatment.

Assessing and treating child and adolescent mental health problems can be complex because children referred to mental health services often suffer from many difficulties (Costello 1989). For more complex problems, a multidisciplinary and multiagency assessment and treatment approach is preferable.

The child in the context of the family

Families affect children's development across a variety of domains that encompass cognitive, emotional and social development (Boyum & Parke 1999). As has already been outlined, children referred to child and adolescent mental health services can have a combination of individual difficulties and problems within the family system. This section will look at the role of the family in the development and maintenance of child psychopathology in more detail.

Families consist not just of individual members but include the relationships of each member to one another, and with the family as a whole, that together constitute the 'family unit' (Frude 1990). The family is therefore a system (Von Bertanlanffy 1968) that strives to maintain stability by balancing the individuality of its members with the cohesiveness of the unit. A change in one part of the system has repercussions for the whole unit as it adapts to that change in order to maintain equilibrium. According to Frude (1990), a family that is well structured and communicates effectively is likely to function well.

Families need to be flexible to manage stressors to the system such as bereavement, illness, divorce or financial difficulties. In addition, the family is a developing unit in which relationships change in response to the developing child. Younger children demand more parental involvement because they seek stimulation from within the family and consequently require greater structure and limit setting. As the child progresses towards adolescence, stimulation is increasingly sought outside the family as peer relationships develop, thus resulting in a renegotiation of boundaries and limits. Problems arise when there is poor communication, deficient structure and poor adaptation to change (Frude 1990).

Elements within the family system that can be potential risk factors for child psychopathology will now be examined, including the parent–child relationship, parental mental health problems and the marital relationship. Following this, some of the factors that can maintain family problems will be reviewed.

The parent–child relationship

The quality of the parent–child relationship significantly affects how children view themselves and the world around them, according to attachment theory (Bowlby 1969). Ainsworth et al (1978) identified different types of attachment relationship based on their assessment tool the Strange Situation Test. If a child receives warm and responsive parenting they develop a secure attachment that produces a positive self-concept and good peer relationships. This secure attachment protects the child against the development of psychological problems. In contrast, children with an anxious/avoidant pattern of attachment are likely to have experienced interaction with an unresponsive, inaccessible or inappropriately responsive caregiver that increases the risk of developing potential problems (Crittenden & Ainsworth 1989). Indeed, parent–child interaction that is characterized by high levels of criticism and lack of warmth/approval can indicate child maltreatment or neglect (Iwaniec 1995).

Parental mental health problems

Parental mental health has also been found to be associated with child adjustment. Maternal anxiety disorder has been found to significantly predict the presence of anxiety disorders in children (McClure et al 2001). Children with psychosocial problems are more likely to have mothers who are depressed (Downey & Coyne 1990). Parental problems such as depression, alcohol abuse or criminality can increase the child's vulnerability to psychological problems by affecting the quality of the attachment relationship and by modelling dysfunctional coping strategies (Carr 1999).

Recent research on parental beliefs has highlighted the relationship between these beliefs and parenting behaviour. For example, the ability to take a child-centred perspective has been found to be related to greater parental responsiveness (Landry et al 1996). Abusive parents have been found to hold unrealistic expectations of their children, thus triggering abusive behaviour when children fail to meet these expectations (Azar et al 1984). Bugental & Shennum (1984) demonstrated that parental beliefs about their own power in caregiving situations influenced their perceptions of children and parenting behaviour.

The marital relationship

The quality of the marital relationship has also been found to be a significant predictor of childhood disorders such as depression, withdrawal, aggression and poor academic performance (Katz & Gottman 1994) and is strongly associated with conduct disorder (Kazdin 1995). Boys who witnessed parental abuse in their early years have been found to be more likely to instigate marital abuse as adults (Egeland 1988).

Family maintenance factors

Some of the family factors that can lead to psychological problems have been looked at. How the family unit responds to psychological problems can also be crucial in keeping the problems going. Carr (1999) outlines various family interaction patterns involved in the maintenance of children's problems. Four of these will be outlined: inadvertent reinforcement, coercive interaction patterns, disengagement and triangulation.

Parents or siblings can unwittingly reinforce the child's problem behaviour by offering attention to it, a process called inadvertent reinforcement. Coercive interaction patterns can develop in which the child's aggression is negatively reinforced as the parent's behaviour becomes increasingly aversive and they then withdraw when the child's agression escalates. Parental disengagement can occur, resulting in low levels of parental supervision and consequently there is increased susceptibility to peer pressure and delinquency (Steinberg 1986). Triangulation is a process in which there is an alliance between one parent and the child, resulting in marginalization of the other parent. This pattern is common in families with unacknowledged marital problems because the child's difficulties can serve as a useful distraction from the parents' relationship.

Summary

- Mental health services are available within the NHS for children and adolescents with a range of methods for assessment and intervention.

- Children and adolescents develop mental health problems within the context of the family unit.

- Factors within the family system predispose the child to develop psychological problems and are essential components of both assessment and intervention.

- How families respond to these difficulties will affect prognosis and outcome of any intervention.

References

Abidin R R 1995 Parenting stress index. Psychological Assessment Resources, Odessa, FL

Ainsworth M D, Blehar M C, Waters E, Wall S 1978 Patterns of attachment. Lawrence Erlbaum Associates, Inc., Hillsdale, NJ

Angold A, Prendergast A, Cox R et al 1995 The child and adolescent psychiatric assessment (CAPA). Psychological Medicine 25:739–753

Axline V 1989 Play therapy. Houghton Mifflin, Boston, MA

Azar S T, Robinson D R, Hekimian E, Twentyman C T 1984 Unrealistic expectations and problem-solving ability in maltreating and comparison mothers. Journal of Consulting and Clinical Psychology 52:687–691

Bayley N 1993 Bayley scales of infant development, 2nd edn. Psychological Corporation, San Antonio

Bene J, Anthony J 1957 Manual for the family relations test. National Foundations for Education Research, London

Binney V, Wright J C 1997 The bag of feelings: an ideographic technique for the assessment and exploration of feelings in children and adolescents. Clinical Child Psychology and Psychiatry 2:449–462

Blatt S J, Zohar A, Quinlan D M et al 1996 Levels of relatedness within the dependency factor of the Depressive Experiences Questionnaire for Adolescents. Journal of Personality Assessment 62:52–71

Bowlby J 1969 Attachment and loss, vol 1: Attachment. Basic Books, New York

Boyum L A, Parke R D 1999 Family. In: Silverman W K, Ollendick T H (eds) Developmental issues in the clinical treatment of children. Allyn & Bacon, Boston, p 141–155

Bugental D, Shennum W A 1984 Difficult children as elicitors and targets of adult communication patterns: an attributional–behavioural transactional analysis. Monographs of the Society for Research in Child Development 49:1–69

Carr A 1999 The handbook of child and adolescent clinical psychology: a contextual approach. Routledge, London

Conners C K 1997 Conners' Parent Rating Scale – Revised. Multi-Health Systems, Inc., North Tonawanda, NY

Connor D F, Fisher S G 1997 An interactional model of child and adolescent mental health clinical case formulation. Clinical Child Psychology and Psychiatry 2:353–368

Costello E J 1989 Developments in child psychiatric epidemiology. Journal of the American Academy of Child and Adolescent Psychiatry 28:836–841

Crittenden P M, Ainsworth M D S 1989 Child maltreatment and attachment theory. In: Cicchetti D, Carlson V (eds) Child maltreatment. Cambridge University Press, New York, p 432–463

Downey G, Coyne J C 1990 Children of depressed parents: an integrative review. Psychological Bulletin 108:50–76

Egeland B 1988 Breaking the cycle of abuse: implications for prediction and intervention. In: Browne K, Davies C, Stratton P (eds) Early prediction and prevention of child abuse. Wiley, Chichester

Frude N 1990 Understanding family problems: a psychological approach. Wiley, Chichester

Geldard K, Geldard D 1997 Counselling children: a practical introduction. Sage, London

Graham P 1998 Cognitive behaviour therapy for children and families. Cambridge University Press, Cambridge

Iwaniec D 1995 The emotionally abused and neglected child. Wiley, Chichester

Katz L F, Gottman J M 1994 Patterns of marital interaction and children's emotional development. In: Parke R D, Kellam S G (eds) Exploring family relationships with other social contexts. Lawrence Erlbaum Associates, Inc., Hillsdale, NJ, p 49–74

Kazdin A 1995 Conduct disorders in childhood and adolescence. Sage, Thousand Oaks, CA

Landry S H, Garner P W, Swank P R, Baldwin C D 1996 Effects of maternal scaffolding during joint toy play with preterm and full-term infants. Merrill-Palmer Quarterly 42:177–199

Lang M, Tisher M 1978 Children's depression scale CDS (9–16 years), research edn. Hawthorn Vic, Australian Council for Educational Research

McClure E B, Brennan P A, Hammen C, Le-Brocque R M 2001 Parental anxiety disorders, child anxiety disorders and the perceived parent–child relationship in an Australian high-risk sample. Journal of Abnormal Child Psychology 29:1–10

Sadeh A, Anders T F 1993 Infant sleep problems: origins, assessment and interventions. Infant Mental Health Journal 14:17–34

Steinberg L 1986 Latchkey children and susceptibility to peer pressure: an ecological analysis. Developmental Psychology 22:433–439

Taylor E A 1986 The overactive child. Blackwell Scientific Publications, Oxford

Von Bertanlanffy L 1968 General systems theory. Braziller, New York

Wechsler D 1991 Intelligence scale for children, 3rd edn. Psychological Corporation, San Antonio

Wilkes T C R, Belsher G, Rush A J, Frank E 1994 Cognitive therapy for depressed adolescents. Guilford, London

Part B: A PHYSIOTHERAPIST'S CONTRIBUTION TO A CHILD GUIDANCE CLINIC

Diana Beaven

This part of the chapter describes the innovative contribution of a physiotherapist to a child guidance clinic using an approach that includes creative movement and touch.

Introduction

Children delight in kinaesthetic sensations, thus movement and touch can be potent interventions. Most children enjoy the acquisition of physical skills and, provided that relaxation is taught using a method appropriate to their age group, youngsters will usually be receptive. Awareness of tension, posture and movement, learned through relaxation, will act as a buffer against stress and illhealth in later life and influence vitality and the development of 'self' concept (Gullensten et al 1999).

Relaxation techniques can be worked successfully into physical education periods at school but there is also a place for their application in the classroom, e.g. checking finger tension in writing, drawing and the playing of musical instruments. Older children can usefully talk about stress-provoking situations, e.g. bullying, parental rows and examinations. They enjoy taking their pulse, breathing rate and other objective measures of human functioning and can master the Laura Mitchell method of relaxation (Mitchell 1977).

Infants can feel overwhelmed by rage and need vigorous physical activity to release strong emotion. This activity needs to be followed by a slow and controlled task, e.g. walking along an imaginary tightrope or freezing when the leader 'casts a spell' over the group. It is necessary to have this quietening-down time after the expressive activity to ground children's energy and prevent them from feeling out of control.

Besides the teaching of relaxation to children in mainstream schools, there is an application to individuals with special needs. For 1 year, the author gave sessional input as a physiotherapist to a child guidance clinic, working closely with a multidisciplinary team. Children who demonstrated emotional and behavioural disorder were seen in the context of their families. A child experiencing difficulties might be reflecting problems within the family (see the first part of this chapter). In addition to the family receiving help from the multidisciplinary team, the team asked the author to become involved with children who were experiencing symptoms that were physical in nature or related to body energy. The problems included hyperventilation, migraine, bedwetting, aggression and hyperactivity. The approach involved relaxation, calm breathing and creative movement, supplemented by counselling of the child and family. The interventions for several children are outlined in the following examples.

Individual case studies

Hyperventilation

Case study: Jane

> Jane was 14 and had experienced several panic attacks at school. She was frightened of the sensation of not being able to breathe and concerned by her sickness absence from school. The therapist spent some time listening to Jane, and used her hands to gently release muscular holding in her supine body, encouraging the spine to lengthen and widen. This created greater openness in the chest and abdomen, allowing the diaphragm to move more freely and the breathing to settle. In the third session, diagrams were used to expand the explanation of the symptoms of hyperventilation and related this to her feelings of panic. Jane began to understand how the asthma she had largely outgrown had left her breathing with excessive upper chest movement, which accelerated when she was anxious.
>
> William Reich (cited in Dychtwald 1986) describes the cathartic release of emotion through manipulation of physical tissue. The hands-on approach to releasing muscular tension and freeing the breathing helped Jane to express some of her present worries. She related episodes of bullying at school, which preceded the panic attacks. Jane was happy for this information to be passed on to the team psychologist, who was planning a meeting with Jane's mother and her teacher. Jane was taught some stretching and shaking movements of her body to help her wind down after school. As muscular tension decreased, Jane found that she was better able to discuss her worries with her mother. After five weekly sessions, Jane felt able to cope with school confidently and had learned to relax, breathe freely and express her difficulties.

Hyperactivity

Case study: Karen

Karen was a restless, overactive but endearing 6-year-old. She was eager to please but could not keep still. The team psychiatrist, after meeting Karen and her family, was not able to identify any family dynamics or allergic food reactions that might be influencing the hyperactivity. Indeed, the family seemed stable, loving and healthy. Karen was more at ease when allowed to move freely around the room, sometimes rocking and balancing on furniture and the floor. In her restlessness, she appeared to be searching for rhythms. With her mother's assistance, ways for Karen to enjoy movements that involved steadying rhythms were explored. Sitting back to back on the floor rocking in different directions with the therapist and then with her mother, helped her to settle. The value of using swings, hammocks and rocking chairs was explained. The therapist experimented with different pieces of music to find what rhythms encouraged Karen to express her restlessness in creative movement; slow steady music helped her to find calming movement rhythms for her body.

Dance-type movement, which brings a person's energy down into the lower limbs, is useful. The position of hips and knees bent, as in a Zulu warrior's stamping and in Tai Chi, can be very grounding, i.e. can settle a person's energy. Karen enjoyed lunging and movement, performed very slowly and steadily in the skiing posture. At the end of each session, Karen and her mother lay down for a few minutes, contracting and relaxing different parts of their bodies, then becoming aware of the contact of their floppy bodies with the floor. Karen was encouraged to think of stroking her cat and to capture all the detail of this scene (children have a good visual memory). The stroking of Karen's forehead helped her to settle.

As a result of these sessions Karen and her mother found ways to channel and modify Karen's restless energy; however there was no permanent change. A break in the sessions was agreed while Karen's mother took her to a cranial osteopath. Five treatments proved dramatically helpful in relieving Karen's restlessness. Karen's birth was by forceps, and as a baby she had been distressed and tearful, with an erratic sleep problem. She had been happiest when rocked and carried around. The cranial osteopath defined the problems as a distortion in the cranium that was compromising the normal slight degree of mobility in the bones and meninges. The osteopath viewed this mobility as essential to health. With a very gentle hold of the head and light use of pressure, the cranial osteopath worked to encourage tissue motion and improve fluid dynamics. Six months after the final osteopathic treatment, Karen's mother said her daughter had sustained the improvement in concentration and well-being and seemed much happier and less restless (Harries 2000).

Examples of work with preteens and teenagers

An aggressive teenage girl presented with premenstrual mood swings and irritability leading to violent outbursts. She was seen for five individual sessions of relaxation and movement, weekly at first, then fortnightly. By the last session she described feeling calmer and her parents reported a decline in her destructive and abusive behaviour. Practical work with teenagers in each case included a counselling element. In the author's experience, the release of muscular tension brings the person a greater awareness of feeling and willingness to discuss worries and conflicts.

A teenage boy who regularly wet his bed responded to a similar blend of relaxation and counselling. Although dialogue with the parents is important, the majority of teenagers benefit from having most of their sessions alone with the physiotherapist.

Several aggressive boys, between the ages of 9 and 13 years, needed more robust intervention. Had the referrals been received at around the same time, a group might have been effective, but this was not the case. A group would have allowed the boys to learn from each other in imaginative ways and pit their strength against equals. With the use of a creative movement approach, strong but playful actions can be explored with individuals. Movements were chosen to provide outlets for excessive energy, anger and frustration. The need to be masterful and expressive was also acknowledged. On one occasion, the young person and therapist sat on the floor back to back, while they both tried to push the other across the floor. Pushing in pairs in the standing position with the back, the arms, the side and hips provided opportunities to express strength and resistance. Where possible, siblings were allowed to join in these games; stamping to African rhythms, punching pillows and using the voice, movement and breathing proved exhilarating and cathartic. After vigorous expression, it was sometimes appropriate to teach the young people a quiet relaxation technique. There was a need to explore opportunities, to express this unbridled energy at home and school – sport, drumming and the martial arts were found to be helpful, especially when these provided a context for father and son to be involved together.

A multidisciplinary approach to sexual abuse

Multidisciplinary working can link together the psychological and the practical. For example, the author and a clinical psychologist jointly facilitated a group of three sexually abused girls, sharing professional skills. Some elements of the treatment report by the author and psychologist describing this group are included in this section. The group dynamic developed from verbal disclosure of the problems to practical exercises chosen to provide the opportunity to work through the difficulties. Relaxation and breathing helped to release contracted pelvic muscles and to free diaphragmatic breathing when upper chest breathing was precipitating panic and insomnia. The therapist's touch, a stretch of taut neck muscles or a hand to guide breathing helped to convey acceptance of the body and the person and a welcoming of physical sensations. Creative movement in pairs was used to explore the roles of leading and following; this led to a discussion of the girls' fear of being out of control when not being in charge of a situation. Assertiveness role-plays were enjoyed, with feedback given to the girls on voice and posture to help them understand the signals conveyed by their body language. The theme of making choices and saying 'no' was explored in this way. The girls' facial expressions changed as they moved with ease into games resisting physical pressure. The girls described feelings of empowerment and appeared to gain confidence in approaching the theme of power and choice through movement and voice work. They gained a sense of how posture could convey purpose and how to feel less like victims through assertion of their needs. Ways in which body language could unwittingly play a part in eliciting further abusive behaviour were discussed.

Physical and psychological approach

There are advantages in non-verbal approaches in abuse work. An insistence that the abused person uses words to disclose the experience may echo the intrusiveness and pressure experienced in the original abuse (see Chapter 23). Non-verbal approaches can feel less intrusive. They create a space for these young people to move through their difficulties and become more mentally and physically agile.

A common feature of most forms of therapy for physiological difficulties is the bringing of order out of a debilitating sense of uncertainty or chaos, and a regaining of an empowering sense of control. Non-verbal therapies increase confidence in the ability to bring order out of chaos by allowing a means of expression and the experience of control, mastery and achievement non-verbally. There might also be an inherent human awareness of a need for order, balance and rhythm. Meeting this need and restoring balance and rhythm is both healing and empowering; non-verbal therapies can facilitate this process more easily than verbal methods (Beaven & Tollinton 1994).

Dissociation

Violation of boundaries can lead to a loss of the sense of the individual as a separate self. Vizard (1988) described an abused girl adapting to sexual penetration by splitting her thought processes from her bodily feelings in a way which persisted over years. By sharing the facilitation of the group between disciplines holding knowledge and expertise in the combined fields of the body and the mind, an opportunity was provided for the abused girls to make links between the physical and the psychological and thus avoid the splitting of thinking processes from bodily feelings.

Outcomes   Interestingly, the least verbal member of the group was able to participate in practical work with considerable ease; presumably this felt less direct and less threatening than self-disclosure. Her verbal contributions were often banal platitudes, which she appeared to have learned, perhaps as a defence against real emotion and following much legal statutory involvement. Her speech, however, became more spontaneous after expressive movement. Reluctant to push the girls into experiential work, we started sessions by talking, but on reflection felt that this hindered development of the sessions. Practical work freed the child within and led to more authentic discussion earlier in each session. To move is to know, the sense of knowing in one's bones was reached through bodily awareness work even when the mind had forgotten (Foster 1976).

In the work with the girls, the body and mind were viewed as a Gestalt. 'The individual is viewed as an integrated unity . . . Mind and the body reflect and effect each other' (Bernstein 1982).

Freud (1923) described the ego as first and foremost a bodily ego. Perhaps by working through the body to help the mind to remember the trauma, there was less need for the splitting of thought processes from bodily feeling. To use a metaphor (Bentovim et al 1991), the black hole in the memory created by the mind splitting off the trauma had been faced within the comfort and support of a group. This lessened the need for either the body or the mind to focus on the pain and freed the girls to move on with their lives.

In the fifth group session, the girls worked together to write a poem on the theme of 'the mind forgets but the body remembers' (Vizard 1988). An adapted version appears in Box 16.1.

Efforts to make a formal evaluation of the usefulness of the group meetings, although limited to a sample evaluation questionnaire designed for the group and a self-esteem questionnaire (Lawrence 1981), did give support to the hypothesis that helpful changes had occurred. Meetings with the adolescents and their carers after the groups had ended also showed that, in each family, at that time, both

Box 16.1
The mind forgets but the body remembers

> The body is on edge, the mind cannot explain it. Why is the body beyond the control of the mind?
> The mind should be in control, but the mind wants to forget, to be numb to the pain of the past.
> The body takes over as the mind tries to shut off.
> And yet has the mind succeeded or does the memory remain?
> The body bears the scars, the mind too has been ravaged but it tries hard to hide its distress.
> The anguish is locked away in a small room of the mind.
> A password spoken unwittingly opens the door to the pain.
> Deep down the hurt is still there; can it one day be released?
> I think the mind can begin to let go of the pain by talking with other minds. It will help – at least.

the adults and the adolescents were pleased with the improvement. All reported good progress at school and good relationships with friends and within the family. The family members showed confidence in their ability to cope successfully without further professional therapeutic help at that time (the meetings for two families were after 2 months and for the third family after 5 months).

Conclusion

During the course of the group, the therapists saw positive changes in communication patterns, body language, muscle tension, breathing and general demeanour of the group members. This impression of an increased sense of well-being and improved body image and self-image was confirmed by group members' comments expressed in the evaluation that they were coping more effectively with their lives and were more at ease generally. It appeared that movement and touch, in association with psychological therapy, freed the girls to make changes in their lives.

Subsequent follow-up suggested that they were generally more able to take part in life's experiences and friendship and that these influences helped to continue the process of healing.

Summary

- Expressive movement and relaxation training are important therapeutic interventions for disturbed children.

- Therapeutic touch can be of benefit in releasing breathing and reducing panic attacks.

- Movement and body work combined with verbal expression can be used to influence body image and self image following abuse.

References

Beaven D, Tollinton G 1994 Healing the spirit: a psychological approach to working with sexually abused teenage girls. Physiotherapy 80:7

Bentovim A, Vizard E, Hollows A (eds) 1991 Children and young people as abusers. National Children's Bureau, London.

Bernstein P L (ed) 1982 Eight theoretical approaches in dance movement therapy. Kendal/Hunt Publishing Co, New York, p 171

Dychtwald K 1986 Bodymind. St Martin's Press, New York, p 101

Foster R 1976 Knowing in my bones. A & C Black, London, p 13, 112

Freud S 1923 The complete works of Sigmund Freud, vol 19, The ego and the id, 1923–25 (ed Strachey J 1961). Hogarth Press, London, p 26

Gullensten A L, Edahl C, Hansson L 1999 Validity of the Body Awareness Scale – Health. Scandinavian Journal of the Caring Sciences 13:217–226

Harries R A 2000 Craniosacral therapy. In: Charman R (ed) Complementary therapies for physical therapists. Butterworth-Heinemann, Oxford

Lawrence D 1981 The development of a self-esteem questionnaire. British Journal of Educational Psychology 51:245–251

Mitchell L 1977 Simple relaxation. Pitman Press, Bath

Vizard E 1988 Child sexual abuse: the child's experiences. British Journal of Psychotherapy 5(1): 77–91

Further Reading

Madders J 1979 Stress and relaxation. Acro, New York

Thornquist E, Bundan B H 1991 What is psychomotor therapy? Norwegian University Press, Oslo, p 17

Varma V P 1990 The management of children with emotional and behavioural difficulties. Routledge, London

Part C: PLAY AND OCCUPATIONAL THERAPY

Gita Ingram

This part of the chapter aims to give an overview of the concept of play and playing in the growing child. The development of play and its functions will be explored. Finally, some occupational therapy interventions using play will be discussed.

There are many varied definitions of play and playing. Bundy (1996) has described play as being driven by pleasure and fun. In contrast to working, the pleasure comes primarily from the process of playing itself rather than from any achievement or end product. Nevertheless, playing is a highly purposeful activity. For the small child, play is a way of expressing his or her inner feelings and experiences and is as vital to development as eating and sleeping (Steiner 1999).

The explorative nature of play

Through play, young children explore their physical surroundings in terms of space, shapes, textures, what goes in where and what happens when things come apart and are put together. This helps them develop a sense of their own bodies in relation to the external world. Manipulating objects and completing tasks give children a sense of order and a feeling of achievement. They are also exploring their own resources and the nature and extent of their own feelings during play and as evoked by playing. Copley & Forrayan (1987) state that:

> *Children seem to use play from a very early age as a spontaneous means of working out their relationship to the world about them, and to other people, and as a way of overcoming difficulties, whether physical or emotional. Indeed, a child who seems unable to play is usually a cause for concern.*

Winnicott (1971) considered playing to be a way of thinking. He said that in playing, and perhaps only in playing, is an individual free to be creative. Children play in order to think things out in a similar way to the way that adults play with their thoughts as a means of working things out. In play, children's experiences, their wishes, fears and fantasies of love, hate, separation, destruction and power can be explored. The emotionally healthy child knows that play is make-believe and therefore can be interrupted should the anxiety become overwhelming. This might be because of the strength of feeling evoked by the play or in peer play, because of rivalry between the children.

For play to be used in this way it needs to take place in a safe setting. Should the make-believe break down and the fear or the toy fight become real, a trusted adult needs to be available to contain the situation and help restore order. Children need to know that the adult is present in mind as well as in body and can tolerate the strength of feelings expressed without themselves becoming overwhelmed. If children sense that their parents are not emotionally available in this way, maybe because of illness, stress, tiredness or preoccupation with their own worries, they tend to stick to safe activities, such as structured activities or television (Hoxter 1977). This has serious implications for children who experience chronic maternal depression, emotional deprivation or neglect in respect of their ability to utilize play and shared playing for exploration. The ability of children to play and thereby develop healthily both physically and emotionally is therefore closely linked with the nature of early attachment relationships between child and parent or parent figure. A secure enough attachment is a prerequisite for the child to be able to grow through play.

Play as a rehearsal for social learning and mastery of the environment

Play in the young infant starts off as autoerotic and involves sucking or manipulating parts of the self or parts not yet differentiated from the self (Ingram 2001). This gradually helps the infant work out the boundary and relationship between me and not-me. Two early forms of play are the peep-bo game and throwing toys away and getting them back again. Both involve brief separations and reunions and can be seen as the child's way of working through anxieties about separation, loss and abandonment as well as achieving mastery in a situation over which, in reality he or she has no control (Steiner 1999).

The toddler does not yet have a concept of playing with other children. Social play at this stage consists of parallel play in the presence of a trusted adult alongside another child, watching each other, copying each other and sometimes handing toys to one another. Gradually, in the playgroup or nursery setting children learn not only about doing things but also about relationships with other children, about playing together, taking turns and sharing.

By the time children reach school, play themes are expanded to include more excitement and suspense. An increasing amount of negotiation and sometimes fights over rules and fair play take place. By the ages of seven or eight play becomes more elaborate and influences from popular culture such as television, computer games and reading of fiction are woven into play themes to enrich and stimulate them. Playing on the edge of fear and triumph provides a means of expressing and confronting children's own life experiences (Hoxter 1977).

In adolescence, the process of relinquishing the primary attachment to parents begins; this continues into adulthood. Childhood playing is replaced by adolescent group culture where the peer group can provide a major part of a teenager's precarious and rapidly changing identity (Lanyado 1999).

Winnicott (1971) made the link between playing and cultural experience. He stated that cultural experience begins with creative living first manifested in play. This provides a way of seeing play on a continuum towards the development into creative experience and expression of culture in adolescence and adulthood.

Interventions through play

As a child's natural occupation, play is of central importance in occupational therapy with children, whether itself used as a therapeutic tool or whether used as a means of engaging with a child where the process of play is not the primary focus of the intervention. Various forms of play therapy are used by many occupational therapists who often have undergone postgraduate training to equip them with skills in this specialist area.

To understand what makes play therapeutic it is helpful to draw on the components of good enough parenting, i.e. safety and containment, consistency and the permission for free expression.

Some children are not able to play, often because of adverse early experiences or lack of adequate parenting. Winnicott (1971) states that 'where playing is not possible then the work done by the therapist is directed towards bringing the child from a state of not being able to play into a state of being able to play'.

Assessment and treatment through play can span from non-directive or child-centred models to more focused therapeutic or directive play. Whichever approach is used, the value of observation in learning about the child cannot be underestimated. Observing a baby or an older child at home, in nursery or in school, or indeed in the clinic setting, offers an opportunity to think in a meaningful way about the child's communications and subjective experience.

Virginia Axline adapted Carl Rodgers' person-centred counselling technique to working with children. This is based on reflective listening, acceptance, empathy and genuineness (Rodgers 1951). Axline's eight principles of non-directive play therapy (Axline 1989) remain popular with many occupational therapists and offer a useful technique for forming an effective therapeutic alliance with the child (Box 16.2). In today's climate of brief interventions and the need for throughput, therapists might wish to adapt some aspects of the technique to add some focus on the child's particular difficulties. However, the adherence to maintaining a respect for the child's ability to know and solve his or her own problems, to follow where the child leads, will ensure that the child's agenda remains central.

Box 16.2
*Axline's eight
principles of play
therapy*

1. The therapist must develop a warm friendly relationship with the child, in which good rapport is established as soon as possible.
2. The therapist accepts the child exactly as he or she is.
3. The therapist establishes a feeling of permissiveness in the relationship so that the child feels free to express his or her feelings completely.
4. The therapist is alert to recognize the *feelings* the child is expressing and reflects those feelings back in such a manner that the child gains insight into his or her behaviour.
5. The therapist maintains a deep respect for the child's ability to solve his or her own problems if given an opportunity to do so. The responsibility to make choices and to institute change is the child's.
6. The therapist does not attempt to direct the child's actions or conversation in any manner. The child leads the way; the therapist follows.
7. The therapist does not attempt to hurry the therapy along. It is a gradual process and is recognized as such by the therapist.
8. The therapist establishes only those limitations that are necessary to anchor the therapy to the world of reality and to make the child aware of his or her responsibility in the relationship.

Assessment

Using play therapy models, assessment of a child's emotional state will include the following:

- *General presentation.* Physical appearance, physical and emotional developmental level, level of activity, attachment patterns.
- *Emotional response and communication.* This includes ways of communicating, whether verbal or non-verbal, affect, self-esteem, awareness of feelings of self and others.
- *Thought content.* Worries, fears, wishes, fantasies.
- *Play.* Ability to play, content, use of symbolism, age appropriateness.
- *Function of play and activity for the child.* Not all play is creative or therapeutic. Activity that looks like play might be the child keeping busy to avoid thinking or knowing about that which is too difficult (Ingram 2001).

Such an assessment, done over two to four sessions, can be used to inform other members of the multidisciplinary team in their work with the family or larger system, or it can form a basis for longer-term play therapy.

Bundy (1997) considers that it might be playfulness, rather than play activities that, when evaluated, provides therapists with the information they seek regarding the child's development. She developed a Test of Playfulness (ToP), which gives a framework for evaluating playfulness in young children. Each child is observed for internal or external perception of control, intrinsic or extrinsic source of motivation and free or not free suspension of reality in order to give a playfulness profile (Blunden 2001).

Interventions

Play therapy treatment interventions can be time limited or open ended, and aims will vary accordingly. However, it is recognized that play therapy is no quick fix, and it is therefore generally reserved for children with extensive difficulties resulting from acute trauma, loss or chronic emotional deprivation. Often, parallel work with the parents or carers will be offered by another clinician. It is important to give careful thought to when play therapy is indicated. A child who is experiencing abuse will wish for the abuse to stop but will not be ready for therapy. A child who is being scapegoated in his or her family and where parents and other family members have an investment in the child having difficulties, will again not benefit from play therapy, until these issues are addressed. The child's situation should be relatively stable and the child's carers supportive to ensure a feeling of safety and space in mind to explore emotional issues or relationships. Meanwhile, the child's ongoing well-being still needs addressing and some form of safe play is very important.

This well known poem reflects the sense of mastery experienced in play, but also the need to safely be able to return to reality.

Swing song

Here I go up in my swing
Ever so high.
I am the King of the fields, and the King
Of the town.
I am the King of the earth, and the King
Of the sky.
Here I go up in my swing . . .
Now I go down.

A.A. Milne (1927)

Summary

- Play is central to human development and changes with different developmental stages.

- Play provides pleasure as well as a means of learning about the physical environment and relationships, of managing anxiety and of thinking things out.

- Play is closely linked with emotional health, creativity and culture.

- Play offers a unique holistic therapeutic medium for occupational therapists to assess and treat a variety of psychological conditions in children.

References

Axline V M 1989 Play therapy, 2nd edn. Churchill Livingstone, Edinburgh

Blunden P 2001 The therapeutic use of play. In: Longher L (ed) Occupational therapy for child and adolescent mental health. Churchill Livingstone, Edinburgh, p 67–86

Bundy A C 1996 Play, possibilities, problems, paradoxes. National Association of Paediatric Occupational Therapists' Newsletter, Autumn:29

Copley B, Forrayan B 1987 Therapeutic work with children and young people. Robert Royce, London.

Hoxter S 1977 Play and communication. In: Boston M, Daws D (eds) The child psychotherapist and problems of young people. Wildwood House, London, p 202–231

Ingram G 2001 Psychodynamic theories. In: Lougher L (ed) Occupational therapy for child and adolescent mental health. Churchill Livingstone, Edinburgh, p 97–110

Lanyado M 1999 'It's just an ordinary pain': thoughts on joy and heartache in puberty and early adolescence. In: Hindle D, Smith M V (eds) Personality development. Routledge, London, p 92–115

Milne A A 1927 Now we are six. Methuen, London

Rodgers C 1951 Client-centred therapy. Houghton Mifflin, Boston

Steiner D 1999 The toddler and the wider world. In: Hindle D, Smith M V (eds) Personality development. Routledge, London, p 48–70

Winnicott D W 1971 Playing and reality. Tavistock, London

17 Physical activity and falls prevention in older people with dementia

Pam Dawson and Helen Buri

Introduction

Older adults are vulnerable to mental illnesses in the same way as younger people are susceptible. Mental disorders commonly affecting older adults can be classified as organic or functional in nature. The organic disorders include the dementias, of which Alzheimer's disease is the most common cause. Other forms of dementia affecting the older person include dementia with Lewey bodies (DLB), vascular dementia and New Variant Creutzfeldt–Jakob disease (CJD). The most common functional disorder to occur among the older population is depression, which can be either the reactive or the psychotic type. All of these conditions have been well covered by Creek (2002) and Everett et al (1995). This chapter looks at the case for service development in physiotherapy and occupational therapy and the potential for therapists to use physical activity as a tool for falls prevention in older adults with dementia. Findings from multidisciplinary research are presented to illustrate the developing evidence-base for interventions and to highlight the important contribution of the carer in promoting physical activity and preventing falls.

Incidence and prevalence of mental illness in older adults

Dementia is stated as being difficult to diagnose, not least because in a third of cases, it is associated with other psychiatric symptoms such as depression (Eccles et al 1998). In the National Service Framework (NSF) for Older People it is suggested that depression in people over the age of 65 years is underdiagnosed, in addition to which older people and their families might regard mental illnesses as an inevitable part of ageing (Department of Health 2001). All of these factors mean that estimating the incidence and prevalence of mental illnesses is problematic.

Eccles et al (1998) report that the prevalence of dementia is thought to be about 20% at 80 years of age. Similarly, the Alzheimer's Society estimates that one in five persons over 80 years has dementia, compared with one in 50 aged between 65 and 70 years. Both prevalence and incidence increase with age. Ott et al (1998) found that women were twice as susceptible to developing dementia as men. Dementia is associated with an increased morbidity and mortality (Dewey & Saz 2001, Witthaus et al 1999). Kirby et al (1998) found that the death rate per 100 000 population from Alzheimer's disease has increased from less than 1 in 1979 to 19 for men and 21 for women in 1996.

The case for service development in physiotherapy and occupational therapy

The number of people over the age of 80 will increase by 50% between 1995 and 2025 (Department of Health 2001), and this will inevitably be associated with an increase in older people with mental health problems. Physiotherapy and occupational therapy services need to respond to the challenges laid down by the NSF for Older People (Department of Health 2001). Standard 7 of the NSF sets the scene for the development of integrated multidisciplinary services for older people with mental health problems, and standard 8 has an emphasis on modifying risk factors for disease, regardless of age. In particular, programmes for increasing physical activity are listed as key interventions for the promotion of health and active life in older age, and there is no reason for older people with mental health problems to be excluded from such programmes. The NHS Plan (Department of Health 2000) provides for an increase of allied health professionals in the care of older people, which offers further potential for development of physiotherapy and occupational therapy. However, services need to develop in an evidence-based fashion, with research to underpin practice, and physiotherapy and occupational therapy in the care of older people with dementia has not yet been subject to extensive evaluation. In the field of occupational therapy, research has tended to focus on the assessment of the person and on articulating the nature of human occupation for people with dementia (Borrell et al 1994, Perrin 1997), rather than on the effectiveness of interventions. On the other hand, physiotherapy research has begun to focus on the effectiveness of core interventions, such as mobility training (Pomeroy et al 1999) without a fully developed knowledge base of the relationship between behavioural elements of dementia and the mobility of the affected person (Pomeroy 1995).

The case for physical activity

In the social theory of ageing, two opposing explanations are given. Social Disengagement theory suggests that there is a mutual withdrawal of the person from society and *vice versa*. (Creek 2002). By contrast, Activity Theory proposes that there is a positive association between participation in social activity and life satisfaction (Perrin 1997). However, a 'middle ground' explanation may be more realistic.

The use of physical activity as a therapeutic tool is fundamental to both occupational therapy and physiotherapy. In occupational therapy, both 'occupation' and 'activity' are used to describe performance in the areas of self-care, work and leisure, for example cooking or dressing. Physical activity in the form of therapeutic movement and exercise represents the very core of physiotherapeutic intervention. Engagement in occupation or activity is valued as integrally linked to health and wellness, and its absence as a threat to health (Turner et al 1992).

In the care of an older person with dementia, wellness, rather than improvement in health status, is the focus. Traditional models of rehabilitation are rejected (Perrin & May 2000). More favoured are approaches in which therapists maintain prolonged contact with the older person, collaborate with their carers and match activities (and later, simple actions) to their level of cognitive decline (Clark et al 1995, Corcoran 1993, Perrin & May 2000). The concept of ensuring an appropriate level of challenge within the activity, known as the 'person–environment fit', remains central to therapy (Baum 1995).

The use of physical activity as a therapeutic tool in Alzheimer's disease has been described. Teri et al (1998) found that older adults with Alzheimer's disease and their carers were 100% compliant with some activities aimed at improving strength, balance and flexibility. They concluded that physical exercise was necessary and feasible with this group. Rolland et al (2000) found that in a small sample of people with Alzheimer's disease, a programme of physical activity had no effect on increasing a person's autonomy, but reduced nutritional and behavioural complications as well as the risk of falls.

The problem of falls

The problem of falls has been placed on the health and social care agenda by standard six of the NSF for older people (Department of Health 2001), which aims to reduce falls by ensuring that older people who have fallen receive advice and intervention from specialised falls services. The Cochrane Review of interventions for preventing falls in older people suggests that between one-third and one-half of people over 65 years will fall every year (Gillespie et al 2001). In older people with dementia the incidence of falls has been estimated to be twice that of the cognitively normal population (Tinetti et al 1988). Around 20% of fall incidents require medical attention (Gillespie et al 2001) and falls are regarded as a major cause of disability and the leading cause of mortality due to injury in older people aged over 75 in the UK (Department of Health 2001). The consequences of falls are severe for older people with dementia, because they have a much poorer prognosis following the fall, in terms of resulting problems (Baker et al 1978, Morris et al 1987) and excess mortality (Baker et al 1978). Studies focusing on older people with recurrent falls have shown an association between repeated falls and increased resource utilization (Rizzo et al 1998) and increased admissions to long-term care (Tinetti and Williams 1997). In nursing homes, approximately 60% of residents fall each year (Fuller 2000). Older psychiatric inpatients are particularly susceptible to recurrent falls and a recent study has shown that they can contribute to and predict increased length of inpatient stay (Greene et al 2001).

Falling has been attributed to many different factors: some of them intrinsic, such as gait or balance impairment (Lord et al 1996, Maki et al 1994) and others extrinsic, such as environmental hazards (Northridge et al 1995). Risk factors for falls have been covered extensively elsewhere (Gillespie et al 2001, Lord et al 2001) and, when weighing up the evidence, it seems more likely that it is the interaction between factors that contributes to fall risk, as will be discussed later. For example, the behaviour of the individual within the environment produces the risk of falling, rather than the environment itself (Lawton 1980). People with dementia might be at greater risk of falling than those who are cognitively normal. A cognitive impairment *per se* has been shown to be an independent risk factor, along with other factors particular to people with dementia, such as the effects of mood-stabilizing drugs and electroconvulsive therapy (De Carle & Kohn 2001). Although targeted interventions to prevent falls have been tested in several randomized controlled trials (e.g. Close et al 1999, Hornbrook et al 1994, Tinetti et al 1994), these trials have excluded patients with cognitive impairment, thus leaving an important question unanswered: can falls be prevented in older patients with dementia?

For the remainder of this chapter, the focus will be on the authors' experience of quantitative and qualitative multidisciplinary research in the field of dementia and falls, over a 5-year period since 1996. A recurring theme is that in providing structured interventions to prevent falls, multiple views of risk emerge that present ethical dilemmas for professionals. A second important theme is that physiotherapists and occupational therapists need to consider an alternative model of therapy that encompasses evidence-based interventions to improve gait and modify the environment, while at the same time using a collaborative, psychosocial and cognitive approach with patients and their carers.

Risk management of falls in older people with cognitive impairment

In a randomized controlled trial (RCT) of multidisciplinary intervention for older people with cognitive impairment who had fallen, gait and balance impairment (Koch et al 1994, Tinetti 1986), mobility (Smith 1994), environmental hazards (Tideiksaar 1986) and medical fall risk factors were assessed, and individuals kept fall diaries for 1 year. The participants were randomized to either multidisciplinary intervention targeted at the identified fall risk factors, or conventional care. Nearly 80% of those recruited to the trial were resident in institutional care, which presented particular challenges to the team, in terms of maximizing the success of intervention. The results of our trial showed that participants who complied fully or partially with intervention were significantly less likely to fall than the control group (Shaw et al 2000). The term 'compliance' was used to mean whether or not individuals and carers carried out our advice on exercise and mobility, environmental hazard modification and other medical factors, such as medication withdrawal. The finding that compliance influences the success of falls prevention might not be surprising, yet it is important, because it highlights two key issues. First, the role of the carer in falls prevention and, second, the ability of the professional to offer intervention in a way that can be taken up by the person concerned.

Some preliminary findings from the RCT concerning intervention to modify environmental hazards illustrate the pivotal role of the carer in the success of falls prevention strategies.

Environmental hazards and fall risk in dementia

Environmental hazards have been associated with falls in the general population of older adults (Northridge et al 1995, Steinweg 1997). Close et al (1999) demonstrated a significant reduction in the number of falls in older patients, following a combination of medical intervention and strategies to modify identified environmental risk factors. Yet despite the considerable risk of falls in older people with dementia, very little research has been conducted into the importance of interventions to reduce home hazards. Clemson et al (1996) found that the homes of people with cognitive impairment who fell contained more hazards than non-fallers with cognitive impairment. Lowery et al (2000) found that hazards were frequently present in both the homes and the residential care environments of 65 patients with dementia, although they were not significantly associated with falling. However, several hazards, such as loose mats and lack of rails next to the toilet were attributed by carers to 13 (9.7%) of the overall falls on completion of weekly fall diaries. The preliminary findings of our RCT show that hazards were identified as a risk factor for falls in 75 (73%) of those in the intervention group (Buri et al 1999). Seventy-two per cent of participants lived in institutional accommodation, and in only 26% of cases did carers follow specific recommendations for environmental modification. Many factors are thought to account for such poor compliance, including lack of resources and low staffing. However, the dilemma faced by carers in balancing risk against autonomy for people with dementia might also play a significant role. It might not be in the interests of care staff to change the environment, if such changes lead to the potential for independence and with it increased risk of injury and falls.

The role of carers in falls prevention

Qualitative focus group research was undertaken to further explore the role of carers in maximizing falls prevention strategies. The focus groups investigated the perceptions of care staff in nursing and residential homes on their potential contribution to therapy intervention (Dawson et al 2000). Three main issues emerged from the focus group data analysis. First, that care staff knew individual residents well and felt able to predict their reactions to suggestions of exercise or activity. Second, staff could seize immediate opportunities for activity when residents seemed amenable. Third, the context of each home was important, in relation to understanding the preferred routines of the organization and the individual, and making activities fit into these routines. The implications of these findings are that therapists should consider delegating appropriate activity-based interventions to care staff, as they know important information about residents and are well placed to make activity meaningful and relevant within the life of the individual. For example, a care assistant told the physiotherapist that one of the patients in the trial really enjoyed her evening bath. The physiotherapist taught the staff an exercise routine for them to do with the patient whilst in the water, and her mobility increased sufficient for her to be able to walk the short distance from the lounge to the dining room, instead of being taken in a wheelchair.

However, it is important to be mindful of the limits within which unqualified care assistants can work. After observing a physiotherapist (not connected with the trial) encouraging a resident to exercise, a care assistant made the following observation in one of the focus groups:

> *Physio is for certain parts of the body...exercise is for their whole body...I don't think I'd go and do it with somebody who hadn't done it before [physio]...I might be doing more worse than good if I'm exercising an arm...I mean I could pull it out of the bloody socket. Some of the time when you see the physios really making them work you think well if I did that I'd get done for abuse.*

The ethical issues related to persuading someone to mobilize when they do not want to demand serious consideration. Not least that no one has the right to force any individual into doing something they do not want to do. If the person is not amenable to activity then consent to treatment has not been given. The brief time of a therapist's visit to a home might not be long enough to build up a rapport and to gain the resident's trust, whereas the careworker who is there all day long can try again later, when the resident's mood has changed, provided the therapist has taught the worker the necessary skills.

Generally, professionals involved in care and rehabilitation do not sanction strategies that enhance dependency rather than independence. Interestingly, in an exploratory study of informal carers taken from the control group of the RCT referred to above, the opposite was found to be the case (Buri & Dawson 2000). Carers used multiple strategies to avoid falls, which increased the person's dependency and helplessness. They used controlling strategies such as patrolling, monitoring, surveying and checking the person's movements. Carers went to extreme lengths to block the person into a controlled space thus restricting the person's ability to move about freely:

> *I've also got to guard the bottom end of the bed, so I put a chest of drawers at the bottom end, so that she couldn't get out, then I had a table, then I had an armchair, up at the top end of the bed, then*

after she had the fall and bumped her head on the radiator, I put the cushions off the settee along the radiator, so its like Pickford's removal, putting her into bed (daughter).

The use of such strategies is not endorsed in the professional literature. Carers selectively accepted or rejected advice from professionals, depending on its fit with their personal experience. Professionals should adopt the collaborative approach suggested by Corcoran (1993) when advising carers about coping with falls. They must also take steps to discover individual carers' risk management strategies, which might be different from the professional perspective, and based on notions of fatalism and unpredictability. Whereas carers might need support to learn how to relinquish control, professionals must also accept that control strategies will at times be appropriate and necessary for carers' peace of mind.

Perceptual dysfunction as a risk factor for falls

Although the primary focus in both physiotherapy and occupational therapy intervention in dementia is one of promoting physical activity and enhancing independence (Perrin & May 2000, Pomeroy 1995), little attention has been paid in the professional literature to the possible relationship between perceptual dysfunction and an increased risk of falls. For example, wandering is an example of how spatial disorientation deficits are manifested in the behaviour of someone with dementia. The incidence of perceptual deficits, in particular spatial orientation, have been reported in people with Alzheimer's disease (Henderson et al 1989, Hewawasam 1996, Liu et al 1991, Rosswurm 1989, Van Deusen 1992) but perceptual deficits have never been identified as a specific risk factor for falls. Hewawasam (1996) noted that gait clearly altered when a person approached an area of sharp colour contrast.

Buchner & Larson (1987) found a strong association between hip fractures and wandering behaviour. They hypothesized that intervention to improve spatial orientation might prevent injury from falls. In a small-scale qualitative study, nursing home residents known to be at risk from falls were observed, to explore the notion that perceptual dysfunction is an additional risk factor for falls (Buri et al 2000). The observation schedule comprised categories drawn from interview data with therapists working in the field of falls prevention for older adults with cognitive impairment. Interaction with the environment (such as reaction to changes in colours and patterns), movement (including wandering and gait speed) and psychological factors (such as fear) emerged as important markers of perceptual dysfunction in relation to fall risk. The person–environment fit model discussed above, which is traditionally favoured by occupational therapists working with older people with dementia, could therefore be expanded to include interventions to reduce falls. For example, the removal of extraneous objects and the provision of visual cues to aid way-finding could be useful in managing fall risk. It has already been shown that specially designed environments can help to preserve mobility in people with Alzheimer's disease (Saxton et al 1998). Physiotherapists might also look to an expansion of the traditional approach to gait analysis, by incorporating a cognitive–perceptual explanation for movement difficulties into their assessment and intervention for fall risk (Buri et al 2000).

Gait impairment as a risk factor for falls

Previous studies have shown that gait and mobility problems in older people with dementia may be improved by physiotherapy treatment (Pomeroy 1993, 1994). However a more recent trial of physiotherapy versus non-physical activities, for older people with dementia in respite care, did not show any significant change in mobility or walking speed (Pomeroy et al 1999).

In the RCT of multidisciplinary intervention for older people with cognitive impairment who had fallen, Tinetti's performance-oriented assessment of gait and balance (Tinetti 1986) was used to both guide intervention and measure gait changes. The vast majority of participants in the trial (94%) had gait impairment. After 3 months there was a median improvement of two points in gait score in the intervention group, which was significantly better than the control group (Dawson et al 1999). However, the improvement was not maintained at 6 months; this could be linked to the fact that compliance was greater in the earlier part of the study, when the therapy intervention protocol was more intense. It might be that there is a critical point beyond which intervention should be continued, to maximize long-term benefit, but this needs further investigation. Also, it cannot be assumed that physiotherapy intervention alone was responsible for the change in gait performance, as participants received concurrent multidisciplinary intervention. Many other factors may impact on gait, such as medication withdrawal or environmental modification.

Conclusion

This chapter has given a brief overview of mental illness in older adults and referred the reader to key physiotherapy and occupational therapy texts in the field. The predicted rise in the number of people aged 80 years and over, coupled with the increasing incidence and prevalence of conditions such as dementia, provide challenges for service development in physiotherapy and occupational therapy. The NSF for Older People has placed the problem of falls high on the health and social care agenda, and key findings of the authors' work in falls prevention in older people with dementia have been reported. The role of the careworker has emerged as crucial in maximizing the success of environmental modification and other intervention strategies in residential and nursing homes. Family carers face a difficult and demanding task when dealing with fall risk in the home, and the carer's need to balance risk against autonomy when attempting to keep a relative safe must be acknowledged. A link between fall risk and perceptual problems has been proposed, particularly in relation to gait analysis, and it has been demonstrated that gait can be improved in older people with dementia, although we cannot isolate the contribution of physical therapy from other multidisciplinary interventions. The use of 'physical activity', in its various forms, has therefore been highlighted as a valuable therapeutic tool within a model of therapy that encompasses evidence-based interventions while, at the same time, using a collaborative, psychosocial and cognitive approach with patients and their carers.

Summary

■ Key findings of a study on falls prevention in older people with dementia.

■ The role of the careworker in falls prevention in residential and nursing homes, and in the domestic situation.

■ The link between falls risk and perceptual problems in relation to gait analysis.

■ The use of physical activity along with other multidisciplinary team interventions as a therapeutic tool.

References

Baker B R, Duckworth T, Wilkes E 1978 Mental state and other prognostic factors in femoral fractures of the elderly. Journal of the Royal College of General Practitioners 28:557–559

Baum C 1995 The contribution of occupation to function in persons with Alzheimer's disease. Journal of Occupational Science 2(2):59–67

Borrell L, Gustavsson A, Sandmen P, Kielhofner G 1994 Occupational programming in a day hospital for patients with dementia. Occupational Therapy Journal of Research 14(4):219–238

Buchner D M, Larson E B 1987 Falls and fractures in patients with Alzheimer type dementia. Journal of the American Medical Association 257(11): 1492–1495

Buri H, Dawson P 2000 Caring for a relative with dementia: a theoretical model of coping with fall risk. Health, Risk & Society 2(3):283–293

Buri H, Picton J, Dawson P 2000 Perceptual dysfunction in elderly people with cognitive impairment: a risk factor for falls? British Journal of Occupational Therapy 63(6):248–253

Buri H, Shaw F E, Dawson P, Kenny R A 1999 Preventing falls in cognitively impaired elderly patients: effectiveness of environmental modifica-tion by an occupational therapist. Age and Ageing 28(suppl 1):17–18

Clark C A, Corcoran M, Gitlin L N 1995 An exploratory study of how occupational therapists develop therapeutic relationships with family caregivers. American Journal of Occupational Therapy 49(6):587–594

Clemson L, Cumming R G, Roland M 1996 Case-control study of hazards in the home and risk of falls and hip fractures. Age and Ageing 25:97–101

Close J, Ellis M, Hooper R et al 1999 Prevention of falls in the elderly trial (PROFET): a randomised controlled trial. The Lancet 353:93–97

Corcoran M A 1993 Collaboration: an ethical approach to effective therapeutic relationships. Topics in Geriatric Rehabilitation 9(1):21–29

Creek J (ed) 2002 Occupational therapy and mental health, 3rd edn. Churchill Livingstone, Edinburgh

Dawson P, Buswell C, Shaw F E, Kenny R A 2000 Institutional care workers' contribution to therapy in the prevention of falls in elderly cognitively impaired residents – a qualitative study. Clinical Rehabilitation 14(2):220–221

Dawson P, Krys R, Bowles V et al 1999 Can gait be improved in older people with cognitive impairment who fall? Age and Ageing 29 (suppl 1):47

De Carle A J, Kohn R 2001 Risk factors for falling in a psychogeriatric unit. International Journal of Geriatric Psychiatry 16:762–767

Department of Health 2000 The NHS plan. A plan for investment. A plan for reform. HMSO, London

Department of Health 2001 National service framework for older people. HMSO, London

Dewey M E, Saz P 2001 Dementia, cognitive impairment and mortality in persons aged 65 and over living in the community: a systematic review of the literature. International Journal of Geriatric Psychiatry 16(8):751–761

Eccles M, Clarke J, Livingstone M et al 1998 North of England evidence based guidelines development project: guideline for the primary care management of dementia. British Medical Journal 317:802–808

Everett T, Dennis M, Ricketts E (eds) 1995 Physiotherapy in mental health: a practical approach. Butterworth Heinemann, Oxford

Fuller G R 2000 Falls in the elderly. American Family Physician 61:2173–2174

Gillespie L D, Gillespie W J, Robertson M C et al 2001 Interventions for preventing falls in elderly people (Cochrane Review). In: The Cochrane Library, Issue 4. Update Software, Oxford

Greene E, Cunningham C J, Eustace A et al 2001 Recurrent falls are associated with increased length of stay in elderly psychiatric inpatients. International Journal of Geriatric Psychiatry 16:965–968

Henderson V W, Mack W, White Williams B 1989 Spatial disorientation in Alzheimer's disease. Archives of Neurology 46:391–394

Hewawasam L C 1996 The use of two-dimensional grid patterns to limit hazardous ambulation in elderly patients with Alzheimer's disease. NT Research 1(3):217–227

Hornbrook M C, Stevens V J, Wingfield D J et al 1994 Preventing falls among community-dwelling older persons: results from a randomized trial. Gerontologist 34:16–23

Kirby L, Lehmann P, Majeed A 1998 Dementia in people aged 65 years and older: a growing problem? Population Trends 92:23–28

Koch M, Gottschalk M, Baker D I et al 1994 An impairment and disability assessment and treat-

ment protocol for community-living elderly persons. Physical Therapy 74:286–294

Lawton M 1980 Environment and aging. Brooks Cole, Monterey, CA

Liu L, Gauthier L, Gauthier S 1991 Spatial disorientation in persons with early senile dementia of the Alzheimer type. Canadian Journal of Occupational Therapy 45(1):67–74

Lord S R, Lloyd D G, Li S K 1996 Sensori-motor function, gait patterns and falls in community-dwelling women. Age and Ageing 25:292–299

Lord S R, Sherrington C, Menz H B 2001 Falls in older people. Risk factors and strategies for prevention. Cambridge University Press, Cambridge

Lowery K, Buri H, Ballard C 2000 What is the prevalence of environmental hazards in the homes of dementia sufferers and are they associated with falls. International Journal of Geriatric Psychiatry 15:883–886

Maki B E, Holliday P J, Topper A K 1994 A prospective study of postural balance and risk of falling in an ambulatory and independent elderly population. Journal of Gerontology 49(2):M72–M84

Morris J C, Rubin E H, Morris E J, Mandel S A 1987 Senile dementia of Alzheimer's type: an important risk factor for serious falls. Journal of Gerontology 42:412–417

Northridge M E, Nevitt M C, Kelsey J L, Link B 1995 Home hazards and falls in the elderly: the role of health and functional status. American Journal of Public Health 85:509–515

Ott A, Breteler M M, van Harskamp F et al 1998 Incidence and risk of dementia: The Rotterdam study. American Journal of Epidemiology 147(6):574–580

Perrin T 1997 Occupational need in dementia care: a literature review and implications for practice. Health Care in Later Life 2(3):166–176

Perrin T, May H 2000 Wellbeing in dementia: an approach for occupational therapists and carers. Churchill Livingstone, Edinburgh

Pomeroy V M 1993 The effect of physiotherapy input on mobility skills of elderly people with severe dementing illness. Clinical Rehabilitation 7:163–170

Pomeroy V M 1994 Immobility and severe dementia: when is physiotherapy treatment appropriate? Clinical Rehabilitation 8:226–232

Pomeroy V M 1995 Dementia. In: Everett T, Dennis M, Ricketts E (eds) Physiotherapy in mental health:

a practical approach. Butterworth Heinemann, Oxford

Pomeroy V M, Warren C M, Honeycombe C et al 1999 Mobility and dementia: is physiotherapy treatment during respite care effective? International Journal of Geriatric Psychiatry 14(5):389–397

Rizzo J A, Friedkin R, Williams C S et al 1998 Health care utilisation and costs in a Medicare population by fall status. Medical Care 36(8):1174–1188

Rolland Y, Rival L, Pillard F et al 2000 Feasibility of regular physical exercise for patients with moderate to severe Alzheimer's disease. Journal of Nutrition, Health and Ageing 4(2):109–113

Rosswurm M A 1989 Assessment of perceptual processing deficits in persons with Alzheimer's disease. Western Journal of Nursing Research 11(4):458–468

Saxton J, Silverman M, Ricci E et al 1998 Maintenance of mobility in residents of an Alzheimer special care facility. International Psychogeriatrics 10(2):213–214

Shaw F E, Richardson D A, Dawson P et al 2000 Can multidisciplinary intervention prevent falls in patients with cognitive impairment and dementia attending a casualty department? Age and Ageing 29 (suppl 1):47

Smith R 1994 Validation and reliability of the elderly mobility scale. Physiotherapy 80:744–747

Steinweg K K 1997 The changing approach to falls in the elderly. American Family Physician 56(7): 1815–1823

Teri L, McCurry S M, Buchner D M et al 1998 Exercise and activity level in Alzheimer's disease: a poten-tial treatment focus. Journal of Rehabilitation Research Development 35(4):411–419

Tideiksaar R 1986 Preventing falls: home hazard checklists to help older patients protect themselves. Geriatrics 41:26–28

Tinetti M E 1986 Performance-oriented assessment of mobility problems in elderly patients. Journal of the American Geriatric Society 34:119–126

Tinetti M E, Baker D I, McAvay G et al 1994 A multifactorial intervention to reduce the risk of falling among elderly people living in the community. New England Journal of Medicine 331:821–827

Tinetti M E, Speechley M, Ginter S F 1988 Risk factors for falls among elderly persons living in the community. New England Journal of Medicine 319:1701–1707

Tinetti M E, Williams C S 1997 Falls, injuries due to falls, and the risk of admission to a nursing home. New England Journal of Medicine 337(18):1279–1284

Turner A, Foster M, Johnson S E 1992 Occupational therapy and physical dysfunction: principles, skill and practice, 3rd edn. Churchill Livingstone, Edinburgh

Van Deusen J 1992 Perceptual dysfunction in persons with dementia of the Alzheimer's type: a literature review. Physical and Occupational Therapy in Geriatrics 10(4):33–46

Witthaus E, Ott A, Barendregt J J et al 1999 Burden of mortality and morbidity from dementia. Alzheimer's Disease and Associated Disorders 13(3):176–181

Severe and enduring mental illness

Sarah Childs and Caroline Griffiths

The National Service Framework for Mental Health (Department of Health 1999) reports that 15 000 people in England (i.e. between 14 and 200 per 100 000), experience severe and enduring mental illness. However, there is no agreed definition of severe and enduring mental illness (Slade et al 1997). In view of this, the Department of Health (1996), in its document *Building Bridges*, recommends that services use the following framework definition to develop a locally agreed operational definition. The framework definition focuses on five key dimensions of severe mental illness: safety, informal and formal care, diagnosis, disability, and duration (SIDDD). These dimensions offer a frame of reference for local health and social services to develop their own operational definitions of severe and enduring mental illness, in line with local needs and priorities. It is important to note that, for a person to be regarded as severely mentally ill, not all the dimensions need to be met, and on the specific character, relative importance and interrelationship of the dimensions, there is no consensus (Bachrach 1988).

The five key dimensions will be looked at in further detail, as together they provide a comprehensive depiction of this client group:

Safety
Informal and formal care
Diagnosis
Disability
Duration.

Safety

Four components should be considered when referring to this framework dimension for severe mental illness (Department of Health 1996, p. 12):

1. unintentional self-harm, e.g. self-neglect
2. intentional self-harm
3. safety of others
4. abuse by others, e.g. physical, sexual, emotional, financial.

As a result of the disabilities commonly associated with this client group, people with severe mental illness can be seriously at risk from self-neglect and vulnerable to exploitation or abuse from others. It is important to note that 'a person can be severely mentally ill without occasioning significant risk to their own safety or that of others' (Department of Health 1996, p. 11). Suicide amongst this client group is far more likely than homicide (Confidential Inquiry 1994, quoted in Slade et al 1997).

Informal and formal care

This dimension reflects the current trend of treatment in the community, including shorter hospital stays. It includes people who have severe disabilities but have minimal or no contact with psychiatric services, those who require long-stay hospital admission and those discharged to the community either in supported accommodation or with support from paid or voluntary organizations or from their social networks.

The Department of Health (1996, p. 12) defined this dimension using two components:

1. help from informal carers, including friends and relatives
2. help from formal services, such as day centres, paid staff, voluntary services, hospital admissions, medication and detention under the Mental Health Act.

Diagnosis

Bachrach (1988) states that diagnosis is a necessary, but not a sufficient, criterion for putting an individual into the category of severe and enduring mental illness. Individuals with schizophrenia and bipolar affective disorder make up the majority of those with severe and enduring mental illness and the remaining 25–30% have a primary diagnosis of personality disorder or organic disorder ranging from dementia to drug or alcohol abuse (Repper & Cooney 1999).

Disability

The World Health Organization (WHO) does not have a formal definition for severe and enduring mental illness but suggests that the focus be on disability rather than diagnosis (Slade et al 1997). Bachrach (1988) states that the disability dimension has emerged as the most important criterion in the definition. When working with this client group, it becomes evident that it is the extent of the disability that often distinguishes them from other mental health service users. As therapists seeking to enable individuals to reach their maximum level of function, it is important that we first fully understand the extent of the dysfunction or disability. For these reasons, it is felt appropriate to devote a large proportion of this chapter to describing the disabilities that this client group experiences.

The disability dimension will be explored using the following subheadings:

- clinical disability
- social disability
- institutionalization
- cognitive disability.

Clinical disability

People with enduring mental health problems, despite being treated with appropriate medication regimes, can retain residual symptoms of their illness. Those with schizophrenia might experience auditory hallucinations, paranoid ideas or hold delusional beliefs. These symptoms can be ongoing or episodic, associated with acute phases. The negative symptoms of the illness can often be even more debilitating. 'Marked apathy, paucity of speech, and blunting or incongruity of emotional responses' (WHO 1992, p. 88), along with lack of motivation to perform day-to-day tasks, disable this client group markedly.

Durham (1990) refers to Wing's (1978) 'clinical poverty syndrome' when describing this population. This is characterized by underactivity, slowness of thought and movement, flattening of affect, apathy, poverty of speech and social withdrawal. The experience of having these symptoms, either continuously or periodically, has a major impact on an individual's ability to function in all areas.

Social disability

Much research has been conducted into the poor social networks of people in this group (Brewer et al 1994, Cresswell et al 1992, Segal & Holschuh 1991) and their exclusion from the mainstream community. Creek (1990) highlights two behavioural disturbances that contribute to this process:

1. *Social withdrawal*: difficulty in relating to others and a preoccupation with own thoughts.
2. *Loss of social awareness*: lack of sensitivity to others, sometimes leading to socially inappropriate behaviour.

Allen et al (1992) believe impairment in cognitive functioning leads to social disability. A low cognitive level, so often present in this group of people, means that the person is not able to process the information required to meet the social expectations of others. In summary, people with enduring mental health problems tend to be severely disabled in their social functioning. They can become withdrawn and isolated and, despite being able to make simple conversation on very familiar topics, can find it difficult to initiate social contact.

These problems are often compounded by the existence of limited opportunities for social interaction. People in this group are also more likely to experience occupational deprivation (Mee & Sumsion 2001). Studies have shown that, as well as meeting clients' needs and improving their quality of life, occupation provides a way of relating to others, being a vehicle for non-threatening and non-judgemental interactions (Mee & Sumsion 2001).

Institutionalization

No discussion about this client group could overlook the well-researched effects of institutionalization, or the marked effects that the institutional environment has on its residents. Although only a small proportion of this client group is currently treated in inpatient facilities, a large number of people have been discharged into supported accommodation in the community, following years of treatment in institutions.

Cognitive disability

The final area of the disability dimension to be explored is cognitive disability. The Cognitive Disabilities model defines a cognitive disability as a 'restriction in voluntary motor actions originating in the physical or chemical structures of the brain and producing observable limitations in routine task behaviour' (Allen 1985, p. 31). In short, dysfunction of the brain means that people's performance of all daily life tasks will be impaired. Allen devised six cognitive levels: level 1 being profoundly disabled and level 6 normal cognitive functioning. Although cognitive level can change in many acute conditions, it is remarkably stable in most chronic conditions (Allen 1985). Patients with severe and enduring mental health problems commonly function at level 4. The full implications of functioning at this low level will be discussed later.

Duration

Historically, 'chronicity' was equated with continuous hospital stay of 2 or more years. However, the trends of community care, and the deinstitutionalization that followed, resulted in huge reductions in long-stay hospital populations, so that by 1989 only 3–5% of patients spent more than 1 year in hospital (Jukubasenk & Kopp 1989). Patients were being kept out of hospital, or being discharged earlier and/or receiving treatment in the community. Consequently, chronicity as a measure has been abandoned. Duration was defined by the Department of Health (1996) in the SIDDD framework as the occurrence of any of the other four dimensions for periods that vary between 6 months and more than 2 years.

Poor health status

Morbidity and mortality rates in people with severe and enduring mental illness are, as they have always been, higher than the general population (Koran et al 1989, Phelan et al 2001). Research in many countries suggests that a major factor in the high rates of physical illness is not the severity of the psychiatric symptoms but the usual effects of eating poorly, smoking more and taking less exercise (Brown et al 1999). It has been shown that those people with severe and enduring mental illness have a higher level of tobacco use, alcohol use, obesity and a reduced prevalence of moderate exercise (Davidson et al 2001). Not only is the rate of mortality due to heart disease and smoking increased but there is also a higher level of deaths that could have been avoided by medical intervention (Brown et al 2000).

Some of the defining symptoms of schizophrenia contribute to the poor health status of this group; reduction of cognitive function, apathy and social withdrawal, all of which can lead to a lack of reporting of physical illhealth at an early stage, if at all. These obstructions to the reporting of illhealth are compounded by the lessening of social skills, which can inhibit clear expression of problems to the primary health-care team (Jeste et al 1996). The reaction of members of the primary health-care team if inexperienced in dealing with patients with enduring mental illness might be to avoid actively searching for symptoms in a physical examination and to rely upon self-reporting, which, as stated, is likely to be poor. In mental health settings it has been shown that inexperienced junior psychiatrists often perform inadequate physical assessments of psychiatric inpatients (Rigby & Oswald 1987) and many mental health professionals have little training in physical medicine.

The National Service Framework for Mental Health (Department of Health 1999) promotes the assessment of the physical needs of people with severe mental illness but, along with the reduced ability of patients to report illhealth, the lack of medical time for physical assessment and the emphasis on psychiatric diagnosis rather than the patient's physical needs, there are the overarching effects of social exclusion, homelessness and poverty.

Research into the effects of homelessness has rarely matched samples from similar backgrounds and so it is difficult to separate cause and effect but Sullivan et al (2000), in a study of the quality of life of homeless persons with mental illness, found that those with severe mental disorder were significantly worse-off in terms of physical health and subjective quality of life.

Women with severe and enduring mental illness can have specific health-care needs around reproductive and sexual health, substance abuse and victimization (Mobray et al 1998). Increased HIV-risk behaviour by women with severe mental illness suggests the need for those working with these clients to have awareness of HIV-prevention interventions (McPherson 1999).

However, for both men and women the most important health factors appear to be good housing and social support (Weinhardt et al 1998). The health professional's contribution must be seen in terms of prevention and education. To ensure that patients in both community and inpatient settings have their physical healthcare needs met, research on effectiveness of screening and proactive prevention programmes must be carried out. Future health planning must bring true holistic assessment of people with severe mental illness. If the physical and mental health of the population continue to be perceived as separate entities, we will continue to see people with mental illness dying 10 to 15 years earlier than the general population (Farnam et al 1999).

Assessment and treatment approaches

Occupational therapy

Intrinsic to all occupational therapists is the use of activity. As previously highlighted in this chapter, people with severe and enduring mental health problems commonly experience significant disabilities that affect their performance of day-to-day activities. It is essential that these disabilities are assessed, and their implications fully understood by therapists, so a realistic and clinically sound intervention process can be implemented. Claudia Allen created a model for occupational therapists that relies on the performance of a sensory motor task to predict performance in all activities of daily living. The Cognitive Disabilities model is particularly valuable with people with severe and enduring mental health problems because it highlights the poor cognitive functioning so often present in this client group. It also provides the therapist with a clear guide of the appropriate level of assistance the client will need to successfully and safely perform tasks.

The Cognitive Disabilities model

A cognitive disability is a restriction in voluntary motor action originating in the physical or chemical structures of the brain and producing observable limitations in routine task behaviour.

(Allen 1985, p. 31)

In short, dysfunction in the brain results in impaired performance of routine tasks, or activities done on a daily basis. Claudia Allen describes six cognitive levels, or levels of cognitive disability, ranging from level 1 (automatic actions) indicating severe disability requiring 24-hour nursing care, to level 6 (planned actions) indicating an absence of disability. Response to medications and/or spontaneous improvement in acute psychiatric illness often produces rapid improvement in cognitive level. However, when the acute condition is stabilized, as is the case for most people with severe and enduring mental health problems, the cognitive level remains remarkably stable and we can then predict how these people will function in all areas of their lives. People with severe and enduring mental health problems commonly function at level 4. Box 18.1 summarizes functioning at cognitive level 4.

Box 18.1
Cognitive level 4 (Allen 1988)

- Goal-directed actions are performed spontaneously in response to clearly visible cues.
- Action complies with the steps required to achieve a goal.
- No independent or new learning occurs. New things can be taught by rote learning only. This involves memorizing the steps to do an activity, without the flexibility to understand verify or change steps.
- Attention can be sustained for about 1 hour.
- Reliance on visible cues – objects with striking appearance (colour and shape) are dealt with successfully whereas others, e.g. make-up skin tones mismatched, missed whiskers when shaving, are ignored.
- Fire and burn risk as heat, chemical reactions and electrical hazards are not visible and therefore not recognized.
- Disability is often concealed by the successful performance of many day-to-day activities, but coping with new events and anticipating needs requires caregiver assistance.
- Requires a social support system to assist with general problem solving and to protect from unanticipated hazards.
- Requires competent support on a daily basis.
- Commonly seen in patients with mild dementia, acute manic or depressive episodes, and chronic schizophrenia.

A person functioning at cognitive level 4 will be unable to learn new tasks and problem-solving ability will be poor. When working with these people, step-by-step assistance from the therapist is required when performing activities such as following a recipe and doing the laundry. Ongoing guidance throughout the steps of each task is required and the person cannot be expected to retain information or to generalize information from one situation to another. For example, a person functioning at cognitive level 4, doing the laundry, might require prompting from the therapist to initiate the task, sort the clothes according to colour and fabric type, use the appropriate amount of detergent and place this correctly within the machine, press the appropriate buttons, and to initiate removing clothes when cycle is completed.

It is imperative that cognitive disabilities are recognized and people are given the appropriate level of support they require to successfully perform day-to-day tasks. The disabilities are so often mistaken for laziness or poor motivation when, in reality, the individual simply cannot, as opposed to will not, perform tasks unsupported.

A person's cognitive level can be assessed quickly and accurately by the therapist using one of the two standardized evaluation instruments: the Allen Cognitive Level (ACL) Test–90 or the Routine Task Inventory (RTI).

Intervention

Once the cognitive level has been established, a programme of intervention can be prescribed by the therapist. Traditionally, occupational therapists have used activity to prevent illness or to restore health. Allen's theory and model challenges this idea, and moves from 'trying to change the patient to changing the activity' (Allen 1985, p. 27).

Therapists must recommend adaptations to the environment, including the provision of an appropriate level of assistance, so that persons with impairments can function safely and optimally in the community with their remaining abilities (Henry et al 1998). Matching the task demand to the person's current cognitive level seems to produce an experience that is within a person's comfortable range of tolerance. A task demand that is above the person's current cognitive level elicits reluctance, resistance and sometimes stubborn refusal to participate in tasks. 'Successful performance occurs when the task demands and directions match the patient's cognitive level' (Allen 1988, p. 81).

Physiotherapy

Assessment

Physiotherapists will base their assessment and treatment on a bio-psychosocial model that will encompass the physical disease of the patient within the context of his or her psychological disorder and social circumstances.

Physical assessments should be performed as appropriate with any patient but the time required to achieve a comprehensive assessment can be a few sessions rather than one, and the skills required will include awareness of the patient's possible communication and cognitive loss and will be enhanced by knowledge of cognitive–behavioural techniques.

Treatment   The aim of treatment will be to improve function both physically and mentally and to offer strategies designed to develop healthy lifestyle practices. A physiotherapist engaged in treating musculoskeletal injuries or physical disease in individuals with enduring mental illness might also be part of a team dealing with the effects of long-term mental disorder.

Swift interventions can be most useful – acupuncture, ultrasound and minimal massage can all be performed quickly enough to prevent the patient getting restless before completion of treatment. People with severe and enduring mental disorder can also suffer from stress/anxiety and the physiotherapist can offer relaxation training, massage and exercise to reduce stress, and can work within the multidisciplinary team to provide anxiety management regimes suitable for this client group.

Mutrie (1999) has shown evidence of the positive effect of exercise as an adjunct to medication in the treatment of mental disorders. Chastain & Shapiro (1987) demonstrated the positive effects on the self-esteem of their group, which included patients with schizophrenia, following a programme of aerobic exercise for 6 weeks. Exercise can be offered in many ways, from formal multigym sessions to Tai Chi, and from swimming to dancing. Although the evidence-base is narrow with regards to specific treatments for this population, the research into best practice in management suggests that assertive community treatment is effective, if expensive (Marshall et al 1999). Physiotherapists might find that they can be most effective by working within the community mental health team, where the benefits of physiotherapy intervention can be seen by both patients and colleagues.

Motivation   If it is conceded that exercise can be of benefit to those with severe mental disorder what methods should we adopt to enhance motivation and improve the likelihood of adherence? Box 18.2 gives some jump-off points for physiotherapy intervention with reference to motivation.

All of these pointers can be linked with motivational and cognitive–behavioural techniques, which will aid physiotherapists in providing a service designed to encourage independence and development for their clients.

Box 18.2
Motivational pointers

- *Starting where you are*: what does the client enjoy already and where could that lead? Walking, swimming, gardening, dancing?
- *Environment*: is the place pleasant? Do we have the right equipment? Would a community setting be most appropriate?
- *Client-led realistic (but challenging) goal setting*: use of the client's goals will increase the likelihood of adherence to any programme. Our role is to guide the client towards realistic intermediate steps.
- *Positive feedback*: let people know how they are progressing towards their goal.
- *Peer approval*: adherence is much more likely if the activity is found to be enjoyable and effective by immediate acquaintances.
- *Access equality*: ensure that all clients have equal access to activities. This might require negotiation with local leisure centres, colleges, swimming pools.

Moving towards social inclusion

Now that the majority of people with serious mental health problems exist outside institutions, the challenge for services is to facilitate their access to valued roles within society: to combat exclusionary attitudes and practices and engender acceptance and support (Repper 2000, p. 340).

Causes of social exclusion

The 1998 White Paper *Modernising mental health* (Department of Health 1998, cited in Evans & Repper 2000) highlights how the prejudice attached to mental illness and the failure to understand its causes leads to discrimination and social exclusion. The general public's understanding of mental illness comes largely from the media. Despite the fact that the risk of violence from people with mental health problems is very low (Repper 2000), the media magnifies any incident out of all proportion, leading to a fear of mental illness.

Evans & Repper (2000) feel that poverty, poor housing or homelessness, unemployment, social exclusion and mental health are intricately linked. People with severe and enduring mental illness are often unable to work, because of their poor cognitive functioning or ability to cope with pressure, and hence will commonly be receiving benefits and living in government-funded housing in the poorer areas of their towns or cities.

Reducing social exclusion

As professionals working with people with severe and enduring mental illness, we need to be creating opportunities for inclusion. Sayce & Measey (1999) suggest legal reform, education of the community using the media and film, local initiatives to promote people as 'contributors' and not 'burdens', and increasing familiarization between service users and the rest of the local community. We can support people to become involved in their local communities by enabling them to attend local events, churches, adult education schemes and work. Evans & Repper

(2000) argue that employment plays a crucial role in being accepted or included in society. They feel that we should be moving away from service-based initiatives towards the provision of supported employment in the community, to increase clients' chances of genuine social inclusion. To do this we need to start thinking about how we can alter work to make it ready for the people who need it, rather than changing people to get them ready for work.

Summary

■ People with severe mental illness have a much greater level of disability than other users of mental health services.

■ People with severe mental illness can be seriously at risk from self-neglect and self-harm, and vulnerable to exploitation and abuse.

■ The most important health factors appear to be good housing and social support.

■ The Cognitive Disability model is a useful guide for assessment and treatment intervention.

■ Therapy intervention needs to accept brief attention span and motivational factors.

■ Social exclusion needs to be reduced in the local community, by employers and the media.

References

Allen C K 1985 Occupational therapy for psychiatric diseases: measurement and management of cognitive disabilities. Little Brown and Company, Boston

Allen C K 1988 Functional assessment of the severity of mental disorders. Hospital and Community Psychiatry 39(2):140–142

Allen C K, Earhart C A, Blue T 1992 Occupational therapy treatment goals for the physically and cognitively disabled. The American Occupational Therapy Association Inc., Bethesda, MD

Bachrach L 1988 Defining chronic mental illness: a concept paper. Hospital and Community Psychiatry 39(4):383–388

Brewer P, Gadsden V, Scrimshaw K 1994 The community group network in mental health: a model for social support and community integration. British Journal of Occupational Therapy 57(12):467–470

Brown S, Birtwistle J, Roe L, Thompson C 1999 The unhealthy lifesytle of people with schizophrenia. Psychological Medicine 29:697–701

Brown S, Inskip H, Barraclough B 2000 Causes of excess mortality of schizophrenia. British Journal of Psychiatry 177:212–217

Chastain P B, Shapiro G E 1987 Physical fitness programme for patients with psychiatric disorders. A clinical report. Physical Medicine 67 part iv:545–548

Creek J 1990 Occupational therapy and mental health: principles, skills and practice, 3rd edn. Churchill Livingstone, Edinburgh

Cresswell C M, Kuipers L, Power M J 1992 Social networks and support in long-term psychiatric patients. Hospital and Community Psychiatry 42(11):1125–1131

Davidson S, Judd F, Jolley D et al 2001 Cardiovascular risks for people with mental illness. Australian and New Zealand Journal of Psychiatry 35(2):196–202

Department of Health 1996 Building bridges: a guide to arrangements for interagency working for the care and protection of severely mentally ill people. Department of Health, London

Department of Health 1999 National service framework: mental health. Department of Health, London

Durham T 1990 Long stay. In: Creek J (ed) Occupational therapy and mental health: Principles, skills and practice. Churchill Livingstone, Edinburgh, p 313–331

Evans J, Repper J 2000 Employment, social inclusion, and mental health. Journal of Psychiatric and Mental Health Nursing 7:15–24

Farnam C R, Zipple A M, Tyrell W, Chittinanda P 1999 Health status and risk factors of people with severe and persistent mental illness. Journal of Psychological Nursing and Mental Health Services 37(6):16–21, 44–45

Henry A D, Moore K, Quinlivan M, Triggs M 1998 The relationship of the Allen cognitive test to demographics, diagnosis, and disposition among psychiatric inpatients. American Journal of Occupational Therapy 52(8):638–643

Jeste D V, Glasjo J A, Lindamer L A, Lacro J P 1996 Medical comorbidity in schizophrenia. Schizophrenia Bulletin 22:413–427

Jukabaschk J, Kopp W 1989 On characterising new psychiatric long-stay patients. Social Psychiatry and Psychiatric Epidemiology 24:88–95

Koran L M, Sox H C, Marton K I et al 1989 Medical evaluation of psychiatric patients. Results in a state mental health system. Archives of General Psychiatry 46:733–740

Marshall M, Gray A, Lockwood A, Green R 1999 Case management for people with severe mental disorders. Cochrane Library Issue 2. Update Software, Oxford

McPherson H 1999 The impact of severe mental illness on a woman. In: Romans S E (ed) Folding back the shadows: a perspective on women's mental health. University of Otago Press, Dunedin, New Zealand, p 251–256

Mee J, Sumsion T 2001 Mental health clients confirm the motivating power of occupation. British Journal of Occupational Therapy 64(3):121–128

Mobray C, Oysterman D, Saunders D, Rueda-Riedle A 1998 Women with severe mental disorders: issues and service needs. In: Leviv B L (ed) Women's mental health services: a public health perspective. Sage Publications, Thousand Oaks, CA, p 175–200

Mutrie N 1999 A review of randomised controlled trials for the use of exercise in clinically defined depression. In: Biddle S J H, Fox K R (eds) A review of the relationships between mental health and exercise. Somerset Health Authority, Taunton

Phelan M, Stradins L, Morrison S 2001 Physical health of people with severe mental illness. British Medical Journal 322(7284):443–444

Repper J 2000 Social inclusion. In: Thompson T, Mathias P (eds) Lyttle's mental health and disorder, 3rd edn. Ballière Tindall, London, p 339–358

Repper J, Cooney P 1999 Meeting the needs of people with enduring mental health problems. In: Thompson T, Mathias P (eds) Lyttle's mental health and disorder, 2nd edn. Ballière Tindall, London, p 385–406

Rigby J C, Oswald A G 1987 An evaluation of the performing and recording of physical examinations by psychiatric trainees. British Journal of Psychiatry 177:212–217

Sayce L, Measey L 1999 Strategies to reduce social exclusion for people with mental health problems. Psychiatric Bulletin 23:65–67

Segal S P, Holschuh J 1991 Effects of sheltered care environments and resident characteristics on the development of social networks. Hospital and Community Psychiatry 42(11):1125–1131

Slade M, Powell R, Strathdee G 1997 Current approaches to identifying the severely mentally ill. Social Psychiatry and Psychiatric Epidemiology 32:177–184

Sullivan G, Bernam A, Koegel P, Hollendberg J 2000 Quality of life of homeless persons with mental illness: results from the course-of-homelessness study. Psychiatric Services 51(9):1135–1141

Weinhardt L S, Bicham N L, Carey M P 1998 Sexual coercion among women living with a severe persistent mental illness; review of the literature and recommendations for mental health providers. Aggression and Violent Behavior 4:307–317

Wing J K 1978 Schizophrenia: towards a new synthesis. Academic Press, London

World Health Organization 1992 ICD-10. Classification of mental and behavioural disorders. Clinical descriptions and diagnostic guidelines. World Health Organization, Geneva

19 Forensic psychiatry

Margaret Nicol

Introduction

Forensic psychiatry has been defined in different ways. Chiswick (1994) suggests 'forensic psychiatry is concerned with the application of the law to psychiatric practice, the relationship between crime and psychiatry and the treatment of mentally abnormal offenders'. Whereas Mullen (2000) offers a broader definition that forensic mental health 'is an area of specialisation that, in the criminal sphere, involves the assessment and treatment of those whose behaviour has led, or could lead, to offending'. Both of these definitions have several common features: offending behaviour, the law and treatment of mentally abnormal offenders.

However, Gunn & Taylor (1995), in their textbook on forensic psychiatry, argue for a different perspective, one that they hope will lead to better therapy, and suggest that 'forensic psychiatry is the prevention, amelioration and treatment of victimization which is associated with mental disease'. They contend 'the principal interest for forensic psychiatry in victims is in the identification and treatment of disorder as a form of preventive medicine'. Gunn & Taylor maintain that many mentally abnormal offenders were victims before they became offenders, and that many carry out the same crimes that they experienced as victims.

So an extra dimension – that of prevention – has been added to the concept of forensic psychiatry.

Forensic psychiatry is a growth area in many parts of the world and, within the UK context, mentally disordered offenders have high priority status within mental health services.

The need for forensic mental health services has been well demonstrated, with the first special hospitals being established around 1850. In more recent times the Butler report (Home Office 1975) became an influential factor in providing specific funding for forensic psychiatry and in the establishment of medium-secure settings within the sector. This was followed in 1992 by the Reed Report, which reviewed health and social services for mentally disordered offenders and others requiring similar services (Department of Health 1992). This report was commissioned to review the current services available to mentally disordered offenders and identify areas for improvement. The final summary produced 276 recommendations. Flood (1993), an occupational therapist, highlighted the following from the Reed Report as being fundamental:

- to take a positive approach to individual need
- to take a multidisciplinary and multiagency approach to care and treatment
- to provide an improved range of community services
- to increase medium-secure services related to forensic psychiatry
- to provide adequate health care for prisoners, which would be contracted-in from the NHS
- to provide forensic psychiatric training of both a general and specialized nature.

More recently, the Scottish Office has published its own policy for mentally disordered offenders in Scotland (Scottish Office/DoH 1999). It sets out steps that require services:

- to provide care under conditions of appropriate security with due regard for public safety
- to have regard to quality of care and proper attention to the need of individuals
- where possible, to provide care in the community rather than institutional settings
- to provide care that maximizes rehabilitation and the individual's chance of an independent life.

The most recent development within forensic psychiatry is the setting-up of pilot units to assess and treat dangerous people with severe personality disorders.

Forensic settings

There is a variety of forensic settings, as follows:

- maximum-secure settings (special hospitals)
- medium-secure settings (regional secure units)
- low-secure settings (intensive psychiatric care settings)
- prison.

Each of the above has different characteristics and provides differing levels of supervision.

Special hospitals

These provide assessment and treatment for patients who require maximum security because of their assessed level of dangerousness. There are currently four special hospitals in the UK; three in England (Ashworth, Broadmoor and Rampton) and one in Scotland (The State Hospital, Carstairs), which also caters for patients from Northern Ireland. Special hospitals have a high level of security with perimeter fencing or walls, personal alarms, surveillance cameras, locked doors, monitoring of patient movements and security checks on all persons entering the hospital. Checks of equipment are also maintained at all times.

Historically, special hospitals tended to work in isolation from other parts of the health service but they are now making stringent efforts to liaise with other sections of the NHS so that they participate in an integrated framework for forensic provision within the UK. The culture within special hospitals has changed from a purely custodial role to one where there is a strong emphasis on therapy. Special hospitals, although having to consider the security risks of their residents, have developed flexible rehabilitation programmes that allow residents ground parole, visits to the local community and visits to family. Standards of care, the patient's charter and new therapies have all been introduced. Quality-of-life issues also are being addressed and healthy lifestyles are promoted with better diets, exercise facilities and smoking cessation programmes.

Badger et al (2000), in an international systematic review of the epidemiology of disordered offenders, found the following:

- There are 100 patients in special hospitals per 3 million population.
- There are four times as many men as women.
- There is a wide age range but the average age is in the 30s.
- Average length of stay is 8 years.
- About two-thirds have an index offence of violence against the person.
- About half the population do not require the highest level of security.
- About 50 people per 3 million of the population require high security provision.
- Many require long-term care in medium or low security settings.
- About one-third of those discharged to less secure settings return to special hospitals.

Regional secure units

In 1974, two reports were published that recommended that each regional health authority should develop regional secure units (DHSS 1974, Home Office 1975). The first interim regional secure unit was set up in Middlesbrough in 1976 and Freeman (1982), an occupational therapist, provides an overview of the set-up of the unit and the occupational therapy programme. This remained the only regional secure unit until 1983, when other such units began to be developed (Rogowski 1997). Indeed, at the time of the Reed report 17 years after the Butler report, only 600 beds were available in regional secure units. Currently, there are approximately 1600 beds. Regional secure units vary in size from 30–100 beds and they primarily meet the needs of those patients who are too dangerous for psychiatric units but not so dangerous as to warrant admission to special hospitals.

The level of security at regional secure units is less intense than that within the special hospitals. As patients progress through the system and demonstrate appropriate behaviour, they tend to move through the following parole system:

- no ground parole
- varying intensity of escorted ground parole
- unescorted ground parole
- escorted community visits
- unescorted community visits
- overnight leave
- weekend leave.

Intensive psychiatric care units

These units provide modest security by having a locked door policy and a higher than average skilled staff/resident ratio. Generally, the residents are acutely disturbed, causing disruption and discomfort to others or harming themselves seriously. Smith (1997), in a survey of intensive psychiatric care settings in Scotland, found the largest group of residents were in the units first because of violence to others and second because of absconding. The majority of the patients had a diagnosis of schizophrenia or affective disorders; 70% stayed less than 2 weeks and 23% stayed less than 24 hours. The Mental Welfare Commission for Scotland (1999–2000) also studied this group and reported that nursing staff estimated that 20% of patients did not require the high level of care provided but that there was a lack of facilities within the acute care wards. Best (1996) described the role of the occupational therapist in a psychiatric intensive care unit. She indicated that this setting had emerged from acute psychiatry but required additional skills in risk management and in negotiating and establishing boundaries.

Prisons

Mental disorders in the prison setting are increasing and a recent report suggests that nine out of ten adults in prison suffer from some type of mental illness (Office for National Statistics 1998). Approximately 750 prisoners are transferred each year to hospital for psychiatric treatment. This has been recognized by the government and a recent joint report on the future of the prison health service recognized the need for a developed health service with close links to the NHS (Prison Service/NHS Executive Working Group 1999). It proposed that 300 extra staff be recruited to provide inreach mental health facilities.

Other joint projects between the Prison Service and the NHS are the pilot projects that have been set up to assess and treat dangerous people with severe personality disorder (DPSPD). These projects have been set up to establish an evidence-based approach to the assessment and treatment of DPSPD before any final decision about the structure of new service in this area will be made. The two initial pilot sites are Her Majesty's Prison Whitemoor and Rampton High Security Hospital. Over the next 3 years these, and other pilot projects, will develop and evaluate new approaches to the assessment and interventions for DPSPD. New multidisciplinary teams are being developed to implement these projects.

The multidisciplinary team within the forensic setting

Although the forensic settings described above might differ (with the exception of the Prison Service) there are similarities in the professions who make up the multidisciplinary team. The core team consists of nurses, occupational therapists, psychiatrists, psychologists and social workers, who generally work on a day-to-day basis with patients. Additionally, there are other members of staff who contribute in different ways to the treatment of patients. Their role will vary depending on the needs of the patients and they might not work with all patients but provide a specialized service. This group varies from setting to setting but could be made up of the following:

- art therapist
- dance and movement therapist
- dentist
- dietician
- drama therapist
- health education worker
- librarian
- music therapist
- physiotherapist
- podiatrist
- teacher
- technical instructor.

Mental health legislation

Most patients entering mental health services do so voluntarily. However mental health legislation in the form of the Mental Health Act is required for anyone needing compulsory treatment.

It is important for anyone employed in the forensic setting to have knowledge of the Mental Health Act and how it applies to their residents. Within the UK there are three different Mental Health Acts. The Mental Health (Scotland) Act 1984 and the Mental Health (Northern Ireland) Act 1986 are broadly similar in nature to the Mental Health Act 1983, which relates to England and Wales. It is not the intention of this chapter to deal with the Mental Health Act in great detail. Readers are recommended to study the Act itself or refer to Chapter 2 of Gunn & Taylor's (1995) text *Forensic psychiatry*.

The Mental Health Act 1983 was largely based on a review of the mental health legislation that took place in the 1950s. Within this current mental health legislation the only power to treat compulsorily is within the hospital setting. Since the 1983 Mental Health Act there have been major changes within mental health services. With the advent of community care there has been an awareness that mental health legislation should reflect these major advances, while at the same time providing adequate protection for the public. With this in mind, the government issued a white paper in December 2000 outlining its proposed changes in mental health legislation. It is hoped that a new

Mental Health Act will be in force by 2005. Alan Milburn, the then English Health Minister, in introducing the white paper, stated 'These changes amount to the biggest shake up in mental health in four decades'.

Part 1 of the new proposed Act sets out a legal framework for when and how treatment should be provided without consent of the person with a mental disorder but in his or her own interests or in the interest of public safety. All the multitude of sections will be replaced with a single care and treatment order, which will be authorized by two doctors and one other mental health professional. This order will specify where the care and treatment is to be provided. New powers will be implemented to allow for care and treatment orders for people outside hospital.

The safeguards that will be put in place include:

- a new independent tribunal to determine a longer term use of compulsory powers
- a new right to independent advocacy
- new safeguards for people with long-term mental incapacity
- a new commission for mental health
- statutory requirement to develop care plans.

Part 2 of the new proposed act has created more controversy because it deals with high-risk people. It outlines plans to broaden the definition of what constitutes mental health so as to include dangerous people with severe personality disorders. Care and treatment orders will be applied to this group using specific criteria to determine levels of dangerousness and places of detention and dangerous people with severe personality disorders can be detained indefinitely in specialist services. The major controversy is that the white paper suggests that dangerous people with severe personality disorders who have committed no crime but are thought to be dangerous can be detained. The government has recognized the concerns that many mental health workers and members of voluntary organizations have about the evidence-base that currently exists around the diagnosis and treatment of people with personality disorder. They have accepted that this area needs much more research and have put in place a number of pilot projects within the NHS and the Prison Service to test appropriate models before these will be implemented in the whole service (see the 'Website addresses' section at the end of the chapter).

Scotland is also reviewing its Mental Health Act and has set up the Millan Committee to undertake a comprehensive review and make recommendations. It has currently just completed its second draft consultation and hopes to make recommendations in the near future (see 'Website addresses').

Risk assessment and management

Mullen (2000) suggests that 'risk assessment and risk management have emerged as central elements not just in forensic practice but in all mental health practice'. Mental health services need to be able to care and treat people with a mental illness who have a tendency to violent behaviour. The main aim of risk assessment is to identify and manage people with such behaviour before the violent behaviour manifests itself.

Lindqvist & Skipworth (2000) identify two types of risk variables: static and dynamic. They suggest that the static variables, such as personal demographics and personality characteristics, are less amenable to rehabilitation and that 'a person who has a history of persistent antisocial behaviour and falls ill with a major mental disorder will be an ongoing risk to the public even after the mental disorder is controlled'. They identify the following four dynamic variables with varying resistance to change:

1. the disorder itself, where active psychotic symptoms can lead to violent behaviour
2. family problems and poor sociocultural circumstances
3. substance misuse
4. antitherapeutic regimes, which create violent behaviour.

They go on to suggest that any assessment must take into consideration both the person and the forensic setting that the person is detained in. They therefore contend that forensic psychiatric rehabilitation should focus on two elements – the person and the rehabilitative environment – and suggest the following environmental factors are important:

- shared values and goals
- staff continuity
- timing of the start of the rehabilitation process
- family relationships
- social networking/peers
- process insight (challenging the view that hospital order is a punishment and a sentence to serve)
- the views of the patient on his or her future.

Rogowski (1997), while presenting material from an occupational therapy perspective, provides a helpful overview of risk assessment and identifies a list of practical questions useful to any staff member working with patients within a forensic setting.

Summary

- There is no one recognized definition of forensic mental health.
- There are several different types of forensic mental health settings.
- Many different professionals contribute to the assessment and treatment of mentally disordered offenders.
- The mental health act is changing.
- Risk assessment and management are essential in forensic mental health.

References

Badger D, Nursten J, Williams P, Woodward M 2000 Systematic review of the international literature on the epidemiology of mentally disordered offenders. CRD report 15. NHS Centre for Reviews & Dissemination, University of York, York

Best D 1996 The developing role of occupational therapy in psychiatric intensive care. British Journal of Occupational Therapy 59(4):161–164

Chiswick D 1994 Forensic psychiatry. In: Kendall R E, Zealley A K (eds) Companion to psychiatric studies. Churchill Livingstone, Edinburgh, p 793–817

DHHS 1974 Revised report of the working party on security in NHS psychiatric hospitals (Glancy Report). HMSO, London

Department of Health 1992 Report of health and social services for mentally disordered offenders and others requiring similar services (the Reed Report). Department of Health, London

Flood B 1993 Implications for occupational therapy services following the Reed Report. British Journal of Occupational Therapy 56(8):293–294

Freeman M 1982 Forensic psychiatry and related topics. British Journal of Occupational Therapy June: 191–194

Gunn J, Taylor P J 1995 Forensic psychiatry. Butterworth Heinemann, London

Home Office 1975 Report of the committee on mentally abnormal offenders (the Butler Report). HMSO, London

Lindqvist P, Skipworth J 2000 Evidence-based rehabilitation in forensic psychiatry. British Journal of Psychiatry 176:320–323

Mullen P E 2000 Forensic mental health. British Journal of Psychiatry 176:307–311

Office for National Statistics 1998 Prison population and accommodation, 1971–1998. Social Trends 30

Report of Mental Welfare Commission for Scotland 1999–2000. Scottish Office, HMSO, Edinburgh

Prison Service/NHS Executive Working Group 1999 Report of future organisation of the prison health service.

Rogowski A 1997 Forensic psychiatry. In: Creek J (ed) Occupational therapy and mental health. Churchill Livingstone, Edinburgh, p 459–479

Scottish Office/DoH 1999 Report of health, social work and related services for mentally disordered offenders in Scotland (1999) Scottish Office, Edinburgh

Smith A 1997 Survey of locked facilities in Scottish psychiatric hospitals. Psychiatric Bulletin 21:77–79

Website addresses

www.doh.gov.uk/mentalhealth/summary
www.scotland.gov.uk/lib2

20 Substance misuse

Part A: PROBLEM DRINKING

Marie Donaghy

Introduction

Alcohol has been used for centuries to increase enjoyment within societies. For the majority of people, the widespread use and acceptability of this drug brings only benefits; for others, overuse of alcohol can lead to problem drinking with detrimental social, medical and psychological consequences (Cooper 2000). The focus of this chapter is to provide a definition of problem drinking and a summary of recent social trends in drinking behaviour highlighting the most at-risk age groups and the associated health problems linked to excessive alcohol consumption. Following this, an outline of assessment and intervention is presented alongside arguments to support the inclusion of physical activity and acupuncture as therapeutic adjuncts in the rehabilitation of the problem drinker.

Defining problem drinking

An individual who, as a result of prolonged heavy drinking, experiences physical or psychological harm, including impaired function or dysfunctional behaviour that can lead to disability, or have adverse consequences for interpersonal relationships, is identified as a problem drinker (Royal College of Physicians 2001). The problem drinker usually consumes alcohol daily, at levels recognized to be dangerous to health. Males drinking in excess of 50 units of alcohol a week are defined as heavy drinkers and are likely to endanger their health (Royal College of Physicians 2001). For females, the level is lower at 35 units per week; a unit being equivalent to one-half pint of beer or a single measure of spirit (8 g of ethanol alcohol per unit). Problem drinkers are usually drinking well in excess of these amounts, however, they are recognized to be in relapse drinking when consuming 56 units a week or more (J Chick, personal communication, 1996). Not all heavy drinkers become problem drinkers. The difference between the two categories is in relation to the number of units consumed and the physical, psychological and behavioural consequences of the drinking behaviour. The problem drinker is usually unable to stop for long periods of time, despite repeated effort, and there might be evidence of withdrawal phenomena, nausea and vomiting, tremors and shaking, and hallucinations when the individual stops drinking (American Psychiatric Association 1992).

Prevalence, morbidity and mortality

It is estimated that 90% of the population in the UK are drinkers, of whom four million are heavy drinkers and one-fifth of those are problem drinkers (Paton 1994). Current advice on sensible drinking advocates consideration of daily consumption levels of two to three units a day for females and three to four units a day for males, with one or more alcohol-free days (Department of Health 1995). These guidelines are being exceeded by 40% of men over the age of 16 and 20% of women (Office for National Statistics 2001). The heaviest drinkers are in the age group 16–24 with 50% of men and 40% of women exceeding these guidelines on one or more days of the week (Office for National Statistics 2001).

Several studies have examined the drinking behaviour of adolescents and young adults (Goddard 1996, Miller & Plant 1996, Newbury-Birch et al 2000). The findings suggest that the teenagers in the UK are more often binge drinking (more than five drinks consumed in a row) and displaying high levels of intoxication than teenagers in most other European countries (Hibell et al 1997). Recent evidence from an update of a UK survey undertaken with 7722 schoolchildren, which indicated that 50% of those surveyed (aged 15 years or less) had regularly consumed alcohol in the past 30 days, suggested that although these high levels are being maintained, they have not increased further in the last 5 years (Miller & Plant 2001).

There is evidence to support the view that alcohol use in preadolescents and adolescents is increasing; in 1996, 29% of 12–13-year-old boys and 26% of girls admitted drinking alcohol in the past week, these figures increased to 38% and 30%, respectively, in 1999 (Royal College of Physicians 2001). This is of concern, early-age onset of regular drinking is associated with heavy consumption and alcohol-related problems in later life (Newbury-Birch et al 2000, Paton 1994). Both males and females are at risk, with recent studies providing evidence of binge drinking among university students (Norman et al 1998, Pickard et al 2000, Underwood & Fox 2000), with the two most recent studies reporting high levels of binge drinking among female students, who are at least three times more likely to exceed weekly guidelines than their counterparts in the general population. The general household survey (National Statistics 2001) indicates that 13% of men and 6% of women in the 16–24 age group are heavy drinkers. The conclusions from these recent surveys suggest a pattern of drinking in the UK that starts in school, with one-third of 12–13-year-olds regularly consuming alcohol. This increases at age 15 to 50%, with binge drinking prevalent among teenagers and an at-risk group of males and females who are heavy drinkers in the early years of adulthood. These patterns suggest that the number of young problem drinkers is likely to increase for the foreseeable future, leading to health and social problems that require cost-effective programmes of intervention.

Alcohol consumption in the UK is a significant contributor to morbidity and mortality and the cost of providing medical and social services runs into billions of pounds, accounting for as much as 12% of total NHS expenditure on hospitals (Royal College of Physicians 2001). In the year ending 1999 in Scotland alone, there were 4060 alcohol-related admissions to psychiatric hospitals and 6602 alcohol-related admissions to non-psychiatric hospitals (Scottish Health Statistics 1999). Alcohol abuse was directly responsible for the deaths of 5796 males and 3371 females in the UK (Office for National Statistics 2000, Registrar General for Scotland 2000). However, the link between alcohol abuse and other causes of mortality in the UK is estimated to be far greater at 25 000–40 000 deaths per year (Royal College of General Practitioners 1986). Alcohol-related mortality is highest with regard to chronic liver disease, followed by increased risk of cancer of the larynx and oesophagus, cerebrovascular disease and injuries through accidents (Ritson 1994). Morbidity includes the above diseases and also respiratory disease, neurological deficits, cognitive impairment including dementia, circulatory and respiratory problems, pancreatitis, ulcers and digestive problems (Royal College of Physicians 2001). Poor physical fitness has been reported among problem drinkers (Donaghy et al 1991), along with evidence of negative effects of chronic alcohol consumption on skeletal muscle (Preedy & Peters 1990), loss of bone mass and associated incidence of fractures (Peris et al 1992, Rico 1990). Alcohol-related harm is also associated with common psychopathologies, these include depression (Davidson & Ritson 1993), anxiety (Stockwell & Bolderston 1987), lowered self-esteem (McMahon & Davidson 1986), lowered physical self-perceptions (Donaghy 1997) and lowered self-efficacy (Heller & Krauss 1991). The relationship between alcohol use and mental illness is complex, with both causal links and outcomes from alcohol abuse reported in American epidemiological studies (Clenaghan 2000). There is evidence that people with mental illness are more vulnerable to problem drinking and problem drinkers have a higher incidence of mental illness (Cooper 2000).

Assessment and intervention

The recommendations from the Royal College of Physicians (2001) include the need for alcohol misuse to be given a higher profile, to distinguish it from drug misuse and to tackle prevention. Clinical guidelines for the management of addiction are now available (Department of Health 1999). However, interventions have had only limited success, with 57% of those receiving treatment for alcohol-related problems in psychiatric hospitals being readmissions (ISD 2000).

The growing body of research from the disciplines of genetics, social science and psychology indicate that problem drinking has a multifaceted aetiology (Donaghy & Mutrie 1999a). It would also seem likely that every problem drinker's addictive behaviour has arisen as the result of a different interaction of various aeteological factors (Fig. 20.1). These include environmental, cultural, genetic and social factors. For a fuller discussion of these factors, see Cook (1994). Rehabilitation programmes since the early 1990s have attempted to take these factors into account, moving away from the traditional approach encompassing one model of care to a newer, more collaborative approach that offers a range of options for the patient (Bartu 2000). Options can include family or group therapy, alcohol and general health education, cognitive–behavioural strategies, cue exposure, practical life skills and relationship enhancement. There remains a need to provide intervention for both acute and chronic care needs of the problem drinker. Three major stages have been identified in the management of individuals and their families. Stage 1: detoxification, emergency treatment and screening. Stage 2: rehabilitation, evaluation and assessment; primary care and extended care. Stage 3: maintenance aftercare, relapse prevention and domiciliary care (Institute of Medicine 1990). Activities including exercise, acupuncture, social skills training, relaxation, assertiveness training have been used within rehabilitation mostly during stage 2, with only a few studies including follow-up through to stage 3 (Donaghy 1997).

The use of prescribed drugs as an adjunct to psychosocial and behavioural interventions still plays a major role in treatment, with initial trials in the use of acamprosate suggesting that this drug is useful in maintaining post-detoxification abstinence (Wilde & Wagstaff 1997). For a review of medical and cognitive–behavioural approaches to treatments, see Margolis & Zweben (1998).

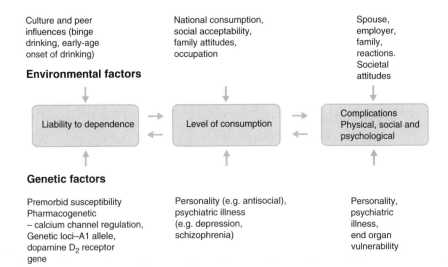

Figure 20.1 *Model of environmental and genetic factors in the aetiology of alcoholism (adapted from Cook 1994)*

Physiotherapists are involved in the assessment and treatment of musculoskeletal and neurological problems that can result from long-term abuse of alcohol, for example, osteoporosis, muscle weakness, peripheral neuropathy, impaired balance and gait, and injuries resulting from trauma. Interventions provided by physiotherapists and occupational therapists working in alcohol rehabilitation can include; the application of exercise, transcutaneous electrical nerve stimulation (TENS), massage, acupuncture, instruction in relaxation techniques, assertiveness training and social skills training. The rationale for treatment and the therapeutic benefits associated with these interventions in the rehabilitation phase of treatment for alcohol addiction are similar to those for illicit drug addiction. The therapeutic benefits for acupuncture, TENS and massage are outlined in the second part of this chapter and are not reiterated here; this part focuses on the evidence and rationale to support the use of acupuncture and physical activity as therapeutic interventions.

Acupuncture

A number of studies, including four randomized controlled trials conducted during the 1990s were reviewed at a national conference on acupuncture (NIH 1998). The consensus statements indicated that there is sufficient evidence to support the use of auricular acupuncture as an adjunct in the treatment of patients with addiction to alcohol. The short-term benefits include relief of symptoms associated with withdrawal, such as craving, anxiety, restlessness and pain. There are several different types of acupuncture cited in these studies including laser, electroacupuncture, stud and sutured bead. The evidence at this time does not appear to favour one approach over another, with most studies reporting positive results. The results of these studies, although supporting an earlier review of 13 studies, eight of which were randomized controlled trials (Moner 1996), provide only tentative evidence.

There is no evidence that acupuncture is effective in primary rehabilitation, or in relapse prevention. Studies had high drop-out rates and this is a recurrently reported problem in addiction research (Stark 1992). The inconsistency in type and dose of acupuncture and outcome measures make comparisons of findings across studies and conclusions difficult. In conclusion, the evidence supports the use of acupuncture for reducing symptoms associated with withdrawal but provides no evidence for extending treatment aimed at influencing lifestyle change or relapse prevention. These behaviours are more amenable to change through physical activity and cognitive–behavioural approaches. The latter is discussed in detail in Chapter 10.

Physical activity

Physiotherapists, occupational therapists and exercise specialists have been involved in the planning and delivery of physical activity programmes for problem drinkers delivering both generic structured programmes (Donaghy 1997) and tailored lifestyle programmes that provide purposeful self-selected activities (Golledge 1998, Ussher et al 2000).

In a review of key international studies highlighting exercise in the rehabilitation of problem drinkers (Donaghy & Mutrie 1999a) the authors conclude that there is unequivocal support for the positive benefits of exercise on aerobic fitness and strength. More importantly, people with low levels of aerobic fitness can improve their fitness in just 3–4 weeks by participating in 30–40 min exercise three times a week, and this can be maintained for up to 12 weeks by following an exercise programme at home. Strength as measured by muscular endurance has also been shown to improve and problem drinkers have been found to be more physically active. Self-report by problem drinkers indicates that getting back to fitness, having more energy and being less breathless are important in making changes in smoking, eating and drinking behaviours (Ussher et al 2000), and in getting back to previously enjoyed activities such as hill walking, running, boxing and cycling to work (Donaghy 1997).

In discussing the quality of the research, Donaghy & Mutrie (1999a) suggest that there is high external validity in relation to physical outcomes, given that the studies have been conducted in North America, Japan and the UK. However, internal validity is less convincing with several studies having poor methodological design. These design limitations include:

- Small sample size with inadequate statistical power increasing the probability of type 2 statistical errors where 'no between group difference' has been reported.
- Failure to ensure that personal contact with professionals is equalized across the different treatment conditions, including controls.
- Failure to ensure that follow-up measures are taken and that participants lost to follow-up are fully accounted for.
- Failure to ensure that reliable and valid means of measuring outcomes are included for both physiological and psychological variables and that studies are consistent in using these measures.
- Failure to avoid resentful demoralization by keeping the treatment and control group procedures as similar as possible.
- Failure to provide theoretical underpinning of studies, making it difficult to forecast what theories might predict results obtained – the links between what was found and psychological theories are poor in most of the studies.

The evidence for psychological benefits in relation to changes in self-esteem, anxiety and depression is not so conclusive. It is not clear whether exercise can have an effect in reducing anxiety and depression over and above that of psychotherapy and whether it can strengthen abstinence behaviour and reduce the likelihood of returning to excessive drinking. We don't know whether the current research findings, where the mean age is 35–45 years, will apply to those aged 16–24, who have been identified as an at-risk group. In their conclusions, Donaghy & Mutrie (1999a) stress that health professionals can, with confidence, promote exercise and increased levels of physical activity, in the knowledge of the established physical benefits and that the potential psychological benefits far outweigh the potential risk of no change.

There is an urgent need to undertake further quantitative research, to evaluate physical activity interventions, and also qualitative research, to determine how physical activity, as part of rehabilitation in different age groups, is perceived by clients, their families and medical staff. Only Ussher et al (2000) and Donaghy (1997) have attempted to integrate physical activity into community activities and only Donaghy (1997) has looked at home-based exercise as a follow-up intervention. Ussher et al (2000) used cognitive–behavioural techniques for promoting exercise adherence including goal setting, self-monitoring decision balance sheets and relapse prevention. The concept of using exercise as a self-control strategy and as an alternative to excessive alcohol consumption is not new (Marlatt & Gordon 1985) however, it could become increasingly attractive to the 13% of men and 6% of women in the 16–24 age group who have been identified as heavy drinkers (National Statistics 2001), particularly when considered alongside the evidence that increasing physical activity can lead to positive changes in perceptions of the physical self and identity (see Chapter 6). What still needs to be explored is how improvements in physical self-perception and physical well-being from exercise participation can best be integrated into the development of cognitive coping strategies aimed at dealing with high-risk situations in the long term (Donaghy & Mutrie 1999a). Although there is some evidence that acupuncture can be used to reduce uncomfortable symptoms of withdrawal, including cravings, and physical activity has been linked to a reduction in cravings in smokers (Ussher et al 2000), there has been no similar research for alcohol. There is a need for physiotherapists and occupational therapists to work with other team members to promote alcohol education and healthy lifestyle as part of prevention and intervention strategies to achieve an overall reduction in hazardous drinking in the population, particularly in the most at-risk groups.

Underpinning mechanisms

It is important to consider explanations of why physical activity might be beneficial as a therapeutic adjunct for this population. Previously described physiological explanations have linked increases in enzyme levels and capilliarization of the muscles, with negating some of the deficit in type IIb muscle fibres found as the direct effects of alcohol on muscle protein. This suggests that the capacity of the muscle to undertake work without fatigue is enhanced (see Donaghy & Mutrie (1999a) for a full explanation). In addition, positive cardiovascular and respiratory changes associated with aerobic exercise will provide the same health benefits to this clinical population as to those in the general population. A number of possible mechanisms to explain the psychological benefits associated with physical activity have been proposed (see Chapter 7 for a full discussion). It is likely that both physiological and psychological explanations are linked to changes in aerobic fitness, strength, independence, self-esteem and health improvement, as evidenced when exercise is used as an adjunctive therapeutic intervention.

Prescribing exercise

In prescribing exercise for this group, consideration should be given to individual preference, encouraging participants to make choices in light of their perceived and actual needs. This might include the desire to feel stronger, to be able to walk further or climb stairs without getting out of breath, to increase confidence regarding participation in physical activity, to induce feelings of well-being or to improve sleep patterns. An initial assessment of fitness strength and flexibility can be linked to exercise counselling and this has been found to be useful in assessing needs and preferences and for setting initial goals (Ussher et al 2000). Integrating physical activity with cognitive–behaviour therapy strategies to assist in the maintenance and progression of the programme is recommended (see Chapters 8 and 10). The frequency, duration and intensity of activities required for optimum physiological and psychological change is not clear at this time. The evidence from the author's multisite randomized controlled study (Donaghy 1997) suggests that 3–4 weeks of moderate-intensity exercise of 30–40 min duration undertaken three times a week will improve physical fitness and physical self-perceptions of strength and condition. Home- and community-based programmes offer the potential of integrating physical activity into daily routines and they can be linked to social integration and family activities. Adherence to exercise is problematic for all populations (Dishman 1994) and practical considerations in prescribing exercise outlined in Chapter 8 are relevant to this population. In addition, Donaghy & Mutrie (1999b) suggest that strategies to increase adherence for problem drinkers could include the following:

- initial exercise counselling to explore personal aims and set appropriate goals
- fortnightly telephone support to see what goals have been achieved and which new ones are being set
- return visits for reassessment at appropriate intervals
- linking with key workers to explore what local facilities are available.

Conclusion

Problem drinking is costly to society in terms of damage to health and recurring treatment costs. Research in the last 5 years indicates that whereas binge drinking can be observed in all age groups, it is prevalent among adolescents, with the highest percentage of heavy drinkers in the

16–24 age group. It is likely that this shift towards earlier regular heavy drinking will increase the number of young males and females who become problem drinkers. The links between early-age-onset drinking, personal identity and the physical self need to be explored alongside other social and cultural factors to gain a greater understanding of those adolescents most likely to be at risk of long-term abuse and to determine the most appropriate interventions.

There is unequivocal support that the inclusion of physical activity in rehabilitation programmes for problem drinkers has a positive effect on aerobic fitness and strength. These benefits, when considered in conjunction with preliminary support for improvements to physical self-perceptions and feelings of well-being, offer the potential to facilitate behavioural and lifestyle change and, as such, should be included routinely in rehabilitation programmes and highlighted as preventative measures for at-risk groups.

For the moment, therapists should feel confident that they have a key role to play in promoting exercise and physical activity for both prevention and intervention. This can be offered as part of a therapeutic package integral to medical and social care and may include interventions such as acupuncture to reduce symptoms experienced during withdrawal, and social skills and occupational training to facilitate lifestyle change.

Summary

■ Problem drinking has a multifaceted aetiology, which includes environmental, cultural, genetic and social factors.

■ Recent social trends in drinking behaviour indicate that teenagers in the UK are more often binge drinking and displaying high levels of intoxication than their European peers, with evidence of early age onset of regular drinking among 12–15-year-olds. The heaviest drinkers are in the age group 16–24.

■ People with mental illness have been found to be more vulnerable to problem drinking and problem drinkers have a higher incidence of mental illness.

■ There is evidence of physical impairment among problem drinkers related to low physical fitness, skeletal muscle damage, loss of bone mass and associated incidence of fractures.

■ Auricular acupuncture can provide short-term benefits for problem drinkers in rehabilitation programmes, including relief of symptoms associated with withdrawal, such as craving, anxiety, restlessness and pain.

■ There is unequivocal support for the positive benefits of exercise delivered as part of a rehabilitation programme for problem drinkers in regard to aerobic fitness and strength with some evidence for improved self-esteem, and a reduction in anxiety and depression.

> ■ Occupational therapists and physiotherapists have a key role to play in promoting exercise and physical activity as part of a therapeutic package aimed at reducing symptoms experienced during withdrawal, improving social skills and facilitating lifestyle change.

References

American Psychiatric Association 1992 Diagnostic and statistical manual of mental disorders, 4th edn. American Psychiatric Association, Washington DC

Bartu A 2000 Treatment and therapeutic interventions. In: Cooper D B (ed) Alcohol use. Radcliffe Medical Press, Abingdon, p 185–193

Clenaghan P 2000 Mental health and mental illness. In: Cooper D B (ed) Alcohol use. Radcliffe Medical Press, Abingdon, p 93–109

Cook C 1994 Aetiology of alcohol misuse. In: Chick J, Cantwell R, (eds) Alcohol and drug misuse. College Seminars Series, Royal College of Psychiatrists, Gaskell, London

Cooper D B 2000 Alcohol use. Radcliffe Medical Press, Abingdon

Davidson K, Ritson B 1993 The relationship between alcohol dependence and depression. Alcohol and Alcoholism 28(2):147–155

Department of Health 1995 Sensible drinking. The report of an interdepartmental working group. DoH, London

Department of Health 1999 Drug misuse and dependence. Guidelines on Clinical Management. DoH, London

Dishman R K 1994 Advances in exercise adherence. Human Kinetics, Champaign, IL

Donaghy M E 1997 An investigation into the effects of exercise as an adjunct to the treatment and rehabilitation of the problem drinker. PhD Thesis. Medical Faculty, Glasgow University, Glasgow

Donaghy M E, Mutrie N 1999a Is exercise beneficial in the treatment and rehabilitation of the problem drinker? A critical review. Physical Therapy Review 4:153–166

Donaghy M E, Mutrie N 1999b Adherence to class-based and home-based exercise as part of a rehabilitation programme for problem drinkers. Journal of Sport Sciences 17:50–51

Donaghy M, Ralston G, Mutrie N 1991 Exercise as a therapeutic adjunct for problem drinkers. Journal of Sport Sciences 9(4):440

Goddard E 1996 Drinking in 1994. HMSO, London

Golledge J 1998 Distinguishing between occupation, purposeful activity and activity, part 1: review and explanation. British Journal of Occupational Therapy 61:100–105

Heller M C, Krauss H H 1991 Perceived self-efficacy as a predictor of aftercare treatment entry by the detoxification patient. Psychology Report 68: 1047–1052

Hibell B, Andersson B, Bjarnason T (eds) 1997 The 1995 ESPAD report. Alcohol and other drug use among students in 26 European countries. Modin Tryck AB, Stockholm

Information and statistics division, National Health Service in Scotland. ISD 2000, Edinburgh

Institute of Medicine 1990 Broadening the base of treatment for alcoholism. Wiley, New York

Margolis R D, Zweben J E 1998 Treating patients with alcohol and other drug problems: an integrated approach. American Psychological Association, Washington DC

Marlatt G A, Gordon J R 1985 Relapse prevention: maintenance strategies in the treatment of addictive behaviours. Guildford, New York

McMahon R C, Davidson R S 1986 An examination of depressed vs nondepressed alcoholics in inpatient treatment. Journal of Clinical Psychology 42:177–184

Miller P, Plant M 1996 Drinking, smoking and illicit drug use among fifteen and sixteen year olds in the United Kingdom. British Medical Journal 7054(313):394–397

Miller P, Plant M 2001 Drinking and smoking among 15–16-year-olds in the United Kingdom: a re-examination. Journal of Substance Use 5:285–289

Moner S E 1996 Acupuncture and addiction treatment. Journal of Addicitive Diseases 15(3):79–100

Newbury-Birch D, White M, Kamali F 2000 Factors influencing alcohol and illicit drug use amongst medical students. Drug and Alcohol Dependence 59:125–130

NIH 1998 Consensus Conference Acupuncture. Journal of the American Medical Association 280:1518–1524

Norman P, Bennett P, Lewis H 1998 Understanding binge drinking among young people: an application of the Theory of Planned Behaviour. Health Education Research 13:163–169

Office for National Statistics 2000 1999 mortality statistics. The Stationery Office, London

Office for National Statistics 2001 Social trends 31. The Stationery Office, London.

Paton A 1994 ABC of alcohol, 3rd edn. British Medical Association, London

Peris P, Pares A, Guanabens N et al 1992 Reduced spinal and femoral bone mass and deranged bone mineral metabolism in chronic alcoholics. Alcohol and Alcoholism 27(6):619–625

Pickard M, Bates L, Dorian M et al 2000 Alcohol and drug use in second-year medical students at the University of Leeds. Medical Education 34:148–150

Preedy V R, Peters T J 1990 Alcohol and skeletal muscle disease. Alcohol and Alcoholism 25: 177–187

Registrar General for Scotland 2000 1999 Annual Report. Common Services Agency, Edinburgh

Rico H 1990 Alcohol and bone disease. Alcohol and Alcoholism 25:345–352

Ritson B 1994 Epidemiology and primary prevention of alcohol misuse. In: Chick J, Cantwell R (eds) Alcohol and drug misuse. College Seminars Series. Royal College of Psychiatrists, Gaskell, London

Royal College of General Practitioners 1986 Alcohol, a balanced view. Royal College of General Practitioners, London

Royal College of Physicians 2001 Alcohol, can the NHS afford it? Recommendations for a coherent alcohol strategy for hospitals. Royal College of Physicians/Sarum Colour View Group, Salisbury, UK

Stark M J 1992 Dropping-out of substance abuse treatment: a clinically orientated review. Clinical Psychology Review 12:93–116

Stockwell T, Bolderston H 1987 Alcohol and phobias. British Journal of Addiction 82: 971–979

Underwood B, Fox K 2000 A survey of alcohol and drug use among UK based dental graduates. British Dental Journal 189:314–317

Ussher M, McCusker M, Morrow V, Donaghy M 2000 A physical activity intervention in a community alcohol service. British Journal of Occupational Therapy 63(12):598–604

Wilde M, Wagstaff A 1997 Acamprosate: a review of its pharmacology and clinical potential in the management of alcohol dependence after detoxification. Drugs 53(6):1039–1053

Part B: ILLICIT DRUG MISUSE

Catherine Pope

Defining drug misuse

At its most literal, 'illicit drug misuse' could be interpreted as the taking of any illegal drug. This chapter concentrates more on the features of dependency and addictive behaviour, specifically related to heroin abusers, as these are the clients more typically seen in rehabilitation by physiotherapists and occupational therapists.

'The essential feature of substance dependence is a cluster of cognitive, behavioural and psychological symptoms indicating that the individual continues use of the substance despite significant substance-related problems' (American Psychiatric Association 1994, p. 176). To expand, these would include evidence of tolerance and withdrawal (physiological dependence) and compulsive drug-taking behaviour, linked to cravings (psychological dependence). Not all illicit drugs cause dependence, and many people remain 'social users'. The World Health Organization (1993) defines harmful use as persisting for at least 1 month, or occurring repeatedly over 12 months.

Prevalence, morbidity and mortality

Official figures support public perception that the use of illicit drugs is rising. The number of people addicted to drugs notified to the Home Office rose from 7052 in 1985 to 37164 in 1995, and whereas the percentage dependent on heroin fell from 82% in 1990 to 66% in 1995, those dependent on methadone rose from 28% to 47% in the same period (Home Office 1986–1996). However, notified people addicted to drugs represent only a small proportion of the problem. The total number of users presenting to drug misuse services for the first time increased to 28 559 in the 6 months ending September 1998, of whom 16 081 were heroin users, mostly in their twenties. This had risen from 17 864 and 8 456 in March 1994 (Department of Health 1999a). In one survey, 29% of 16–24-year-olds reported using a non-prescribed drug in the past year (1998), the vast majority naming cannabis (Office of National Statistics 2000a). Miller & Plant (1996) surveyed 10–15-year-olds in the UK and found that 39.8% of girls and 45% of boys had used illicit drugs at any time. Sutherland & Shepherd (2001a) surveyed 9742 English adolescents and found the prevalence of illicit drug use increased from 0.9% of 11-year-olds to 14.5% at age 16; there was no gender difference. They further found that 18.8% of these pupils were likely to have been in trouble with the police, compared with 1.6% of the non-drug users (Sutherland & Shepherd 2001b). Other social indicators included perceived poor academic performance, lack of religious belief, non-intact family, favouring peer over family opinion and having been suspended from school.

Drug dependence has been reported at two or three times higher amongst men than women (Department of Health 1999a, Office of National Statistics 1997). Although there is no clear class pattern for women, there is a definite increased risk of dependence for men of lower social classes, with a more than 15-fold increase from 5 to 73 per 1000 population from class I to class V (Office of National Statistics 1997).

Illicit drug use is a criminal activity. Home Office (1992) figures showed drug seizures rise from 296 to 1087 per 1 000 000 population between 1981 and 1991, and 96 per 10 000 of the male population were found guilty of drug offences in 1998, almost doubling amongst 16–24-year-olds (Office of National Statistics 2000a).

Health costs associated with drug misuse are almost impossible to quantify, as they include not only the costs of detoxification and relapse prevention but also treatment of drug-related medical problems, overdoses and accidents. There are also the preventative costs of health education and measures to prevent the spread of infectious diseases such as hepatitis or HIV (Health Advisory Service 1996). Mortality figures are also difficult to assess because of the many different causes used in recording deaths, but there appears to be an increase in both direct and underlying drug-related deaths. Oppenheimer et al (1994) found that people addicted to heroin had a 12-times greater mortality risk than the general population, whereas Frischer et al (1997) reported that those injecting heroin had a 22-times greater mortality risk than their non-injecting peers. Totalling those recorded as drug- or morphine-dependent, non-dependent and poisoning where dependent drugs are mentioned, there were 1711 male and 260 female drug-related deaths in 1999, but this still excludes those recorded as suicide, accidents or HIV related (Office of National Statistics 2000b). There is a fourfold greater risk of mortality in social class V than IV, and a 20-times greater risk than class I (Office of National Statistics 1997).

Assessment and intervention

The government guidelines state that 'Drug misusers have the same entitlement as other patients to the services provided by the NHS' (Department of Health 1999b, p. 1). However, this remains a controversial area, with many arguing that methadone prescriptions prolong dependence, and even cause dependence amongst non-heroin users, through the illegal sale of prescriptions (Gossop 2000). To prevent this, good practice dictates supervised medication (Department of Health 1999b). The use of pharmacological agents, particularly methadone, to treat heroin addiction arose from the belief that dependence is a medical disorder, with many studies reporting successful detoxification, but without claims for continued abstinence (for a full discussion, see Stine & Kosten 1997). There is further disagreement surrounding the practice of providing sterile needles to prevent HIV spread, and the provision of NHS-funded rehabilitation placements (Gossop 2000).

Current medical guidelines suggest the use of methadone in liquid form to aid withdrawal, and naltrexone to prevent relapse (Department of Health 1999b). A multidisciplinary approach is encouraged. 'Prescribing should be seen as an enhancement to other psychological, social and medical interventions' (Department of Health 1999b, p. 27). Non-pharmacological approaches are now increasing in popularity, aiming more at relapse prevention than with easing withdrawal, including behavioural therapies (Marlatt & Gordon 1985, National Institute on Drug Abuse 1995).

Physiotherapy

There is a distinct lack of literature supporting the role of physiotherapists in this field, although the growing evidence to support physiotherapy in treating alcohol abuse is transferable to people with other addictions (Donaghy & Durwood 2000). Many people undergoing detoxification regimes report increased pain from old musculoskeletal injuries and those arising from their lifestyle, and much physiotherapy time is spent in traditional forms of assessment and intervention. The injuries encountered are diverse. Injection errors can lead to nerve damage, and even amputation where arteries are mistakenly used. Physiotherapists are known as the physical experts in many mental health units, and certainly 'hands on' skills such as massage, mobilization and therapeutic touch can be important in improving body image and self-esteem among a client group frequently portrayed as undesirable by the media (Gossop 2000) (for a full discussion on the links between self-perceptions and identity, see Chapter 6). There is also an important role in offering non-pharmacological forms of pain relief, such as TENS, acupuncture and exercise.

Increasingly, however, physiotherapists and occupational therapists are using their skills to directly affect the detoxification and relapse prevention process. The cognitive–behavioural approach emphasizes the importance of positive addictions in overcoming the vicious cycle of daily stress and poor coping skills seen in many people addicted to drugs (Marlatt & Gordon 1985).

Physical activity

Although there is now a growing body of evidence to support the use of exercise in mental health (see Chapter 9), and more specifically amongst problem drinkers (see Part A, Chapter 20), there is a scarcity of published data concerning its benefits amongst illicit drug users (Donaghy & Durwood 2000). A review of 11 randomized controlled trials (RCTs) suggesting a causal link between exercise and mental health concluded that moderate exercise was as beneficial as vigorous, and that those with an addictive lifestyle were less likely to exercise sufficiently (Glenister 1996). Glasser (1976) reported that physical activity should be encouraged because aerobic exercises can become positively addicting and rewarding. Others have described the benefit of physical activity in improving sleep patterns (important in the withdrawal stage), and how continuing addiction is incompatible with exercise due to its effect on performance (Marlatt & Gordon 1985).

On a practical level, exercise should be tailored individually and supported to ensure compliance and lasting benefit (Marlatt & Gordon 1985). Exercise counselling is beneficial to ensure that the client's own needs are identified and joint goals set (see the discussion on this in Chapter 9). Successful completion of early goals is important in assisting motivation and increasing periods of activity and this can be enhanced by using behavioural strategies to increase awareness and activation of energy levels (Jacobson et al 2001). Anecdotally, badminton and multigym use have been found to be very popular with clients. Although evidence supports a structured, regular programme (American College of Sports Medicine 1998), there is often a balancing act between providing this and maintaining clients' interest and participation and in achieving their goals.

Acupuncture

Wen & Cheung (1973) are most commonly cited as the first to link acupuncture with the treatment of drug addiction, albeit accidentally, finding that when used for anaesthesia in people addicted to opium their withdrawal symptoms improved. Acupuncture is used in all stages of treatment, with claims that it can decrease withdrawal symptoms, induce relaxation and relieve cravings (Moner 1996). Auricular acupuncture has been reported as the most effective in treating withdrawal (Smith 1988) and electroacupuncture in reducing cravings (McLellan et al 1993, Rampes et al 1997). In a review article, Moner (1996) discusses several possible mechanisms. These include evidence to suggest acupuncture can reduce levels of adrenocorticotrophic hormone (ACTH) and cortisol in withdrawing opiate mice. These hormones rise in response to stress, and are also raised during opiate withdrawal. Opiate abuse affects opiate peptide receptors, thus preventing the activation of endogenous opiate mechanisms during withdrawal. Higher beta-endorphin levels have been found in morphine-dependent mice treated with acupuncture, decreasing symptoms of physical withdrawal. Another theory is that acupuncture activates the parasympathetic nervous system via the auricular lung point, where the vagus nerve is closest to the skin, thereby blocking symptoms (see Moner (1996) for a full discussion). Unfortunately, most studies suffer from poor design and high drop-out rates, and there is less success than in trials involving problem drinkers. Furthermore, sham acupuncture might just be bad acupuncture, leading to similar effects, and therefore will not be a good control (Moner 1996).

TENS

Some patients decline acupuncture, or it might be inappropriate, particularly if needles induce cravings. TENS has been shown to have similar, although possibly less effective, mechanisms (Thompson 1989), and has the benefit of being self-administrative, offering a patient-controlled intervention.

Massage

Despite its popularity and long history, there has been little research on the effectiveness of massage as a therapeutic intervention. A recent review of its possible mechanisms highlighted massage resulting in decreased levels of adrenaline, noradrenaline and cortisol (Lund 2000). These substances are raised in response to stress, and in opiate withdrawal, so we can speculate that by their reduction, massage can reduce withdrawal symptoms. Lund also described how massage can induce relaxation, and raise pain threshold via the release of oxytocin. As oxytocin plays a role in mother–baby bonding, this effect could explain why patients enjoy massage and request it again. The danger here is that the patient might become too dependent on the therapist, and long-term relapse prevention needs self-reliance.

A study of patients with fibromyalgia compared massage, TENS and sham TENS in 30-min sessions, twice a week for 5 weeks (Sunshine et al 1997). The massage group reported decreased levels of depression, anxiety, pain, stiffness and fatigue. Sleeping patterns improved and reduced cortisol levels were found. Both the described symptoms and benefits in this study are transferable to treating those suffering withdrawal symptoms. Other studies have also shown that massage can relieve various musculoskeletal symptoms, and benefit depression and anxiety (Andrade & Clifford 2001, Field 1998), all of which can coexist in this client group.

Massage has long been used to improve blood flow and lymphatic drainage (Andrade & Clifford 2001), so it would seem logical that this should aid the detoxification process, although no specific studies appear to have been carried out on withdrawing patients.

Relaxation

Relaxation can also be effective in reducing the levels of hormones raised during detoxification, and there are many available methods (see Payne (2000) for a full discussion). Drug use can be associated with relaxation, and some patients find relaxation techniques produce an induced 'high', which is useful in controlling craving (Glasser 1976).

Conclusion

Anecdotally, the therapeutic interventions described in this chapter are certainly popular among clients, and as they provide cheap and relatively safe adjuncts to traditional medical treatments, they have a valid and frequently overlooked place in the treatment of illicit drug misuse. The growing evidence to support their use is encouraging but still too small to be conclusive. Although these measures alone will not prevent relapse, they are useful tools to combine with behavioural strategies in promoting a healthier lifestyle.

Summary

- Illicit drug use is a growing health and social problem.

- Medical treatment of people addicted to drugs is controversial.

- There is a need to focus on relapse prevention and improving coping skills.

- There is some evidence to support the use of therapeutic interventions, including exercise, acupuncture and massage, but there is an identified need for further research to further inform the selection of therapeutic interventions with this client group.

References

American College of Sports Medicine 1998 Position stand: the recommended quantity and quality of exercise for developing and maintaining cardio-respiratory and muscular fitness and flexibility in healthy adults. Medicine and Science in Sports Exercise 30(6):975–991

American Psychiatric Association 1994 Diagnostic and statistical manual of mental disorders (DSM IV). APA, Washington DC

Andrade C K, Clifford P 2001 Outcome-based massage Lippincott, Williams and Wilkins, Baltimore, M A

Department of Health 1999a Health and personal social services statistics for England. The Stationery Office, London

Department of Health 1999b Drug misuse and dependence – Guidelines on clinical management. The Stationery Office, London

Donaghy M, Durwood B 2000 A report on the clinical effectiveness of physiotherapy in mental health. CSP, London

Field T M 1998 Massage therapy effects. American Psychologist 53:1270–1281

Frischer M, Goldberg D, Rahman M, Berney L 1997 Mortality and survival amongst a cohort of drug injectors in Glasgow 1982–1994. Addiction 92:419–427

Glasser W 1976 Positive addictions. Harper and Row, New York

Glenister D 1996 Exercise and mental health: a review. Journal of the Royal Society of Health 116(1):7–13

Gossop M 2000 Living with drugs, 5th edn. Ashgate Publishing Ltd, Aldershot, UK

Health Advisory Service 1996 Children and young people. Substance misuse services. The Stationery Office, London

Home Office 1986–1996 Statistics of drug addicts notified to the Home Office, UK (annual reports). Home Office, London

HMSO 1992 Statistics of drug seizures and offences dealt with, UK 1991. HMSO, London

Jacobson N S, Martell C R, Dimidjian S 2001 Behavioral activation treatment for depression: returning to contextual roots. Clinical Psychology, 8:255

Lund I 2000 Massage as a pain relieving method. Physiotherapy 86(12):638–639, 654

Marlatt G A , Gordon J R 1985 Relapse prevention. Guilford Press, London

McLellan A T, Grossman D S, Blaine J D, Haverkos H W 1993 Acupuncture treatment for drug abuse: a technical review. Journal of Substance Abuse 10:568–576

Miller P, Plant M 1996 Drinking, smoking and illicit drug use among 15 and 16 year olds in the UK. British Medical Journal 7054 (313):394–397

Moner SE 1996 Acupuncture and addiction treatment. Journal of Addictive Disorders 15(3): 79–100

National Institute on Drug Abuse 1995 Integrating behavioural therapies with medication in the treatment of drug dependence. US National Institute of Health, Washington DC

Office of National Statistics 1997 Health inequalities: decennial supplement. The Stationery Office, London

Office of National Statistics 2000a Social trends 30. The Stationery Office, London

Office of National Statistics 2000b 1999 mortality statistics. Cause. The Stationery Office, London

Oppenheimer E, Tabutt C, Taylor C, Andrew T 1994 Death and survival in a cohort of heroin addicts from London clinics: a 22-year follow-up study. Addiction 89:1299–1308

Payne R 2000 Relaxation techniques, 2nd edn. Churchill Livingstone, Edinburgh

Rampes H, Pereira S, Mortimer A et al 1997 Does electroacupuncture reduce craving for alcohol? Complementary Therapies in Medicine 5:19–26

Smith M O 1988 Acupuncture treatment for crack: clinical survey of 1500 patients. American Journal of Acupuncture 16:241–247

Stine S, Kosten T 1997 New treatments for opiate dependence. Guilford Press, London

Sunshine W, Field T M, Quintino O et al 1997 Massage therapy and transcutaneous electrical stimulation effects on fibromyalgia. Journal of Clinical Rheumatology 2:18–22

Sutherland I, Shepherd J P 2001a The prevalence of alcohol, cigarette and illicit drug use in a stratified sample of English adolescents. Addiction 96(4):637–640

Sutherland I, Shepherd J P 2001b Social dimensions of adolescent substance use. Addiction 96(3): 445–458

Thompson J 1989 Pharmacology of transcutaneous electrical nerve stimulation (TENS). Journal of the Intractable Pain Society 7(1):33–34

Wen HL, Cheung SYC 1973 Treatment of drug addiction by acupuncture and electrical stimulation. Asian Journal of Medicine 9:138–141

World Health Organization 1993 ICD-10. Classification of mental and behavioural disorders. WHO, Geneva

21 Eating disorders

Linette Whitehead, Louise Montague-Jones and Tina Everett

Introduction

This chapter covers a spectrum of eating disorders that affect both psychosocial and physical functioning. Particular attention is given to anorexia nervosa and bulimia nervosa, as research on other syndromes is at an early stage.

This chapter provides definitions of the different eating disorders and describes provision of care for them. It also presents a rationale for intervention strategies, from both occupational therapy and physiotherapy perspectives, and highlights the importance of self-perception and self-esteem within the context of these interventions. Therapeutic interventions can be offered in a range of contexts, including outpatient, day patient and inpatient settings.

Definition and classification

Fairburn & Walsh (1995, p. 135) define an eating disorder as:

A persistent disturbance of eating or eating-related behaviour that results in the altered consumption or absorption of food and that significantly impairs physical health or psychosocial functioning. This disturbance should not be secondary to any recognised general medical disorder or any other psychiatric disorder.

Palmer (1989, p. 34) suggests that:

Eating disorders may be thought of as arising when there is an inappropriate and ultimately maladaptive entanglement of ideas about weight and eating control with wider personal issues especially emotional control and self-evaluation.

There are two classificatory systems currently in use: the fourth revision of the Diagnostic and Statistical Manual of the American Psychiatric Association (APA), abbreviated as DSM-IV (APA 1994) and the tenth edition of the International Classification of Diseases, abbreviated as ICD-10 (World Health Organization 1992). The DSM-IV system seems to be more widely used in the field of eating disorders. Within DSM-IV, the main categories are anorexia nervosa (Box 21.1) and bulimia nervosa

(Box 21.2). In addition, there is a 'provisional diagnosis worthy of further study' included in the appendix of DSM-IV, which is binge eating disorder (Box 21.3). Apart from these three categories there is a loose category called 'eating disorder not otherwise specified', abbreviated as EDNOS, which includes disorders that do not meet the thresholds for the other diagnostic categories, or which are partial syndromes.

Box 21.1
DSM-IV criteria for anorexia nervosa

A. Refusal to maintain body weight at or above a minimally normal weight for age and height.
B. Intense fear of gaining weight or becoming fat, even though underweight.
C. Disturbance in the way in which one's body weight or shape is experienced, undue influence of body weight on self-evaluation, or denial of the seriousness of the current low body weight.
D. Amenorrhoea (i.e. the absence of at least three consecutive menstrual cycles) in post menarcheal females.

Restricting type: during the current episode of anorexia nervosa, the person has not regularly engaged in binge-eating or purging behaviour (i.e. self-induced vomiting or the misuse of laxatives, diuretics or enemas).

Binge-eating/purging type: during the current episode of anorexia nervosa, the person has regularly engaged in binge-eating or purging behaviour (i.e. self-induced vomiting or the misuse of laxatives, diuretics or enemas).

Box 21.2
DSM-IV criteria for bulimia nervosa

A. Recurrent episodes of binge eating.
B. Recurrent inappropriate compensatory behaviour to prevent weight gain.
C. The binge eating and inappropriate compensatory behaviour occur, on average, at least twice a week for 3 months.
D. Self-evaluation is unduly influenced by body shape and weight.
E. The disturbance does not occur exclusively during episodes of anorexia nervosa.

Purging type: During the current episode of bulimia nervosa, the person has regularly engaged in self-induced vomiting or the misuse of laxatives, diuretics or enemas.

Non-purging type: During the current episode of bulimia nervosa, the person has used other inappropriate compensatory behaviours, such as fasting or excessive exercise, but has not regularly engaged in self-induced vomiting or the misuse of laxatives, diuretics or enemas.

Box 21.3
DSM-IV criteria for binge eating disorder

A. Recurrent episodes of binge eating.
B. The binge eating episodes are associated with three (or more) of the following:
   1. eating much more rapidly than normal
   2. eating until feeling uncomfortably full
   3. eating large amounts of food when not feeling physically hungry
   4. eating alone because of being embarrassed by how much one is eating
   5. feeling disgusted with oneself, depressed or very guilty after overeating
C. Marked distress regarding binge eating is present.
D. The binge eating occurs, on average, at least 2 days a week for 6 months.
E. The binge eating is not associated with the regular use of inappropriate compensatory behaviours (e.g. purging, fasting, excessive exercise) and does not occur exclusively during the course of anorexia nervosa or bulimia nervosa.

Epidemiology

It is difficult to establish accurately the prevalence of eating disorders in the community, in part because most individuals are reluctant to admit that they have these conditions. Palmer (2000) quotes an estimated point prevalence of between 10 and 30 per 100 000 total population for anorexia nervosa, and approximately 100 per 100 000 for bulimia nervosa and binge eating disorder. Eating disorders are particularly prevalent among young women, and are found less commonly among males.

Societal influences

There has been a great deal of interest in the impact of our societal context on the incidence of eating disorders. Any theory has to be able to account for the gender imbalance (approximately 10 females to each male in clinical samples) as well as the relative rarity of the disorders. Thus, our societal emphasis on the importance of slimness for women is likely to account for the widespread prevalence of dieting, but seems unlikely on its own to cause a small number of women to develop eating disorders. Similarly, theories about women's role in our society, although of interest, do not take us far enough in understanding the onset of eating disorders in a minority of the female population. It seems that the incidence of eating disorders is more likely to be the outcome of the interaction of a number of personal and social factors, including genetic make-up, temperamental characteristics, family and peer group influences, early trauma and social and cultural pressures (see Fairburn et al's comprehensive studies on risk factors (1997, 1998, 1999)).

Comorbidity

Many people with an eating disorder have additional problems, of which the most common are mood disorders, and treatment needs to take account of these. A number of people with bulimia nervosa have comorbid substance abuse and borderline personality disorder, which can complicate their treatment.

Assessment

Assessors should endeavour to identify the person's motivation for seeking help from the outset to avoid potential conflicts and misunderstandings that can later undermine planned intervention. This is particularly likely to arise with younger people, who might have been brought by their families or spurred on to seek treatment by a teacher or GP, without themselves being committed to change. It is important to seek to understand the aspects of the eating disorder that have been important to and valued by the individual, as well as the aspects that are experienced as aversive and which the person wishes to relinquish. It is vital to be sensitive to the person's feelings of embarrassment or shame in revealing thoughts or behaviours that they might regard as reprehensible.

A comprehensive assessment of an eating disorder calls for examination of the individual's current physical health; dieting; food-related behaviours; attitudes towards eating, weight and shape; mood; social and occupational functioning as well as the onset and development of the problem. Assessment is typically carried out by a range of different professionals depending on the treatment setting. In some inpatient units, the entire multidisciplinary team is involved in the assessment process. For a full discussion of the assessment process in eating disorders, see Palmer (2000).

Intervention

As indicated in the introduction to this chapter, planned intervention for people with an eating disorder can take place in a number of different settings. By far the majority of individuals with eating disorders will be seen in outpatient settings, by a variety of different practitioners including GPs, practice counsellors, dieticians, counselling and clinical psychologists, family therapists, psychotherapists and psychiatrists. Palmer (1989, p. 38) summarizes the tasks of recovery from an eating disorder as follows:

> *The individual needs to restore both weight and eating to levels which allow the natural regulatory mechanisms . . . to resume their normal function. Furthermore, she must separate ideas about weight and eating control from the wider personal issues with which they have become entangled. Lastly, the individual must begin to find other ways of thinking about and acting upon the problems of self-esteem (or whatever) which have previously been rendered insoluble by this entanglement.*

A range of treatment modalities have been offered to people with eating disorders, including nutritional counselling, psychodynamic counselling and psychotherapy, family therapy, interpersonal therapy and cognitive–behavioural therapy. To read more about these approaches, see Garner & Garfinkel (1997). It is certainly worth considering involving the family when the individual is still a teenager and living at home, particularly when there is high expressed hostility or criticism expressed by the family towards the adolescent, or where there is perceived over-involvement of one or more family members in the adolescent's problems. To read more about family therapy for eating disorders, see Dare & Eisler (1995).

There is some evidence for the effectiveness of a family approach, coming particularly from centres highly experienced and practised in its use, and with good access to skilled supervision. The best evidence for the efficacy of a particular intervention for eating disorders is for cognitive–behavioural therapy when applied to people with bulimia nervosa (see Wilson & Fairburn (1998) for a comprehensive discussion of outcome research in the field of eating disorders).

Where a particular individual has not been responsive to outpatient work, or where the person has become severely ill, it might be appropriate to offer a more intensive level of intervention as a day-patient or inpatient. Many day-patient or inpatient units include provision of occupational therapy or physiotherapy or both to augment the other interventions on offer. The contributions of the occupational therapist and physiotherapist to the eating disorders team will be discussed further below.

The occupational therapist

Occupational therapy provides an opportunity to address an individual's life roles and functional skills whilst within hospital care and beyond.

The therapeutic relationship

People with eating disorders can often feel ashamed, undervalued and generally not in control of their lives, and thus easily feel blamed, judged or criticized. The therapist needs to use skills of empathy, positive regard and patience when working with them (Martin 1998). Fear of change will affect motivation to change. It is of paramount importance that health professionals form a collaborative therapeutic relationship with each individual to enable the identification of agreed goals. The person with the eating disorder needs to feel ready to make a decision to start to give up the behaviours associated with the problem and commit themselves to making changes.

Promote healthy eating

The occupational therapist can assess an individual's skills and difficulties and expected goals associated with planning meals, shopping, meal preparation, cooking and eating. Strategies to help overcome difficulties experienced at any stage of the process are then actively practised. Clear communication with other members of the multidisciplinary team, in particular the dietician and the individual therapist/key worker, ensures that all personnel work toward the same goals.

Promote a healthy balance of activities

A key aim of occupational therapy is to address the balance of activities in three main occupational components of an individual's life:

1. leisure
2. productivity
3. self care.

Often, people with an eating disorder present with an imbalance of activities both between and within these occupational components. Some might be neglected or avoided, e.g. leisure or social activities. Others might become excessive, taking up an overwhelming amount of time, e.g. exercise or academic work.

Martin (1998, p. 183) explains this by saying '...eating disordered individuals are dysfunctional not only in their attitudes and habits regarding eating and weight control but also in pursuing and engaging in meaningful activity (occupation).'

Individual work or a group approach can be utilized to help address these needs. The advantage of a group approach, e.g. activity scheduling and life-skills planning group, is the opportunity for individuals to share past experiences and ideas, and explore information on community resources together. This process can provide a sense of personal empowerment and independence. The therapist can work in partnership with the individual to identify their needs or changes they want to make in relation to the occupational components of their lives and, through problem solving and goal setting, identify steps to take to reach goals.

For example, goals can focus on looking for employment. This might include returning to previous work but reviewing expectations and roles to address whether they are realistic. It might include looking at new opportunities, exploring options within the local community and devising curricula vitae.

One client described her initial occupational/activity needs as:

To fill my time when not on the treatment programme...I don't want this to result in bingeing and thinking about food. I want to do something constructive with my free time. I need something to replace the anorexia, i.e. a role or skill, which I feel good at other than being thin. I feel completely socially inadequate and scared of the outside world. I need to try and make new friends.

Develop leisure and social interests and activities, and improve social skills

People with an eating disorder might have few leisure interests other than those associated with food or weight loss. They might neglect activities previously enjoyed, finding it difficult to allow themselves to experience fun or pleasure, or seeing such activities as a waste of time, not producing or achieving anything. They can often be described as perfectionists, setting themselves high standards and being viewed as competent. However, they often feel very incompetent and gaining recognition from others for high levels of performance can be a way of feeling valued and accepted (Breden 1992). Engaging in leisure activities for enjoyment's sake can therefore be very difficult to do. Some people can also feel socially inadequate and, having avoided social situations, have poorly developed social skills.

The occupational therapist can assist in identifying an individual's previous leisure pursuits and examining those determined by the eating disorder, e.g. excessive exercise.

The development of new social, recreational and leisure activities is then encouraged within an individual's local community. Within a day- or inpatient treatment programme, recreational activities can be practised, e.g. crafts and games, and also new ways of applying acceptable levels of exercise to one's life, e.g. walking, gardening. People with an eating disorder are encouraged to allocate time within their activity schedules for leisure pursuits.

Provide opportunities for self-expression

Occupational therapists can use creative media such as art, pottery or writing to enable individuals to express their thoughts and feelings in regard to personally relevant issues (Martin 1991). As Creek states '...a capacity for thinking and acting creatively will influence the way in which problems are approached and will enhance the ability to find solutions' (Creek 2002, p. 267).

A creative therapy group can provide opportunity for non-verbal self-expression using art materials. The images that are created can add increased clarity to expression, allowing the individual to develop a greater awareness of themselves and thus foster the development of self-esteem.

Improve self-esteem

Improving self-esteem is an objective inherent within all previously outlined aims. Providing opportunities to enable an individual to explore changes to make, and to try out new ways to manage aspects of life differently can promote a sense of empowerment, independence, confidence and control (see Chapter 6 for a full discussion).

The physiotherapist

The physiotherapist can play a central role in enhancing the body image of a person with an eating disorder via a range of different physical activities. This role will now be explored further.

Exercise addiction and approaches to activity

Eating disorders symptoms are often associated with compulsive exercise and it is therefore debatable as to whether introducing exercise into the treatment programme is advisable. Current research is inconclusive, but it makes sense to offer carefully planned and supervised exercise in a supportive environment. Close (2000) maintains that physiotherapy is the one therapy among many others that is often ignored by the eating disorders team. The physiotherapist is able to offer not just exercise, but intervention for the all too common joint problems that accompany anorexia, as well as relaxation, diaphragmatic breathing and massage.

These interventions can be given individually at first but can later be combined through group work.

Williamson et al (1995) claimed that a more significant predisposer to eating disorder than compulsive exercise is body image disturbance. His study of 98 college athletes supports the theory postulated by himself and others (Rosen 1992, Slade 1988, Thompson 1992, Williamson 1990) that body image disturbance is a primary determinant of anorexia and bulimia nervosa.

Body awareness group

To set exercise into the context of caring for, rather than abusing, the body, it can be introduced within a body awareness group provided for outpatients, or as part of an eating disorders day programme. The need to be 'in control' of losing weight has generally lead to a feeling of being 'out of control' by the obsessive compulsions of diet and exercise (see Chapter 6 for links to physical self, exercise and need for autonomy). One of the main aims of the group is therefore to restore a feeling of control and mastery. Experiencing that gentle toning exercises can reduce feelings of flabbiness and ballooning as weight is gained is one way this can be achieved. It is important that the group is enjoyable and that people with an eating disorder can learn to nurture themselves, and reduce feelings of self-loathing. The establishment of a healthy lifestyle, which incorporates exercise with relaxation and with adequate nutrition, is a key goal.

Leadership

It is best if the physiotherapist can co-lead the group with a member of the eating disorders team. It is vital to have staff time together for preparation, feedback, forward planning and offloading (Everett 1995). It is important, too, that the participants take ownership of the group and are involved in planning and evaluation.

Exercise

Tai Chi-based exercises ('Chi-gong') are recommended because they are gentle, non-aerobic and easy to perform in the standing position. More importantly, they encourage a sense of well-being, postural awareness and enhanced energy. The main clinical research into the benefits of Tai Chi has been in relation to the reduction of falls in the elderly, improving postural awareness, sense of balance and increased confidence (Wolf et al 1997). The results, although not clinically significant, do have some relevance to interventions for eating disorders. Beaumont et al (1994) observe that a malnourished state will accentuate postural difficulties as protein depletion causes muscle, tendon and ligament shortening. McArdle et al (1996) report research that concludes that diminished bone mineral density (BMD) in anorexics, along with small skeletal size, can render them particularly susceptible to osteoparotic fractures at a younger age than expected for comparison groups. The time spent on Tai Chi in the body awareness group is not sufficient to affect BMD but, if individuals choose to pursue Tai Chi as a safe form of regular exercise, it might well have lasting beneficial effects. Tai Chi music can be used to enhance good feelings of enjoyment and relaxation and the group could end with a relaxation session (See Payne 2000). It is essential to address the issue of compulsive exercise and to talk about how it can be avoided in the future, while allowing for a sensible resumption of exercise as weight is gained. Just as people with an eating disorder have a distorted body image, they might well have unrealistic goals regarding weight-training, etc. Page & Fox (1997) state that the poor quality of information on which young people base their decision-making with regard to their bodies is a major problem. Facts must be provided and incorrect cognitions challenged. Team activities and socialization will be encouraged.

Massage

Massage can be introduced as a form of nurturing and caring for the body. Self-massage techniques can be incorporated into the Tai Chi or relaxation, and then massage of the head and hands and feet will be demonstrated and individuals in the group can practice on each other. The wishes of a person who chooses not to participate in the massage must be respected, but opportunity can be given to join in at a later session. There is little evidence for the use of massage in this context, but one randomly controlled study of 24 bulimic females (Field et al 1998) revealed from both self-report and behaviour observation, an immediate decrease in anxiety and depression after massage sessions and improved attitudes to their eating disorder over the 5-week trial period.

Conclusion

Rosen (1995, p. 369) states that 'Of all psychological factors that are believed to cause eating disorders, body image dissatisfaction is the most relevant and immediate antecedent' and 'without significant body image change, maintenance of recovery will be a struggle'. He also states that body image is the most consistent predictor of improvement and relapse after treatment for anorexia and bulimia nervosa. Although Rosen recommends the cognitive–behavioural model for the treatment of eating disorders, he states that a thorough assessment and treatment of body image will greatly facilitate recovery.

Cognitive–behaviour therapy has been shown to be effective in changing cognitions in the difficult areas of low self-esteem and altered physical self-perception. Socialization and self-expression are important for establishing new connections that can facilitate significant life changes and assist the development of self-esteem.

Box 21.4
Sample programme for body awareness group

> 1. Chi-gong (Tai Chi) exercises with music
> 2. Discussion on suitable exercise outside group
> 3. Hand massage with oils on each other
> 4. Relaxation and diaphragmatic breathing.

A body awareness group is a practical way of addressing body image dissatisfaction and the need for individuals with an eating disorder to have an enjoyable and nurturing body experience, replacing negative feelings. Input from a multidisciplinary team within the context of an eating disorders inpatient or day programme can greatly enhance the effectiveness of interventions with more severely affected individuals with eating disorder.

Summary

- Eating disorders affect both psychosocial and physical functioning.

- There are distinct criteria for anorexia nervosa, bulimia nervosa and for binge eating disorders in the DSM-IV classification. Cognitive–behavioural therapy has the best evidence for positive outcome for bulimia nervosa but is a recognized intervention for all eating disorders.

- Occupational therapy aims to promote healthy eating, improve self-esteem, and develop leisure and social skills.

- Physiotherapy aims to improve body image through self-nurturing and balanced exercise programmes.

References

APA 1994 Diagnostic and statistical manual of mental disorders, 4th edn. American Psychiatric Association, Washington DC

Beaumont P, Arthur B et al 1994 Excessive physical activity in dieting disorder patients: proposals for a supervised exercise program. International Journal of Eating Disorders 15(1):21–36

Breden A K 1992 Occupational therapy and the treatment of eating disorders in occupational therapy and psychosocial dysfunction. Occupational Therapy in Health Care 8(2–3):49–68

Close M 2000 Physiotherapy and exercise. In: Laske B, Bryant-Waugh R (eds) Anorexia nervosa and related eating disorders in children and adolescents, 2nd edn. Psychology Press/Taylor and Francis, Hove, UK

Creek J (ed) 2002 Occupational therapy and mental health, 3rd edn. Churchill Livingstone, Edinburgh

Dare C, Eisler I 1995 Family therapy. In: Szmukler G, Dare C, Treasure J (eds) Handbook of eating disorders. Wiley, Chichester, UK, p 333–349

Everett T 1995 The group process as a helping technique. In: Everett T, Dennis M, Ricketts E et al (eds) Physiotherapy in mental health. Butterworth-Heinemann, London, p 51–60

Fairburn C G, Walsh B T 1995 Atypical eating disorders. In: Brownell K D, Fairburn C G (eds) Eating disorders and obesity. Guilford Press, New York

Fairburn C G, Welch S L, Doll H A et al 1997 Risk factors for bulimia nervosa. Archives of General Psychiatry 54:509–517

Fairburn C G, Doll H A, Welch S L et al 1998 Risk factors for binge eating disorder. Archives of General Psychiatry 55:425–432

Fairburn C G, Cooper Z, Doll H A, Welch S L 1999 Risk factors for anorexia nervosa. Archives of General Psychiatry 56:468–476

Field T, Schanberg S, Kubin C et al 1998 Bulimic adolescents benefit from massage therapy. Adolescence 33(131). Libra Publishers, San Diego, CA

Garner D M, Garfinkel P E (eds) 1997 Handbook of treatment for eating disorders, 2nd edn. Guilford Press, New York

Martin J E 1991 Occupational therapy in bulimia. British Journal of Occupational Therapy 54(2): 48–52

Martin J E 1998 Eating disorders, food and occupational therapy. Whurr Publications, London

McCardle W, Katch F, Katch V 1996 Exercise physiology. Williams and Wilkins, Baltimore, MD

Page A, Fox K 1997 Adolescent weight management and the physical self. In: K Fox (ed) The physical self from motivation to well-being. Human Kinetics, Champaign, IL

Palmer R L 1989 The spring story: a way of talking about clinical eating disorders. British Review of Bulimia and Anorexia Nervosa 4(1):33–41

Palmer B 2000 Helping people with eating disorders: a clinical guide to assessment and treatment. Wiley, Chichester, UK

Payne R 2000 Relaxation techniques, 2nd edn. Churchill Livingstone, Edinburgh

Rosen J 1992 Body-image disorder: definition, development, and contribution of eating disorders. In: Crowther J, Tennenbaum D, Hobfalls S et al (eds) The aetiology of bulimia nervosa: the individual and familial context. Hemisphere, Washington DC

Rosen J 1995 Assessment and treatment of body image disturbance. In: Brownell K, Fairburn C (eds) Eating disorders and obesity. Guildford Press, New York

Slade P 1988 Body image in anorexia nervosa. British Journal of Psychiatry 153:20–22

Thompson J 1992 Body image: extent of disturbance, associated features, theoretical models, assessment methodologies, intervention strategies, and a proposal for a new DSM-IV category – body image disorder. In: Progress in behaviour modification Vol. 28. Sycamore Publishers, Sycamore, IL, p 3–54

Williamson D 1990 Assessment of eating disorders: obesity, anorexia and bulimia nervosa. Pergamon Press, New York

Williamson D, Netemeyer R, Jackman L et al 1995 Structural equation modelling of risk factors for the development of eating disorder symptoms in female athletes. International Journal of Eating Disorders 17(4):387–393

Wilson G T, Fairburn C G 1998 Treatment of eating disorders. In: Nathan P E, Gorman J M (eds) Psychotherapies and drugs that work: a review of the outcome studies. Oxford University Press, Oxford

Wolf S, Barnhart H, Ellison G et al 1997 The effect of Tai Chi Quan and computerized balance training on postural stability in older subjects. Physical Therapy 77(4):371–381

World Health Organization (1992) The ICD-10 classification of mental and behavioural disorders: clinical descriptions and diagnostic guidelines. WHO, Geneva

Further reading

Crisp A, Hsu L, Harding B et al 1980 Clinical features of anorexia nervosa. Journal of Psychosomatic Research 24:179–191

Doktor D (ed) 1994 Art therapies and clients with eating disorders = fragile board. Jessie Wigley Publishers, London

Fox K, Corbin C 1989 The physical self-perception profile: development and preliminary validation. Journal of Sport and Exercise Psychology 11: 408–430

Griffiths R, Beaumont P, Giannakopoulis E et al 1999 Measuring self-esteem in dieting disordered patients: the validity of the Rosenburg and Coopersmith contrasted. Wiley, Chichester, UK

Johnson K, Parkinson S 1999 There's no point raging on your own: using art therapy in groups for people with eating disorders. Group Analysis 32:87–96

22 Chronic fatigue syndrome

Tina Everett

Beliefs and misunderstandings associated with this condition are discussed following an introduction to the topic, and a summary of the evidence for interventions. The role of therapeutic intervention is highlighted in relation to a cognitive approach to graded exercise, with particular reference to chronic fatigue syndrome (CFS) in young people and its effects on education.

Introduction

Chronic fatigue syndrome was recognized formally as a medical condition around the middle of the nineteenth century (Wessely et al 1998). Since then it has been studied as a disease under the names of neurasthenia, fibromyalgia, Royal Free disease, Iceland disease and later as myalgic encephalomyelitis, commonly known as ME or postviral fatigue syndrome (PVFS). Up to the late 1950s, it was seen as an epidemic and it has been associated with anxiety surrounding the threat of polio (Wessely et al 1998). In the 1960s and 1970s the apparent epidemics were replaced by the wider problem of sporadic cases of chronic fatigue. The self-help group The ME Association started in 1976 and, along with Action for ME, became prominent in the media in the 1980s. The ME Association still wishes the term ME to be used, but substituting encephalomyelitis with encephalopathy, meaning abnormality of brain function (Shepherd & Chaudhuri 2001). The term chronic fatigue syndrome (CFS) has been widely accepted in healthcare since the early 1990s.

Wessely & Powell (1989) proposed that several factors (including the patient's belief in a physical disease, inactivity and depressive disorder) interact to perpetuate the illness. According to this theory, the symptoms are caused at least in part by depression and decreased physical fitness known as deconditioning. Wessely et al (1998) state that normal and abnormal fatigue should be seen not in terms of aetiology but instead via concepts of help-seeking behaviour and functional impairment. Research initially focused largely on the cause and pathology of CFS (Pemberton et al 1994) and less on rehabilitation. In the late 1990s, emphasis has been more focused on intervention, and the benefits of cognitive–behavioural therapy (CBT) have been widely researched (Clements et al 1997, Price & Couper 1999).

Diagnosis

The 1995 Oxford consensus meeting agreed to establish a set of diagnostic criteria for CFS and they have become known as the Oxford criteria. The definition is:

- 6 months duration
- a definite onset (not lifelong)
- impaired function
- physical and mental fatigability
- myalgia, mood and sleep disturbance.

There are also American criteria, which differ slightly in that four somatic symptoms (chosen from a list of eight) must be present, e.g. sore throat, inflamed lymph nodes (Wessely et al 1998). The exclusion criteria are:

- extensive list of known physical causes
- psychosis
- bipolar disorder
- substance abuse.

A patient is usually seen by a physician and a psychiatrist before being given a diagnosis of CFS. History of psychiatric illness (apart from the above criteria) does not come into the Oxford exclusion criteria for diagnosis but it was agreed it should be recorded for research purposes. Katon & Russo (1992) demonstrated that the greater the number of somatic symptoms in subjects with CFS the greater the probability of psychiatric disorder. Results from published epidemiological studies indicate at least two per thousand of the adult population have the diagnosis of CFS (Shepherd & Chaudhuri 2001).

Young people

Presentation

Reports have indicated that CFS is less common in children than adults (Jordan et al 1998). Fatigue amongst adults is one of the most common complaints in the GP surgery (Wessely et al 1998). By contrast, tiredness in children as a reason for consultation is much less common (OPCS 1985). Reporting of somatic symptoms, including fatigue, increases during adolescence and early adulthood (Eminson et al 1996).

A case-controlled study by Carter et al (1995) found that young fatigue subjects scored higher on somatization than healthy or depressed matched controls. Somatization is characterized by physical symptoms suggestive of an organic disorder, in the absence of demonstrable pathology (Rose 1994).

Effects on education

It has been suggested that CFS is the most common current cause of long-term school non-attendance (Wright et al 1999). Marcovitch (1997) states that children with other serious illnesses including malignancies, cystic fibrosis and rheumatoid arthritis can have surprisingly little time off school in comparison. Home tuition is often made available for children with chronic fatigue. Although this might be helpful in the short term, many clinicians recommend a return to school as early as possible. This is because home tuition can increase dependency and slow down rehabilitation (Garralda 1999). In fact, clinicians feel that the 6-month duration criteria is too long for the application of a diagnosis of CFS in childhood and adolescence. If this is shortened, it might allow earlier recognition and reduced risk of long-term school absenteeism with prolonged disability (Garralda 1999).

Sources of information

The internet

Adults with CFS and parents of children with the condition often present practising clinicians with print-outs from the internet (Wright et al 1999). Wright et al studied all available information on the internet and found a very wide variation in the quality of this information. Some of the advice is either contrary to current research evidence or not supported by it. Of the 13 websites found, only six discuss rest and activity and only two of these recommend graded activity; two even recommend prolonged bed rest, which is known to be positively harmful (4–6 weeks bed rest has been shown to result in 40% of loss of muscle strength; Bloomfield 1997). Almost half of the websites make no mention of psychological support and one actively discouraged psychiatric input. Many give details of diet, complementary therapies and pharmacological treatment but there is limited research evidence on the benefits of these approaches.

Self-help groups

Another source of information about CFS is to be found in the literature provided by the self-help groups, Action for ME and The ME Association. Although an attempt is made in this literature to concur with medical opinion and to quote from research, not all the literature is substantiated and some is anecdotal. The Action for ME current fact sheet *Living with ME* (Action for ME 2001) claims that ME is a potentially chronic and disabling disorder. It no longer attributes the cause to a persistent viral infection or an overactive immune system, but the condition is said to be preceded by a viral illness in two-thirds of cases. The ME Association, in its latest book *ME/CFS/PVFS* (Shepherd & Chaudhuri 2001) also now questions evidence for persisting viral infection as a cause for CFS.

It is considered important by the present author to critically analyse and compare the information from self-help groups and medical research, as this can have direct bearing on the attitudes and beliefs of people with CFS towards recommended treatment. Whether or not a virus is the original trigger for the condition, there is no evidence of organic disease continuing long term, nor, indeed, is viral infection found consistently across everyone with CFS (Fry & Martin 1996). Some studies question the link between infection and CFS (Wessely et al 1998), and Shepherd and Chaudhuri (2001) discuss the case for immune dysfunction. However, the concept of a continuing or reactivating viral infection is still very common in the minds of many people with CFS and should be discussed at assessment.

It is well known that bed rest and inactivity reduce muscle bulk and strength and, as this is the case, bed rest will only increase the impaired muscle function. However a recent study (Bazelmans et al 2001) disputes the theory that deconditioning is a perpetuating factor in CFS/ME. Although there were only 26 subjects, a comparison of physical fitness of CFS subjects and healthy matched controls (i.e. unfit people) found no significant difference in physical fitness, using standardized measures, despite marked differences in levels of function.

Treatment for CFS

Bed rest and activity levels

The ME Association (Shepherd 1995, Shepherd & Chaudhuri 2001) claims that some clinicians advise a graded exercise regime, regardless of how the indiviual feels, and they warn that this can result in further relapse. Graded exercise was advocated by Fulcher & White (1998) – who recommend a graded increase in activity but with full cooperation of the individual and opportunity given for slowing the pace or remaining static if symptoms increase. In this randomized controlled trial, a daily exercise programme was negotiated with the study participants and increased by 1 or 2 minutes each week up to a maximum of 30 minutes. It was then increased in intensity up to 60% of peak oxygen consumption. The 66 participants who completed the study were given ambulatory heart rate monitors to ensure that they reached, but did not exceed, target heart rates. The main exercise was walking, but swimming and cycling were also encouraged. Fatigue, functional capacity and fitness were significantly better after exercise than after flexibility treatment when measured after 3 months and again after 1 year. A later audit (White & Naish 2001) on the success of this treatment regime concluded that graded exercise therapy should be more widely available in general physiotherapy departments by specially trained therapists and that cognitive techniques for chronic pain are equally useful for people with CFS (see Chapter 12).

Case Study: Susan

Susan has been unwell with CFS for 4 years. She is waiting to start the CBT programme with a clinical psychologist. Meanwhile, she is gradually increasing her daily walking distance with the fortnightly telephone support of a physiotherapist. Her illness beliefs remain as yet unchallenged, although concerns about the dangers of exercise have already been discussed.

Shepherd (2001) quotes from an ME Association audit of people with CFS (2338 respondents) involving self-reported outcomes from a wide range of treatments. Around 50% stated that graded exercise had made their condition worse and Shepherd suggests this might be because of inflexible exercise programmes, disregarding the person's feelings. This could indicate that there was no partnership between the therapist and the people with ME/CFS who were engaged in the intervention programme. It demonstrates the necessity for exercise counselling and appropriate joint goal setting so that people with CFS can take ownership of their exercise programmes. In the author's experience, some people with CFS are already functioning at their maximum capacity with a strong sense of duty regarding work and/or family commitments. Exercise can then be introduced as recreational and enjoyable space for self, e.g. a gentle walk or cycle ride, or attendance at a Tai Chi class. Relaxation techniques can be as important as graded exercise. In the MDT from which the author takes CFS referrals, 'mindfulness meditation' (Kabat-Zinn et al 1985) has been recently introduced and is proving both popular and therapeutic. Mindfulness meditation has been shown to be a valid intervention for people with chronic pain (Kabat-Zinn et al 1985), depressive relapse (Teasedale et al 1995) and as a stress reduction intervention in the treatment of anxiety disorders (Miller et al 1995). It is now being researched in relation to CFS.

Cognitive–
behaviour
therapy (CBT)

In CBT the individual is helped to recognize patterns of distorted thinking and dysfunctional behaviour that reinforce negative thoughts about the past, self and the future. This is done by detailed systematic discussion of the problem and, for example, by giving behavioural assignments to the client, so that thoughts and behaviour are evaluated and modified. The goal of therapy is to bring about desired life changes, and quantitative research has been used to assess if this actually occurs (see Chapter 10). The most recent Cochrane review of CBT (Price & Couper 1999) systematically reviewed randomized controlled trials of CBT for adults with CFS. They tested the hypothesis that CBT is more effective than orthodox medical management or other interventions for adults with CFS. Only three relevant trials of adequate quality were found (Deale et al 1997, Lloyd et al 1993, Sharpe et al 1996) and these all demonstrated that CBT significantly benefits physical functioning in adult outpatients with CFS when compared to orthodox medical management or relaxation. The Lloyd et al study (1993) was used by Shepherd to devalue CBT (Shepherd 1995) but, according to the Cochrane review (Price & Couper 1999), it has a small effect size on outcome. This is, first, because CBT is combined with placebo medication, and second, because the CBT was carried out for only 6 hours, as opposed to 15 in the other two studies. All three studies follow-up participants for only 6 months after the treatment intervention. The study by Fulcher & White (1998), which provided good quality evidence that graded exercise and activity is an effective treatment for CFS, was excluded from the Cochrane review of CBT because the experimental intervention did not include a specific cognitive element. The Cochrane reviewer, while providing convincing evidence that CBT in adults improves physical functioning and other relevant outcomes such as mood, when compared to orthodox medical management, concludes that there is no evidence of high quality that suggests that CBT is any more effective than graded exercise and activity.

Beliefs and behaviours

Surawy et al (1994) examined the beliefs of adults with CFS regarding their condition and found that psychological problems, such as depression, were regarded by people with CFS as indicating weakness, fault or blameworthiness. Rest was always regarded as the best way to hasten recovery and a repeated oscillation between rest and bursts of activity was observed. Although people with CFS generally report that the onset occurred with a viral illness, further enquiry often revealed major psychosocial stressors and difficult life events preceding the onset of the illness. They found that people with CFS set themselves up for failure by having targets well beyond their capabilities. In this study the researchers psychologically assessed 100 people meeting the criteria for CFS and more than 50 of these were treated using a cognitive–behavioural approach. Study participants were selected on the basis of the symptoms of physical and mental fatigue – the fatigue having the quality of being exacerbated by activity. They found that the explanation of a physical illness can in some ways protect individuals from feelings of failure and low self-esteem, and prevent them from resolving the problems of over commitment, excessive demands and the emotions associated with loss. They advocate the cognitive approach to treatment involving the negotiation of small and attainable goals, with as high an emphasis on reducing striving as on reducing rest in the early stages of treatment.

CBT is, however, costly in staff time, can have waiting lists up to a year and also carries the risk of deterring individuals who are fearful of contact with mental health workers. Cognitive techniques can, however, be used by general health workers. A recent study of patient education to encourage graded exercise in CFS demonstrated that this approach

Case Study: Kate

> *Kate, a sporty university student, became ill following glandular fever and had to take 2 years out from her studies. Thanks to sensible advice, she avoided prolonged bed rest and managed to maintain low levels of activity. She is now increasing her stamina, combining travelling to and from college with regular walks using a pedometer.*

can be as effective as CBT but is shorter and requires less therapist skill (Powell et al 2001).

Everett (2000) undertook a qualitative study to explore secondary school teachers' beliefs and attitudes about CFS, to discover their sources of information and to look at their needs for support in relation to adolescents with CFS. Results suggested the presence of confusion among teachers from the available information, but some understanding of the physical and psychological components of CFS. An acute awareness of the complexities of management, and the need both to support the student and to be informed and supported by health professionals was also apparent. The mental health physiotherapist can have a key role to play in liaison with schools, offering expert advice on exercise and activity, and in supporting students with CFS and their families as well as teachers. Further study is needed to see if these conclusions are supported nationally, and to ascertain if further information and support for teachers affects outcome of CFS for students.

Conclusion

There has been confusion regarding the nature, origin and course of CFS, which comes in part from the very real conflict between some information given by self-help groups and internet advice, and information arising from controlled medical and psychological research. CFS is a common and serious illness, which greatly affects the lives of many people and their families. There are both physical and psychological factors relating to onset, course and outcome so effective treatment must take account of both sets of factors, emphasizing those most relevant to the individual. Physiotherapists can work together with cognitive therapists to support people with CFS with a common-sense approach to recovery, using similar approaches to those advocated for chronic pain (Chalder 1999) (Box 22.1). Listening skills and empathy need to be combined with education, practical advice and support.

Box 22.1
Interventions in CFS

- Clear explanation of the cycle of fatigue.
- Define targets and write down up to 10 steps to achieve each target.
- Encourage use of weekly activity diary.
- Discuss sleep patterns and regular bed times.
- Teach and encourage use of suitable relaxation techniques.
- Challenge and reframe negative thoughts.
- Aim towards increasing heart rate/stamina for 20–30 minutes three times a week.
- Where suitable, test fitness and encourage use of heart rate monitors, pedometers, etc.

Summary

■ There are clear diagnostic criteria for CFS.

■ A person's beliefs and attitudes about CFS can affect their outcome.

■ Literature on CFS from the media, the internet and the self-help groups can be in conflict with medical research.

■ There is clear evidence for the use of graded exercise and CBT as key interventions in CFS.

■ Physiotherapists and cognitive therapists can together support people with CFS towards recovery.

References

Action for ME 2001 Living with ME. Action for ME, Wells, UK

Bazelmans E, Bleijenberg G, Van der Meer J W M et al 2001 Is physical deconditioning a perpetuating factor in chronic fatigue syndrome? A controlled study on maximal exercise performance and relations with fatigue, impairment and physical activity. Psychological Medicine 31:107–114

Bloomfield S 1997 Changes in musculo-skeletal structure and function with prolonged bed rest. Medicine and Science in Sport and Exercise 29:197–206

Carter B, Edwards J, Kronenberger W et al 1995 Case control study of chronic fatigue in pediatric patients. Pediatrics 95(2):179–186

Chalder T 1999 Family orientated cognitive behaviour therapy for adolescents with CFS. In: Garralda E (ed) Chronic fatigue syndrome. Association for Child Psychology and Psychiatry Occasional Papers 16, London

Clements A, Sharpe M, Simkin S et al 1997 Chronic fatigue syndrome: a qualitative investigation of patients' beliefs about the illness. Journal of Psychosomatic Research 42:615–624

Deale A, Chalder T, Marks I et al 1997 Cognitive behaviour therapy for chronic fatigue syndrome: a randomized controlled trial. American Journal of Psychiatry 154:408–414

Eminson M, Benjamin S, Shortall A et al (1996) Physical symptoms and illness attitudes in children and adolescents: and epidemiological study. Journal of Child Psychology and Psychiatry 37:519–528

Everett C 2000 An exploration of secondary school teachers' beliefs and attitudes about adolescent children with chronic fatigue syndrome. Unpublished MSc thesis. Queen Margaret College, Edinburgh

Fry A, Martin M A 1996 Fatigue in the chronic fatigue syndrome: a cognitive phenomenon? Journal of Psychosomatic Research 45:414–426

Fulcher K, White P 1998 Chronic fatigue syndrome a description of graded exercise treatment. Physiotherapy 84(5):223–226

Garralda E 1999 Chronic fatigue syndrome: helping children and adolescents. Association for Child Psychology and Psychiatry, Occasional Papers 16, London

Jordan K, Landis D, Downey M et al 1998 Chronic fatigue syndrome in children and adolescents: a review. Journal of Adolescent Health 22:4–18

Kabat-Zinn J, Lipworth L, Burney R 1985 The clinical use of mindfulness meditation for the self-regulation of chronic pain. Journal of Behavioural Medicine 8:163–190

Katon W, Russo J 1992 Chronic fatigue syndrome criteria: a critique for the requirements for multiple physical complaints. Archives of International Medicine 152:1604–1609

Lloyd A, Hickie I, Brockman A et al 1993 Immunologic and psychologic therapy for patients with chronic fatigue syndrome: a double-blind, placebo-controlled trial. American Journal of Medicine 94:197–203

Marcovitch H 1997 Managing chronic fatigue syndrome in children. British Medical Journal 314:1635–1636

Miller J, Fletcher K, Kabat-Zinn J 1995 Three year follow-up and clinical implications of a mindfulness meditation-based stress reduction intervention in the treatment of anxiety disorders. General Hospital Psychiatry 17(3):192–200

OPCS 1985 Morbidity statistics from general practice: third national morbidity survey, 3rd edn. HMSO, London

Pemberton S, Hatcher S, Stanley P et al 1994 Chronic fatigue syndrome: a way forward. British Journal of Occupational Therapy 57(10):381–383

Powell P, Bentall R, Nye F et al 2001 Randomised controlled trial of patient education to encourage graded exercise in chronic fatigue syndrome. British Medical Journal 322:387–390

Price J, Couper J 1999 Cognitive behaviour therapy for chronic fatigue syndrome in adults. The Cochrane Library, Issue 2. Update Software, Oxford

Rose N (ed) 1994 Essential psychiatry, 2nd edn. Blackwell Scientific Publications, Oxford

Sharpe M, Hawton K, Simkin S et al 1996 Cognitive therapy for chronic fatigue syndrome: a randomised controlled trial. British Medical Journal 312:22–36

Shepherd C 1995 Guidelines for the care of patients, 2nd edn. ME Association, Stanford-le-Hope, Essex, UK

Shepherd C 2001 Pacing and exercise in Chronic Fatigue Syndrome. Physiotherapy 87(8): 395–396

Shepherd C, Chaudhuri D 2001 ME/CFS/PVFS an exploration of the key clinical issues. The ME Association, Stanford-le-Hope, Essex, UK

Surawy C, Hackman A, Hawton K et al 1994 Chronic fatigue syndrome: a cognitive approach. Behaviour Research Therapy 33(5):535–544

Teasedale J, Segal Z, Williams J 1995 How does cognitive therapy prevent depressive relapse and why should attentional control (mindfulness) training help? Behavioural Research and Therapy, 33(1):25–39

Wessely S, Powell R 1989 Fatigue syndromes: a comparison of chronic "post-viral" fatigue with neuromuscular and affective disorder. Journal of Neurology, Neurosurgery and Psychiatry 52: 940–948

Wessely S, Hotopf M, Sharpe M 1998 Chronic fatigue and its syndromes. Oxford University Press, Oxford

White P, Naish V 2001 Graded exercise therapy for chronic fatigue syndrome an audit. Physiotherapy 87(6):285–288

Wright B, Williams C, Partridge I 1999 Management advice for children with chronic fatigue syndrome: a systematic study of information from the internet. Irish Journal of Psychological Medicine 16(2):67–71

23 Childhood sexual abuse

Sally Feaver

Prevalence

Although rarely the primary reason, many people who seek psychological help, and therefore come into contact with occupational therapists and physiotherapists, have a history of childhood sexual abuse (CSA). This chapter identifies some key pointers necessary for sensitive practice for therapists and some of the ways in which therapists can assist in the therapeutic process.

The prevalence of CSA is difficult to determine. This is an inevitable result of society's response to the issue of sexual abuse over the past decade and also in part due to the difficulties with the exact definition of abuse. Repression and denial of the abuse by the victim means a distortion of the figures, reflecting a significant underestimation. Consequently, the true extent of the problem and the resulting impact on people's lives is unknown.

Taking this inaccuracy into account, prevalence is usually stated to be somewhere around 27% for women and 16% for men (Finkelhor et al 1990). The mental health service user population has a higher than expected reported incidence, with 33% commonly cited (Mullen et al 1993, Palmer et al 1993).

Definitions vary, and this has contributed to the distortion of the national picture of prevalence. The common variables include the extent to which the abuse must have involved physical contact and was experienced as physical violation by the victim. Most authors would accept the perception of abuse and resultant trauma on the victim as being the most clinically relevant.

Prevalence however, is academic. Therapists need to know that a proportion of mental health service users who present with a variety of symptoms, are more likely to have a history of sexual abuse than the rest of the population.

Consequences of CSA

The effects of the abuse on adult life are immense. It is impossible to give an accurate prediction of the precise consequences, however the literature is consistent in identifying varying degrees of psychological and psychiatric problems. The risk of victims of CSA developing mental health disorders in adult life are significantly increased (Muenzenmaier et al 1993, Mullen et al 1993).

The effects of abuse have been categorized both in order of severity and the psychological symptomatology. The severity ranges from 'substantial lasting effects' to 'serious pathology' (Bowne & Finkelhor 1986). Meekums (2000), in a review of literature between 1989 and 1995, concludes that a variety of psychological symptomatology is likely to be present, including a significant risk of depression and psychosis. Generally, effects are usually stated to include guilt, low self-esteem and psychosexual problems, relationship difficulties, and a tendency towards self-destructive behaviours including substance misuse, eating disorders and antisocial behaviours.

Several authors characterize the effects of abuse as post-traumatic stress disorder. Post-traumatic stress disorder can be conceptualized as the 'normal response to abnormal situation'. Common symptoms include recurrent and intrusive recollections of trauma, sleep difficulties with associated hypervigilance and an exaggerated startle response (American Psychiatric Association 1994). Herman (1992) overrides these common symptoms with additional features pertinent to survivors of sexual abuse, namely dysphoria, shame, failure of self protection, anxiety, phobias and panic attacks.

Effects on the victim can be conceptualized in many ways, but one useful reference is to Maslow's (1970) hierarchy of needs, in terms of a child's primary need for protection and safety. Victims have not experienced that protection and safety and consequently childhood has not been a safe place from which to develop and grow. Essentially, abuse fundamentally alters the child's self-perception and perception of others and the adult world. Additionally, CSA can be seen as a violation of boundaries, resulting in the individual having difficulties accepting they have a self, that they are separate and that their body is not there to meet other people's needs. Their sense of self is damaged and the betrayal experienced from those responsible for nurturing and protecting, means that distrust of others is inevitable.

It is important for therapists to understand the effects of the trauma and how the psychological defences develop at the time of the abuse to enable the child to survive. Naturally, psychological defences operate to enable an individual, in this situation a child, to continue to get his or her needs met. Children 'reframe' their abuse experience if they believe that they are in danger. This involves a shift of blame onto themselves to allow fulfilment of their need to be looked after. For this to occur, 'disassociation' is employed as the primary defence, which in turn is responsible for a series of behaviours associated with survivors of CSA (Loftus 1994, cited in Malley & Reilly 1999).

Defence mechanisms initiated for survival purposes at the time of the abuse become habitual after many years. Repression and disassociation are common and the experiences commonly reveal themselves as flashbacks, triggered by external current events such as death of the perpetrator.

Trauma also has physiological consequences. Responding to the anticipatory cues, repetitive trauma produces, over time, hyperarousal and hypersensitivity to stimuli because the body has become used to a constant state of vigil. Adults describe reacting to fast movement around them, startling easily, overreacting to physical changes and being very alert to minor changes (Herman 1992). In addition, CSA has been linked with somatic symptoms such as chronic pelvic pain, gastrointestinal disorders, chronic headaches and general medical problems (Schachter et al 1999).

Skills and competencies

So what are the skills and competencies therapists need to acquire to effectively mediate and provide healing in the context of their client–therapist contact?

Therapists need to have an opportunity to deal with their own feelings and dispel any myths associated with gaps in their knowledge about abuse. Common myths include the extent to which the child was or was not in a position to stop abuse; the covert guilt of the victim and abuse occurring only in certain societal groups.

Therapists must also deal with their own denial and disgust. Clinical supervision has an important part to play in providing an environment where the therapist is able to explore some of these issues. The need for regular supervision is highlighted by many authors (Abrahamson 1998, Draucker 1992, Sanderson 1995).

Disclosure

It is recognized that many individuals seek psychological help for other concerns and that the disclosure of CSA can occur 'spontaneously' in the process of therapeutic relation with a therapist. Disclosure to a therapist is likely because of the relationship therapists frequently have with clients – that of therapeutic friend. A therapist might be working with survivors using touch, and the close physical proximity could inadvertently provoke a disclosure, due to the distress that the survivors feel.

Qualitative research by Schachter et al (1999) identified the importance for survivors to feel safe within the relationship with a therapist for disclosure to take place. Schachter makes some recommendations for sensitive practice for therapists:

- establishment of positive rapport and trusting therapeutic relationships
- establishing a sense of partnership
- sharing of information
- working with physical factors (sensitivity to touch, privacy, body positions)
- responding sensitively to disclosure of abuse
- practice holistic health care
- increase knowledge about CSA and the effects
- know about the local community support service.

Frequently, survivors have encountered a range of unhelpful reactions to any disclosure of abuse. Non-supportive responses include 'non belief', 'blame', 'asking intrusive or voyeuristic questions' or 'minimizing' the abuse (Draucker 1992). Particularly unhelpful were the 'oh my God' responses. These research findings were supported by qualitative research by physiotherapists interested in developing guidelines for physiotherapy practice that are sensitive to the needs of survivors. The results of this research showed the least appropriate response was to ignore the disclosure, but also responses such as 'you don't have to tell me this if you don't want to', to some survivors signified lack of interest. 'Pity', 'advice' and 'minimalization' were also seen as unhelpful.

Helpful responses were normalizing and included 'many women have told me something like this before' and general expressions of understanding and support and exploration of the practical issues such as, 'tell me if anything I am doing with you doesn't feel right'.

Later research by Draucker shows the response needs to be 'calm concern' the 'validation of belief' and acknowledgment of the difficulty of disclosure. This can be reinforced with the message that it might be important to talk about the abuse further to help relate the abuse to current presenting problems, and this can be done at a pace that is right and even with another professional if appropriate. The sense of control must remain with the client.

'Victim to survivor'

In most traumatic events, the healing process starts after the immediate numbing. CSA is unique in that trauma can be frozen in shock stage, with memories either lost into unconsciousness or remembered vaguely but deeply influencing future life narrative. Consequently, by the time adulthood is reached, simply telling the story is no longer enough; healing needs to effect a meaningful transition, a 'reframing' of what has happened.

Mary Bratton (1999) has described a staged healing process, which forms a useful framework for therapists to understand their role in part of that healing. Therapists can be involved in each, one, or all of the stages of: 'defining abuse as assault', 'challenging distorted reality', 'recounting', 'reparenting', 'repairing developmental damage', 'integration' and 'transformation'.

'Redefining abuse as assault' is the beginning of the healing process that is the journey from being a victim to survivor. 'Changing the distorted reality' is the beginning of the realization about the adult responsibility for the assault. Survivors need to understand that defences were employed by them to maintain their own survival as children and that these defences are normal and effective coping mechanisms. This helps the transition from the notion of 'weak victim' to 'strong survivor'.

'Recounting' can occur only when changes have taken place in the survivor's self view. Early recounting can reinforce guilt and shame. Recounting in the context of reality, with understanding of accountability and attributable responsibility, form the foundation for part of the healing process.

'Repairing developmental damage' involves letting go, grieving and accepting of responsibility for whom the individual survivor is now. 'Integration' and 'tranformation' are the move beyond surviving and the claiming of a sense of wholeness.

Intervention

Dealing directly with the trauma and memories associated with CSA is not the role of therapists without access to further psychotherapeutic training. However, therapists can make a significant contribution to the total therapeutic package. Therapists can be in a prime position to facilitate life changes made by survivors, a vital element of the integration and transformation stage of healing. Issues around self-esteem and interpersonal functioning are additional domains of concern for therapists.

Creative arts

There is strong support for a range of the creative therapy being offered to adult survivors of CSA. Blantner (1991) suggests that different creative media can be used at different stages of the recovery process and that all therapists work by gradually enabling survivors to share and reveal more meaningful and emotionally significant material, slowly increasing the level of insight. Byrd (1995) suggests there are compelling reasons for the creative arts to provide a vehicle for an alternative expression for events that are too painful for words. Sampson (1999) advocates the use of poems as a means to express memories and feelings that make sense of emotional distress in a way that words fail. Miller (1990, cited in Froehlich 1992), advocates the use of creative media to facilitate expression of thoughts and feelings. Bonder (1991) also supports the use of the creative media and emphasizes the use of relaxation. Quina & Carlson (1989) emphasize the importance of providing opportunities for expression, the reconstruction of self-esteem and the development of coping skills.

Generally, all creative media provide a forum through which to explore feelings and thoughts using client-centred therapy philosophy and looking at issues of trust, self- identity and body image (Bourdon & Cook 1993). Creative arts allow emotional distance and deeper understanding. Survivors can choose a variety of ways to express feelings and to communicate non-verbally the psychological consequences of the abuse: collages designed to reflect the emotion felt as a child or paintings expressing their stage of the healing process. Themes such as 'what you anticipate for the future' or 'how you feel you are now' help put a concrete expression to feelings and assist the development of insight and self knowledge. Painful subjects, in the appropriate therapeutic environment, can be explored from the safety of the 'as if'.

There is also support for the more physically active media such as dance and psychodrama. Bratton (1999) advocates the importance of physically active therapy as the trauma is experienced viscerally, so resolution involves the viscera. Assaults to sensations provoke a fear response. Healthy connection between the individual and his or her body is one of the positive contributions therapists can make to a survivor's healing journey. Provided therapists are aware of the potential issues around physical boundaries and control, they have a vital part to play. Dance provides opportunities for self expression, reducing anxiety, correcting body disturbances and improving self concept.

Anger management   Survivors can have difficulty recognizing, acknowledging and expressing anger. Survivors can learn that anger is an appropriate response to the abuse and be taught to use techniques such as 'dosing', where anger can be expressed in short, 30-minute bursts, or exercises that help to express anger in a safe way, such as punching a ball, throwing clay and any aerobic exercise.

Creative writing   Clients who are experiencing difficulty in talking about aspects of trauma, or simply need to be offered an alternative expressive media, can be introduced to writing. This self-reflective tool can be used either in diary form or as creative writing, in which a series of specific themes appropriate to the individual in the process of rebuilding self-esteem is recorded. A diary can be a 24-hour therapist enabling an individual survivor to record hunches, feelings, dreams, questions and responses after a therapy session. Either carried out as an individual or a group, the writer is given the opportunity to explore and heal by using imagination to act 'as if'. Acting 'as if' produces similar biochemical changes to the actual happening.

Relaxation   Anxiety and tension are commonly experienced by adult survivors. Recent research has improved understanding of how trauma is experienced as a psychological and physiological memory in the body (Perry 1999). Relaxation is a useful technique that enables an individual to gain a greater sense of control and experience a tension-free body. There are many techniques of relaxation; reciprocal inhibition advocated by Mitchell (1977) might be the method of choice for adult survivors. Other methods of relaxation, such as guided imagery or other less structured methods perhaps do not provide the degree of structure and strong boundary issues relating to one's personal body and self awareness.

Self awareness   Increasing self awareness is commonly cited as a goal for therapy intervention. Increased self knowledge comes from listening to ourselves. Reflecting and listening helps us to understand our behaviour and the way others respond to it. In turn, this gives greater sense of control to our lives. Exercises for self awareness are many and varied but a number of them fall into the category of mental relaxation. Mental relaxation provides an opportunity for increasing self awareness in a safe environment. Payne (1995) describes exercises that include a number of 'scripts' which are read internally within an environment in which the individual is practicing relaxation techniques. For example, the script might be:

To focus on the body, noting any sensations or areas of discomfort, allowing yourself to focus on that area and then specifically increase and decrease the tension in that area.

Additional use of imagery as a safe and non-invasive technique, such as 'guided fantasy' can bring about changes in an individual's perception. Images, arising from the guidance of a therapist (as opposed to spontaneously from a deeply relaxed state), form the basis of guided relaxation. Once physical relaxation has occurred, the therapist can introduce images of safety, health, strength, healing and other positive images according to the symptomatology of the survivor. Additional to the perceptual changes, there is some research to suggest that imagery can produce changes to physiology (Dossey 1995).

Conclusion

CSA is a serious and probably underestimated problem that occurrs in approximately 25% of the population, at the conservative estimate. The consequences are various but profound and therapists working in mental health need to have the necessary competencies to enable survivors of CSA to have access to sensitive and therapeutic practice. Although not engaged primarily in dealing with the pathology resulting from the abuse, therapists are key individuals who need to know how to respond to disclosure, the likely sequelae and the appropriate therapeutic environment. Survivors of CSA need the opportunity to disclose, reframe and rediscover themselves. Therapists can, by using a variety of creative mediums, play an important part by providing a permissive safe environment in which healing can occur.

Summary

- Many mental health service users who come into contact with occupational therapists and physiotherapists, have a history of CSA.

- The consequences of the abuse are far reaching and can profoundly affect the survivors in the physiological, psychological and emotional domains.

- Survivors might choose to disclose CSA as part of their everyday interactions with therapists and it is essential that this disclosure is handled in an appropriate way.

- Therapists are not in a position to directly deal with the traumas and memories associated with CSA, but can contribute to the overall healing process.

- Therapists need to be fully aware of the need for sensitivity around issues such as touch, personal space, boundaries and the abuse of power.

■ Specific interventions that can help in the overall healing include creative arts and creative writing, exercise, dance, body image work, anger management and relaxation.

References

Abrahamson V 1998 Do occupational therapists feel equipped to deal with adult legacy of childhood sexual abuse? British Journal of Occupational Therapy 61(2):63–67

American Psychiatric Association 1994 Diagnostic and statistical manual of mental disorders, 4th edn. APA, Washington DC

Blantner A 1991 Theoretical principles underlying creative arts therapies. The Arts in Psychotherapy 18(5):405–409

Bonder, B R 1991 Psychopathology and function: a guide for occupational therapists. Slack, New Jersey, p 111-121.

Bourdon L S, Cook A S 1993 Losses associated with sexual abuse: therapist and clients perceptions. Journal of Childhood Sexual Abuse 2(4):69–82

Bowne A, Finkelhor D 1986 The impact of childhood sexual abuse: a review of the research. Psychological Bulletin 99:66–77

Bratton M 1999 From surviving to thriving. Harworth Press, New York

Byrd K R 1995 The myth of psyche and cupid as an allegory for survivors of childhood sexual abuse. The Arts in Psychotherapy 22(5):403–411

Dossey B M 1995 Holistic nursing: a handbook for practice. Aspen Publishers, Gaithersburg, MD

Draucker, C B 1992 Counselling survivors of childhood sexual abuse. Sage Publications, London

Finkelhor D, Hotaling G, Lewis I A, Smith C 1990 Sexual abuse in a national study of adult men and women: prevalence characteristics and risk factors. Child Abuse and Neglect 14:19–28

Froehlich J 1992 Occupational therapy interventions with survivors of sexual abuse. In: Merrill S (ed) Occupational therapy and psychosocial dysfunction. Haworth Press, New York

Herman J 1992 Trauma and recovery. Basic Books, New York

Loftus E F 1994 The reality of repressed memories. American Psychologist 48(5):518–420. Cited in Malley P, Reilly E 1999 Legal and ethical dimensions for mental health professionals. Taylor Francis, Philadelphia

Maslow, A H 1970 Motivation and personality, 2nd edn. Harper & Row, New York

Meekums B 2000 Creative group therapy for women survivors of childhood sexual abuse. Jessica Kingsley Publishers, London

Mitchell L, 1977 Simple relaxation. John Murray, London

Muenzenmaier K, Meyer I, Stuening E, Ferber J 1993 Childhood abuse and neglect amoung women outpatients with chronic mental illness. Hospital and Community Psychiatry 44(7):666–670

Mullen P E 1990 The long term influence of sexual assault on the mental health of victims. Journal of Forensic Psychiatry 1:13–34

Mullen P E, Martin J I, Anderson J C et al 1993 Childhood sexual abuse and mental ill health in later adult life. British Journal of Psychiatry 163:721–732

Palmer R L, Coleman L, Chaloner D et al 1993 Childhood experiences with adults; a comparison of reports by women psychiatric patients and general practice attendees. British Journal of Psychiatry 163:499–504

Payne R 1995 Relaxation techniques: a practical handbook for the health care professional. Churchill Livingstone, Edinburgh

Perry B D 1999 The memories of states: how the brain stores and retrieves traumatic memories. In: Goodwin J M, Attias R (eds) Splintered reflections: images of the body in trauma. Basic Books, New York, p 9–34

Quina K, Carlson N 1989 Rape, incest and sexual harassment; a guide for helping survivors. Praeger Publishers, New York

Sampson F 1999 The healing word. The Poetry Society, Milton Keynes, UK

Sanderson C 1995 Counselling adult survivors of CSA, 2nd edn. Jessica Kingsley, London

Schachter C L, Stalker C A, Teram E 1999 Toward sensitive practice: issues for physical therapists working with survivors of CSA. Physical Therapy 79:248–261

24 Self harm

Mary Kavanagh

Hilary is 45, and is married to John, a Major in the armed forces. Their life together has involved frequent moves, both in the UK and abroad. They have three children who are all away studying at university. Hilary began cutting herself with pieces of broken china when she was pregnant with her first child. She also started overdosing on paracetamol and has been admitted on several occasions to accident and emergency departments. She has been seen by various counsellors in the past but has always refused formal help. Her husband has never been sympathetic to her behaviour, describing her as histrionic and attention-seeking. After a recent attempt to throw herself through a glass window at their home, following a row with her husband, Hilary has been admitted to an acute ward for assessment.

Therapists encounter many individuals who self-harm, in the course of their work in mental health settings, yet it is worth emphasizing that Hilary and others like her represent only the minority of those who appear regularly at accident and emergency departments: self harm accounts for approximately 150 000 attendances in the UK annually (Hawton et al 1997).

Defining self harm

The whole issue regarding treatment of self harm is not helped by confusing and often misleading terminology associated with the area. Terms like 'parasuicide' and 'attempted suicide' have often clouded the picture by presupposing that death is always the main intended outcome. Similarly, phrases such as 'a cry for help' (Stengel 1964) have done nothing to disabuse the public and professionals that people are just 'acting out' and there is no serious intent to die during an act of self harm. For the purposes of clarity, the definition of self harm used in this chapter will be 'those acts which are intended to cause physical damage to the individual whatever the intended outcome' (Whitehead & Royles 2002, p. 100).

Methods used in self harm

A range of methods can be seen: self poisoning using paracetamol being the most common and accounting for 85% of numbers. Other methods involve swallowing household and garden fluids (such as bleach and weedkiller), carbon monoxide poisoning, burning, picking/scratching at the skin, biting, pulling out hair, inserting objects in body orifices, stabbing, cutting with razor blades, hanging, electrocution and attempted drowning (House et al 1998). On the whole, females tend to use methods such as self poisoning and males tend to choose more violent methods, such as hanging and electrocution.

There are bodies of thought that would include behaviours that ultimately cause damage to the body, such as alcoholism, recreational drug overdose and eating disorders in this whole debate. Neither must we ignore the cultural aspect of ritual self harm in tribal initiation ceremonies and current trends in body piercing and tattooing (all of which inflict certain degrees of pain). However, for the purposes of this chapter, they will not be alluded to except in the context of complex behaviours that people who self harm also engage in, the most common being substance misuse and self-starvation or bingeing.

Prevalence of self harm

The figure of 150 000 attendances at hospital per annum quoted earlier by Hawton et al (1997) refers only to those individuals who present with clear signs of self harm. Many areas do not have a continuous monitoring system of self-harming behaviour and there can therefore be only an estimate of 400 per 100 000 head of population, with the UK having one of the highest rates in Europe. Trends show an increase in self harm among young men and Asian women (Schmidtke et al 1996).

It must be recognized that there are many individuals who conceal, and tend to, their injuries at home or, if they do attend hospital, present with injuries attributable to other causes (domestic and DIY accidents, sports injuries). Experiences of negative encounters with professionals often dictates that people present with 'more socially acceptable injuries', which will be treated sympathetically (Dace). Although some injuries can be extreme, such as attempts at self-castration, and are more associated with coexisting mental health issues, most injuries do not require too much medical intervention, but instead need more specialist input from mental health professionals (see below).

Reasons for self harm and its relationship with mental health

Approximately one-third of those who self harm repeatedly have a concomitant psychiatric diagnosis such as eating disorder, substance misuse, personality disorder or psychosis (Winchel & Stanley 1991). They might have difficulties in managing emotions and behaviours, running parallel with poor problem-solving skills and impulsive behaviour, and consequently require a great deal of input from services.

There is also a significant group of individuals, presenting to the services for the first time, who self harm when experiencing levels of distress and recent life crises such as the breakdown of a relationship. Of these, approximately 40% are given a psychiatric diagnosis ranging from depression (60%) to schizophrenia (10%) and bipolar affective disorder (10%) (Morgan et al 1975). A further 10% will have ongoing substance misuse issues (Merrill et al 1992, Suokas & Lonnqvist 1995).

Self-harming behaviour can have two foci: (1) instrumental (in achieving change in others' behaviour, i.e. persuading a partner to return to a relationship); or (2) expressive (the way the individual feels at the time) (Bancroft & Hawton 1983), which can vary from:

- coping with overwhelming feelings of anger, pain, grief, confusion, distress and finding a way to communicate these
- relieving physical tension
- distracting self from feelings of self-hatred
- achieving a sense of control
- comfort and nurture
- feeling 'real', which can be achieved only by feeling pain
- as a response to voices
- 'blanking' out bad memories, e.g. of abuse.

Circumstances at the time can also be factors (Arnold & Magill 1996):

- abuse
- marital violence
- problems with housing/employment/debt
- poor personal health
- conflict or loss in personal relationships regarding significant others
- inability to conceive a child
- bullying at school or work.

Children and adolescents often self harm because of relationship difficulties within the family and because they have poor problem-solving skills (Brent 1997). For older adults, a change in living circumstances, loss and bereavement and social factors such as isolation and poverty

Case study: Hilary (continued)

When pregnant with her first child, Hilary, a naturally shy person, began to feel more and more anxious about fulfilling the role of an officer's wife. She began to dread social functions. Her husband refused to listen to her concerns and berated her for being histrionic and stupid. Alone in the house one day, she dropped a saucer and cut herself accidentally when trying to pick it up. Although she was in pain, she also felt a sense of release of some pent-up emotion, and immediate relief. That was the start of years of secret cutting first on her arms...

can be trigger factors in self harm (Hepple & Quinton 1997, Whitehead & Royles 2002).

Risk assessment and relation to suicide

Government guidelines indicate that all patients presenting to general hospitals should receive a psychosocial assessment (Department of Health and Social Security 1984). This is not always done, because of staff shortages. It should also be recognized that around 50% of people who present at hospital with self-inflicted injuries have also visited their GP in the month before the episode of self-harm (Morgan et al 1975). Within mental health settings, increasing emphasis has been placed on doing a thorough risk assessment as part of National Service Frameworks for Mental Health (standard 7). Morgan (2000, p. 2) defines this as a 'gathering of information and analysis of the potential outcomes of identified behaviours', including an identification of risk factors specific to the individual. This is often a lengthy process, involving not only detailed documentation but also the building of a therapeutic relationship with the person to identify triggers, strengths and needs. Only by doing this can a comprehensive picture of the individual be gained.

Research has shown a correlation between episodes of self-harm and suicide, regardless of whether a psychiatric diagnosis has been given (House et al 1998). Further acts of deliberate self-harm are common: 6% repeat within 3 months of the initial episode, rising to 30% within 1 year. There are also a small number of individuals whose repeated acts of self-harm account for a larger number of episodes; 1% will die by suicide within 1 year of a self-harming attempt, with the rates increasing to 3% within the following 7 years and, of those who have completed suicide, at least 25% presented at a general hospital in the year preceding the act (Hawton & Fagg 1988). These figures can be contrasted with those with a psychiatric diagnosis, where rates of suicide are much higher (10–20% in schizophrenia and bipolar affective disorder) (Harris & Barraclough 1997).

The use of recognized instruments such as the Suicidal Intent Scale (Beck et al 1974) and comprehensive assessments such as the Clinical Risk Management Tool (Morgan 2000) is vital to identify risk indicators. When carrying out an assessment, the therapist needs to find out whether any of the following are present:

- social factors: living alone, divorced, widowed, separated
- access to means of suicide (medication, weapons, vehicles)
- physical illness, particularly of a long-term and painful nature
- positive family history of suicide or mental health problems: including depression, schizophrenia, personality disorder, substance misuse
- childhood bereavement
- current incarceration in detention centre, young offender institution, prison.

In addition, the therapist needs to discover if there is evidence of:

- recent major life events, including bereavement, redundancy, loss of significant relationship
- anniversaries of loss
- recent escalation of self-harming behaviour
- recent discharge from psychiatric care or change in level of psychiatric care
- loss of usual support systems.

Other important factors include (Morgan 2000):

- evidence of planning and premeditation (no one likely to disturb, note written, pets put into care, will made)
- level of severity of method used
- regret at having survived previous attempt at suicide.

Case study: Hilary (continued)

> Hilary felt that she could tolerate the marriage only until her children left home. After that point she had decided to kill herself, but a row with her husband had precipitated her jumping through the window, and she was distressed at being alive.

Treatment approaches

There has been limited investigation into the effectiveness of specific approaches with people who self harm, and the results of what research has been done prove, on the whole, inconclusive (Garner et al 1996). Interventions such as: dialectical behaviour therapy, consisting of weekly group and individual therapy (Linehan et al 1991); crisis cards detailing sources of help after first initial admission (Morgan et al 1985); and problem-solving work to aid with developing coping strategies have indicated a general reduction in self-harming behaviour in the short term (Linehan et al 1991, McLeavey et al 1987). Women particularly appear to benefit from work on relationship issues (Hawton et al 1998, van der Sande et al 1997). Social skills training (Walsh & Rosen 1988), anger management (Byrt & Reece 1999) and brief family intervention (Kerfoot et al 1997) have also been shown to be effective, and longitudinal studies currently underway might or might not demonstrate if this progress is likely to be upheld in the long-term.

Building the relationship

What becomes apparent from the literature and the experience of people who self harm is the necessity of developing a good therapeutic relationship to work on specific issues around self-harming behaviour (Roberts & Mackay 1999). This will enable a thorough assessment to identify individual contextual and trigger factors, which will help the person develop more life-enhancing coping strategies as part of an overall management plan.

Unfortunately, professional attitudes have been identified as one of the factors impinging on building a good therapeutic relationship. These range from: condemnation and punishment, shock, fear, misunderstanding, reluctance to address the self-harming behaviour directly with the person, treating the person as 'disturbed', and prescribing medication alone without the bigger picture being addressed (Babiker & Arnold 1998). People who self harm have reported professionals being less than helpful, perceiving them as wasting valuable time and resources through attention-seeking and manipulative behaviour (Dunleavy 1992, Pembroke 1994).

Consequently, there is a need for each agency working with this client group to adopt a consistent policy towards people who self harm. Currently there is a range of treatment approaches (the majority of them behavioural in their frame of reference):

■ Close monitoring and prevention of self-harm behaviour by physical restraint if necessary.
■ Placing people on contracts not to self-harm while treatment is taking place, with discharge from service if self-harm continues.
■ Informing the person that self-harm is unacceptable and that he or she should talk to nursing staff instead.
■ Making the person pay for emergency services if he or she is a repeated self-harmer.
■ Withdrawal of attention for self harm, focusing instead on 'appropriate behaviours'.
■ Provision of clean razors as part of a harm minimization programme.
■ Self-harming behaviour not addressed directly in therapy, the view being that it will decrease as the main issues underlying the whole situation are addressed.

Each of the above might have some value in certain settings, but what they represent to the person who self-harms is a confusing message from services as to what is appropriate and what is not.

By far the overriding concern for individuals who self harm is the establishment of a good therapeutic relationship with a significant person involved with their care and support, who is non-judgemental and gives space for the person to talk and express him- or herself (Arnold & Magill 1996).

Areas of intervention

These can be divided into:

■ intervention to look at dealing directly with the urge to self harm
■ more general intervention with other professionals such as physiotherapists and occupational therapists
■ intervention to deal directly with the urge to self harm.

Strategies that might help postpone the actual act of self-injury include the removal of self from the venue for self-injury; having the means of asking for support as so not to self injure and the use of distraction techniques to decrease the desire to self injure. More general intervention with other professionals can address specific areas of need, which include:

- *Problems in communication and self-expression*: these can be addressed in creative work such as art, pottery, drama, writing letters, dance and movement, where feelings can be explored through a variety of media. Groupwork can be used to enhance social skills and assertiveness to enable participants to work on communicating feelings such as anger, sadness and disappointment in a more constructive way than self harming. Self-esteem work in the cognitive–behavioural frame of reference can help the person to build up a realistic self portrait, as well as confidence and coping strategies.

- *Encouraging other methods of releasing emotion cathartically, rather than self-destructively*: some clinical areas have used punchbags; other outlets for the person might be taking bottles to the bottle bank, smashing cracked plates, shouting, screaming in a place where they will not be overheard. However, the above methods need to be used with care and in a contained environment in case the tension increases and the person feels more out of control than they did before.

- *Dealing with stress and tension and the build-up of feelings*: exercise – cycling, gym, weights, swimming – can be used as a means of relieving physical tension. However, many people are sensitive to exposing parts of the body where scars are present and might want to wear extra clothes to hide the scarring. This can cause problems at some public venues, for example, some swimming pools will not allow tee shirts to be worn over bathing costumes. Relaxation and stress management techniques can be taught and self-nurturing encouraged through warm baths, aromatherapy, yoga, massage, music. General activities such as breadmaking and pottery, where kneading dough or clay can be physically demanding, can also encourage the release of frustration and tension.

Case study: Hilary (continued)

Hilary spent 3 months in hospital working with a psychologist who helped her to understand more about her feelings of low self-esteem and her inability to express emotions, particularly towards her husband. She found an outlet for some of her anger in exercise classes and also in pottery and art, where she was able to let go of some of the feelings she had kept pent up for years. She attended an assertiveness group on the ward and developed skills in saying how she felt about particular situations, particularly when she felt angry or upset. She wanted her husband to come to family therapy with her but he was unwilling to do so. Eventually, Hilary decided to separate from her husband and, although this has been very stressful for her, she feels that she is finally able to be herself.

■ *Specialist work to enable people to look at underlying issues about why they self-harm*: referral to clinical psychologists and psychotherapists, in conjunction with the work of the multidisciplinary team.

Training needs for therapists

There is no doubt that working with people who self-harm is a very challenging aspect of any therapist's work. Regular support and supervision is vital to ensure that professional standards are maintained, as well as enabling practitioners to develop therapeutic skills to work with this particular group, who often present with distressing needs. Education and training is also vital in enabling therapists to identify where self-harm has occurred and to carry out appropriate risk assessments to ensure protection for themselves and the individuals they work with. In accordance with looking at effective treatments, there is also a need for ongoing research to look at therapeutic interventions with this particular group of people.

Summary

■ Significant numbers of people self harm without ever presenting to the services.

■ There is not necessarily an intent to die with persons who self harm.

■ There needs to be a comprehensive risk assessment of individuals who self harm.

■ A range of methods can be used in self-harming behaviour.

■ The most important phase of working with individuals who self harm is that of building a non-judgemental relationship.

■ A wide variety of treatment interventions is available to professionals working in this field.

■ This is a stressful area of work and there needs to be comprehensive training and support for those professionals who work with individuals who self harm.

■ Further research needs to take place to look at the effectiveness of interventions with individuals who self harm.

References

Arnold L, Magill A 1996 Working with self-injury: a practical guide. The Basement Project, Bristol

Babiker G, Arnold L 1998 The language of injury – comprehending self-mutilation. BPS Books, Leicester

Bancroft J, Hawton K 1983 Why people take overdoses: a study of psychiatrists' judgements. British Journal of Medical Psychology 56:197–204

Beck A T, Schuyler D, Herman I 1974 Development of suicidal intent scales. In: Beck A T, Resia H, Lettie D (eds) The prediction of suicide. Charles Press, Bowie Maryland

Brent D A 1997 The aftercare of adolescents with deliberate self-harm. Journal of Child Psychology and Psychiatry 38:277–286

Byrt R, Reece J 1999 Patients' perspectives of self-harm in a medium secure unit. Mental Health Practice 3:30–33

Dace E (undated) The hurt yourself less workbook. National Self Harm Network, London

Department of Health and Social Security 1984 The management of deliberate self-harm. HN(84):25. HMSO, London

Dunleavy R 1992 An adequate response to a cry for help? Parasuicide patients' perception of their nursing care. Professional Nurse January:213–215

Garner R, Butler G, Hutchings D 1996 A study of the patterns of planned activity and incidents of DSH within an RSU. British Journal of Occupational Therapy 40:156–160

Harris E C, Barraclough B M 1997 Suicide as an outcome measure for mental disorders – a meta analysis. British Journal of Psychiatry 170:205–228

Hawton K, Fagg J 1988 Suicide and other causes of death, following attempted suicide. British Journal of Psychiatry 152:359–366

Hawton K, Fagg J, Simkin S 1997 Trends in deliberate self-harm in Oxford, 1985–1995: implications for clinical services and the prevention of suicide. British Journal of Psychiatry 171:556–560

Hawton K, Arensman E, Townsend E 1998 Deliberate self-harm: systematic review of efficacy of psychosocial and pharmacological treatments in preventing repetition. British Medical Journal 317:441–447

Hepple J, Quinton C 1997 One hundred cases of attempted suicide in the elderly. British Journal of Psychiatry 171:42–46

House A, Owens D, Patchett L 1998 Effective health care: deliberate self-harm. NHS Centre for Reviews and Dissemination, York, UK

Kerfoot M, McNiven F, Gill J 1997 Brief family intervention in adolescents who deliberately self-harm. Journal of the Royal Society of Medicine 90:484–487

Linehan M M, Armstrong H E, Suarez A et al 1991 Cognitive-behavioural treatment of chronically parasuicidal borderline patients. Cognitive Therapy Research 11:1–12

McLeavey B C, Daly R, Ludgate J W, Murray C 1987 Interpersonal problem-solving training in the treatment of self-poisoning behaviour. Suicide and Life Threatening Behaviour 24:382–394

Merrill J, Milner G, Owens J 1992 Alcohol and attempted suicide. British Journal of Addictions 87:83–89

Morgan S 2000 Clinical risk management: a clinical tool and practitioner manual. Sainsbury Centre for Mental Health, London

Morgan H, Burns C, Pocock H 1975 Deliberate self-harm: clinical and socioeconomic characteristics of 368 patients. British Journal of Psychiatry 127:564–574

Morgan H, Jones E, Owen J 1985 Secondary prevention of non-fatal deliberate self-harm: the green card study. British Journal of Psychiatry 163:111–112

Pembroke L R 1994 Self-harm: perspectives from personal experience. Survivors Speak Out, London

Roberts D, Mackay G 1999 A nursing model of overdose assessment. Nursing Times 95:58–60

Schmidtke A, Bille-Brahe U, De Leo D 1996 Attempted suicide in Europe: rates, trends and sociodemographic characteristic of suicide attempters during the period 1989–92. Results of the WHO/EURO multicentre study on Parasuicide. Acta Psychiatrica Scandinavica 93:327–338

Stengel E 1964 Suicide and attempted suicide. Penguin, Harmondsworth, UK

Suokas J, Lonnqvist J 1995 Suicide attempts in which alcohol is involved: a special group in general hospital emergency rooms. Acta Psychiatrica Scandinavica 91:36–40

van der Sande R, Buskens E, Allart E et al 1997 Psychosocial interventions following suicide attempt – a systematic review of treatment interventions. Acta Psychiatrica Scandinavica 96:43–50

Walsh B W, Rosen P M 1988 Self-mutilation: theory, research and treatment. Guildford Press, New York

Whitehead L, Royles M 2002 Deliberate self-harm: assessment and treatment interventions. In: Regel S, Roberts D (eds) Mental health liaison: a handbook for nurses and health professionals. Ballière Tindall, Edinburgh

Winchel R M, Stanley M 1991 Self-injurious behaviour: a review of the behaviour and biology of self-mutilation. American Journal of Psychiatry 148:306–317

25 Employment for health

Sally Feaver

This chapter explores the important role employment has to play in the perception of health. People with mental health problems are more likely to be unemployed and this can add to a sense of loss of purpose. Good practice guidelines and the results of research that indicates useful models to facilitate return to work are identified.

The World Health Organization has included employment as one of the 12 indicators of health. In this context, health is seen 'not as the absence of organ pathology, but as an encompassing, positive, dynamic state of well-beingness, reflecting satisfaction in one's own activities' (Yerxa 1998, p. 412). This description promotes a concept of health as the ownership of a portfolio of skills that enables individuals to achieve their goals, regardless of their abilities.

Employment and disability

There is evidence to suggest that the large majority of people with mental health and other disabilities want to work (Crowther et al 2001). However, levels of unemployment among people with disabilities in the UK remain at around 60–70% (Crowther et al 2001, Wehman et al 1998). Young people with disabilities are three times more likely to be unemployed than their non-disabled counterparts.

There are powerful arguments for improving employment opportunities for people with disabilities. There is an ethical basis for the human right to work, which was set out in legislation in the 1948 Universal Declaration of Human Rights, and this right has been protected and expanded by the UK Disability Discrimination Act 1995. This, however, has yet to reach its full impact on employment. Two-thirds of UK employers do not believe the Act has any impact on them.

Defining current terms and practices

It has already been established that employment, and thus 'return to work' is a core concern for therapists. Programmes have been implemented under different terms: 'return to work', 'work rehabilitation', 'occupational rehabilitation', 'industrial rehabilitation', 'vocational rehabilitation', 'work hardening' and 'work conditioning' (Jundt & King 1999).

Return to work programmes for people with mental health disabilities have taken various formats, with sheltered employment, supported employment, and the clubhouse movement being the most well known. Despite differences in structure between individual programmes, they share a common goal, facilitating employment for those with disabilities, and common methods, vocational assessment, counselling and training (Schmidt et al 1995).

Research undertaken in North America has shown that the most successful type of programme is supported employment (Crowther et al 2001, Hyde 1998, Parent 1996, Wehman et al 1998). A practical definition of supported employment is competitive paid work with ongoing support from trained job coaches or employment specialists (Crowther et al 2001, Krause et al 1998).

The reported success of supported employment establishes that there has been a shift from therapy in a clinical setting to focusing on the workplace as the therapeutic environment. Crowther et al (2001) provide an overview of the figures in the discipline of mental health. In the UK, prevocational training is still the norm, but there are 80 agencies providing supported employment (Crowther et al 2001, p. 204). As the relevant literature published is dominated by North America, it is therefore likely that the evidence for the role of occupational therapy in enabling people with disabilities to return to work will be within the context of supported employment, as this is currently established as best practice in North America.

The importance of employment

Studies have shown that unemployment results in an increased likelihood of depression, anxiety and general distress, and causes a decrease in self-esteem and confidence (Douthwaite 1994). Symptoms associated with long-term unemployment – social withdrawal, isolation, passivity and lethargy – are very similar to the symptoms of chronic mental health conditions.

First, employment has an important influence on how people see themselves, on their concept of their personal value and identity, and therefore their self-esteem (Wehman et al 1998, p. 42). It is believed that employment can cause improvements in clinical symptoms for people with severe mental illness by increasing self-esteem, increasing independence and lessening psychiatric symptoms (Crowther et al 2001, p. 204).

Employment offers a daily routine, which provides structure and partially enforces activity, which is regarded as highly positive. It provides people with relationships that are not in the context of a family and unites them with their work colleagues in goals that are not personal but are work orientated (Wehman et al 1998).

Unemployment can act as a form of social exclusion for people with disabilities (Crowther et al 2001, p. 204). Potentially, this can compound other difficulties they might have in acceptance and integration into mainstream society. Clearly, there are financial implications to lack of employment, both practical and psychological. Being paid for a job can be very rewarding, to say nothing of the economic advantages. Receiving income and other remuneration can provide opportunities for greater independence and mobility in society (Wehman et al 1998). There is still a stigma attached to receiving benefits.

There is also the argument that society as a whole benefits, not just the individual. There are hefty costs, in financial and workforce terms, in not assisting people with disabilities to gain employment. There are social security costs and injury compensation costs, and costs of non-productive use of potential workforce (Krause et al 1998, Wehman et al 1998).

Factors affecting successful return to work

There is no evidence that the diagnosed condition impacts directly on the person's chances of returning to work. What has been found to have an impact is the length of time the person has had the disability, and the severity of the injury (Niemeyer et al 1994, p. 329). Other factors that have been established as relevant are independent of rehabilitation treatment and the disability (Schmidt et al 1995, p. 953). The review by Niemeyer et al (1994, p. 329) suggested the following variables: age, gender, physical demand level of job, educational level, job skills, marital status and ethnicity. Psychosocial factors were also seen as crucial determinants.

Less positive outcomes were associated with: perception of high pain density, high number of pain descriptors, decreased sense of self-efficacy, depression, emotional vulnerability, hypochondria, additional life stress, anger and frustration, compensation issues and a history of alcohol abuse (Niemeyer et al 1994, p. 333–334). A further underlying factor, related to the above, is the person's motivation to return to work (Hyde 1998, Schmidt et al 1995).

Finally, the results of the study of work rehabilitation programmes by Jundt & King found the workplace to be the prominent concern for therapists (Jundt & King 1999, p. 143). This shift in focus from just looking at the person's 'problems' to looking at the physical, social and cultural issues in the environment, is in keeping with the social model of disability, and reflects a very positive change.

The role of therapists

Employment is an area of occupation that is extremely relevant to therapists. The therapy professions have played a part in the development of work rehabilitation programmes (Jundt & King 1999). Niemeyer et al (1994, p. 335) consider that work rehabilitation programmes are highly representative of therapy values, 'a whole-person, biopsychosocial perspective'.

The therapy perspective places the emphasis on a holistic approach to the person's situation. This prominence of an all-encompassing approach is seen in the therapists' role in the context of the multidisciplinary team (MDT). The best-skilled team comprises occupational therapists, with physical therapists, psychologists and vocational specialists (Niemeyer et al 1994).

Good practice

Stokes (1997) conducted a survey on a multidisciplinary panel, which provided information on what panel members considered most important in the return to work of people with disabilities. The information gathered identified five key issues in successful return to work.

1. Financial assessments to be offered to clients, to explore the implications of employment choices.
2. The importance of a holistic approach in therapy.
3. The necessity for support and information for potential employers, and clarification of the requirements of people with disabilities in the workplace.
4. A need to address the lack of communication between disciplines, services and agencies.
5. New and increased efforts to discover a way to canvas the views of service users.

The views of people with disabilities

There have been relatively few attempts to document the views of the users of work rehabilitation programmes. Parent's 1996 Consumer Satisfaction Survey reported views emerging from users of supported employment. Five steps were outlined, which would improve consumer satisfaction and could support evidence of good practice:

1. Getting to know the person, their lives, and their goals.
2. Sharing all available information so that every aspect can be considered.
3. Ensuring frequent communication and encouraging full participation of ideas.
4. Assessing progress continually and making any necessary changes.
5. Providing fundamental assistance in the form of practical projects to ascertain what the realistic employment options are.

Hyde (1998) identifies some dissatisfaction with work rehabilitation programmes. Specifically, issues with employment in sheltered workshops were:

■ the introduction of incentives for workshop mangers to promote economic efficiency
■ 'unrealistically high' expectations of workers' production capacity
■ significant disruptions to the daily work routine, brought about by the policy changes surrounding sheltered employment.

Concerns with supported employment were:

■ the lack of job security because of the temporary nature of contracts
■ workers did not feel they were as highly regarded, or were treated as well as, able-bodied colleagues
■ there were also 'unrealistic' productivity targets.

Conclusion   It seems apparent that the majority of people with disabilities want to be meaningfully employed, and are progressively more aware of their 'human rights' to fulfil this need. These fundamental issues are set in the current social, political and economic climate of increasing awareness, whatever the motivation, of the advantages of improving the employment options, and ongoing situation in the workplace, for people with disabilities.

The advantageous effects of early intervention have been recognized in this area, as in other areas of concern for therapists. The length and severity of the disability, coupled with previous experience of employment and any familiarity with a particular job skill set, need to be incorporated into the intervention planning. The emphasis is on a holistic approach.

The therapist needs to take into account other relevant factors, from gender, age and ethnicity, to the individual's support networks, to a number of psychosocial factors. The encouragement and incorporation of users' views and input is an essential aspect of client-centred care. An all-encompassing approach requires effective communication between professionals – in the multidisciplinary team and in other relevant services or agencies. It also requires a two-way exchange of information on needs and requirements with employers.

An aspect of work rehabilitation that the therapies are increasingly incorporating into intervention is on-site services. An emphasis on intervention strategies with the person in the work setting has emerged as a decisive factor in future successful employment. Support and training in a clinical environment appear to be effective only up to a point. This is further evidenced by the view that supported employment is the best service option. The position of supported employment as the most successful return to work programme makes it crucial for therapists to look at their role within this context. The role of therapy in on-site intervention, in workplace assessments and in ongoing support, is less advanced in the UK than in North America.

For the therapy professions to play an effective, successful role in work rehabilitation programmes in the UK, it would seem to be essential that there is a dedicated and comprehensive approach to some form of on-site intervention. On-site and ongoing intervention would allow therapists to facilitate the career goals and career fulfilment of their clients to a far greater extent.

Summary

- Employment has an important part to play in the perception of health.

- Employment offers routine, relationships, facilitates social inclusion and has evident economic advantages.

- People with mental health problems are more likely to be unemployed than non-disabled people.

- The length of time the person has had the disability has the most impact on chance of returning to work or successfully finding work.

- Therapists play an important part in enabling individuals to find or return to work.

- Good practice involves supporting and providing information for potential employers.

- Supported employment is the most successful type of work rehabilitation programme.

- Supported employment is competitive paid work with ongoing support from job coaches.

References

Crowther R E, Marshall M, Bond G R, Huxley P 2001 Helping people with severe mental illness to obtain work: systematic review. British Medical Journal 322:204–208

Douthwaite J 1994 Unemployment: a challenge to occupational therapy. British Journal of Occupational Therapy 57(11):432–436

Hyde J 1998 Sheltered and supported employment in the 1990s: the experiences of disabled workers in the UK. Disability & Society 13(2):199–215

Jundt J, King P M 1999 Work rehabilitation programs: a 1997 survey. Work: Journal of Prevention, Assessment and Rehabilitation 12:139–144

Krause N, Dasinger L K, Neuhauser F 1998 Modified work and return to work: a review of the literature. Journal of Occupational Rehabilitation 8(2):113–139

Niemeyer L O, Jacobs K, Reynolds-Lynch K et al 1994 Work hardening: past, present, and the future – the work programs special interest section national work-hardening outcome study.

American Journal of Occupational Therapy 48(4):327–339

Parent W 1996 Consumer choice and satisfaction in supported employment. Journal of Vocational Rehabilitation 6:23–30

Schmidt S H, Oort-Marburger D, Meijman T F 1995 Employment after rehabilitation for musculoskeletal impairments: the impact of vocational rehabilitation and working on a trial basis. Archive of Physical Medical Rehabilitation 76:950–954

Stokes F 1997 Using the Delphi technique in planning a research project on the occupational therapist's role in enabling people to take vocational choices following illness or injury. British Journal of Occupational Therapy 60(6):263–267

Wehman P, Revell G, Kregel J 1998 Supported employment: a decade of rapid growth and impact. American Rehabilitation 24(1): 31–43

Yerxa E J 1998 Health and the human spirit for occupation. American Journal of Occupational Therapy 52(6):412–418

INDEX